5TH EDITION

Infection Control

and Management of Hazardous Materials for the Dental Team

CHRIS H. MILLER, MS, PhD

Professor Emeritus of Oral Microbiology
Executive Associate Dean Emeritus
Associate Dean Emeritus for Academic Affairs and Graduate Education
Indiana University School of Dentistry
Indianapolis, Indiana

ELSEVIER

3251 Riverport Lane
St. Louis, Missouri 63043

INFECTION CONTROL AND MANAGEMENT OF HAZARDOUS
MATERIALS FOR THE DENTAL TEAM, FIFTH EDITION

ISBN: 978-0-323-08257-0

Notices

ISBN: 978-0-323-08257-0

Vice President and Publisher: Linda Duncan
Executive Content Strategist: Kathy Falk
Content Manager: Kristin Hebberd
Content Development Specialist: Joslyn Dumas
Publishing Services Manager: Julie Eddy
Project Manager: Jan Waters
Design Direction: Karen Pauls

Printed in China

Last digit is the print number: 9 8 7 6 5 4 3 2

This edition of Infection Control and Management
of Hazardous Materials for the Dental Team
is dedicated to Dr. David Lee Miller, whose devotion to dentistry
and love of life was matched by few and admired by all.

Preface

Infection control, safety, and proper management of hazardous materials in dentistry are as important as they ever were. In fact, they may be more important because of the increasing demand by our society to document our actions in health care and a variety of other areas. Also, the news media and the Internet have made dental and medical patients more and more knowledgeable about microorganisms and disease occurrence and prevention, and we have to be prepared for their questions. Continuously emerging diseases create new situations in healthcare that require forward thinking based on the basic concepts of disease prevention. Thus, infection control and maintenance of a safe environment for our patients and the dental team continue to be critically important and will continue to be in the future.

Numerous changes in infection control have occurred since the first edition of this book 19 years ago, and we have tried to incorporate these changes in each subsequent edition. These changes have mainly involved the constant appearance of new products and equipment (some of which require the use of new procedures), new regulations and recommendations from governmental agencies and professional groups, and new sources of information (e.g., Internet sites). Even though the discipline has changed, the purpose of this book remains the same, to provide the basic concepts, the step-by-step procedures, and the current regulatory aspects related to infection control and office safety for students and continuing members of the entire dental team.

We've maintained the teaching aids from the previous edition, including a listing of learning objectives, key words, review questions, and selected readings for each chapter. The massive glossary and appendices will hopefully assist the understanding of the subject for all readers.

NEW TO THIS EDITION

In addition to updating all the chapters and adding some new photos, I've included 4 new chapters:
- *Chapter 10: Hand Hygiene*, which addresses its importance in disease prevention and discusses the procedures and products for handwashing and use of alcohol hand rubs.
- *Chapter 18: Preventing Sharps Injuries*, which looks at the occurrence of these injuries and how to establish a culture of safety in the office using a variety of prevention techniques.
- *Chapter 20: General Office Safety and Asepsis*, which describes how to maintain asepsis and safety throughout the office, including the reception area and bathrooms, and how to manage the potential contamination brought into the office by all people, including patients, visitors, delivery persons, family members, trainees, sales representatives, and others.
- *Chapter 22: Cross-contamination Between Work and Home*, which describes the routes of spread of contamination from work to home and from home to work, along with suggestions of infection prevention techniques in the home.

We've added a new Appendix H, which provides the regulatory text of the updated 2012 version of OSHA's Hazard Communication Standard. The use of color photos including several new clinical pictures should enhance the readability of the text.

ABOUT EVOLVE

Another big addition to the 5th edition is the expanded Evolve site, which includes a wealth of helpful information for both faculty and students. Material found on Evolve includes the following:

For the instructor:

- The **TEACH Instructor Resource Manual** is a useful guide for instructors featuring chapter-by-chapter lesson plans, lecture outlines, and PowerPoint slides.
- A **600-question Test Bank** written by author, Chris H. Miller.
- The complete **image collection** in downloadable formats.
- 20 **Case Discussions** to stimulate critical thinking by the student. Each case discussion provides 1) a dental office scenario for the student to read and identify breaches in infection prevention procedures; 2) the potential consequences of those improper procedures; 3) what should have been done to prevent those potential consequences; and 4) the related regulations and recommendations.

For the student:

- **Practice Quizzes,** separated by chapter, with approximately 300 multiple-choice questions for student self-study, with instant-feedback answers, rationales, and page-number references for remediation.

- **Answers for the Review Questions** found at the end of each chapter.
- **Flashcards** created from the book's key terms and glossary.
- **Sequencing Exercises** for students.
- A printable version of **Appendix E** (Exposure Incident Report).
- A variety of **Weblinks** providing avenues for further study.

This book has always been an important reference for the Dental Assisting National Board (DANB) Infection Control Examination (ICE).

FROM THE AUTHOR

I thank Charles John Palenik for his excellent contributions to previous editions of this text. His expertise will long be appreciated. I also thank many other colleagues for sharing their expertise with me and continuing to excite me about infection control (which is also referred to as infection prevention). My interactions with front-line dentists, dental hygienists, dental assistants, laboratory technicians, manufacturers, and distributors continue to challenge me in attempts to answer their questions and concerns. I will be ever grateful to my past students who always stimulated my mind and feelings.

CHRIS H. MILLER

Contents

PART THREE

OFFICE SAFETY

PART ONE

The Microbial World

Scope of Microbiology and Infection Control

OUTLINE

Role of Microorganisms in Infection Control

Discovery of Microorganisms and Infection Control Procedures

Important Activities of Microorganisms

LEARNING OBJECTIVES

After completing this chapter, the student should be able to do the following:

1. Describe the role of microorganisms in infection control.
2. Describe the early beginnings of microbiology as a science and the early procedures used to control microbes and prevent infectious diseases.
3. List beneficial activities of microbes.

KEY TERMS

Bacteriology
Bacteriophages
Infection Control

Mycology
Pasteurization
Prions

Probiotics
Protozoology
Virology

ROLE OF MICROORGANISMS IN INFECTION CONTROL

Microbiology is the study of small life forms, including bacteria, special fungi called molds and yeasts, protozoa, certain algae, and viruses. Several subdisciplines within microbiology, such as bacteriology, mycology (study of fungi), protozoology, and virology, concentrate on specific types of microorganisms or on the activities of selected microorganisms, such as those important in the fields of medical microbiology, dental microbiology, food microbiology, industrial microbiology, and environmental (aquatic, soil, sewage, and space) microbiology. Close relationships also exist between microbiology and the fields of immunology (study of the immune system) and biochemistry (the chemistry of life forms).

The field of infection control (controlling microbial contamination and infection) is seated deeply within the discipline of microbiology. In fact, microbiology had its beginnings as a science concerned with the control and identification of microorganisms in attempts to explain and prevent disease. An understanding of the physical and chemical properties of microorganisms, where microorganisms exist, how they grow, how the environment or special physical and chemical agents influence microorganisms, and how microorganisms cause specific diseases of concern forms the basis for killing microorganisms and understanding and preventing their spread from person to person. Also, a general knowledge of immunology and body defense mechanisms contributes to the understanding of disease prevention through immunization and through reliance on the natural barriers of the body against infection.

DISCOVERY OF MICROORGANISMS AND INFECTION CONTROL PROCEDURES

Diseases were recognized long before their causative agents. The Italian physician Girolamo Fracastoro is generally credited as being the first to recognize, in 1546, the existence of tiny living particles that cause "catching" (contagious) diseases by being spread by direct contact with human beings and animals and by indirect contact with objects. Because microorganisms are too small to see with the naked eye, their actual existence was not established until Antoni van Leeuwenhoek first observed what he called "animalcules" (bacteria, yeasts, and protozoa) in 1667. The microorganisms became visible when he observed tooth scrapings and gutter water under a simple microscope.

The relationship of these "little animals" to disease was not established until "The Golden Age of Microbiology" in the mid to late 1800s by researchers such as Louis Pasteur (France), Robert Koch (Germany), Ignaz Semmelweis (Austria), Oliver Wendell Holmes (United States), Lord Joseph Lister (England), and Willoughby D. Miller (United States), who became known as the "Father of Oral Microbiology."

By 1900, microorganisms known as bacteria had been described and recognized as the cause of numerous diseases, such as anthrax, diphtheria, tuberculosis, cholera, tetanus, leprosy, epidemic meningitis, gonorrhea, brucellosis, pneumonia, abscesses, food poisoning, dental caries, and periodontal diseases.

The Golden Age of Microbiology also brought about the basis for disease prevention through use of infection control procedures. Semmelweis in Vienna and Holmes in the United States first recognized the importance of handwashing to prevent the spread of disease agents. Pasteur and John Tyndall recognized the use of heat to destroy vegetative bacteria and resistant bacterial spores. They used boiling water to kill bacteria, and the process known as pasteurization (destroying pathogens in milk or other fluid by heating it to 63° C [145.4° F] for 30 minutes or to 72° C [161.6° F] for 15 seconds) still is used today. As a surgeon, Lord Lister became concerned about postoperative infections and demonstrated that boiling instruments and washing his hands and surgical linens with phenol before surgery greatly reduced these complications. He also proposed that infections of open wounds were caused by microorganisms in the air, so he sprayed the air around his patients with phenol before surgery. These procedures were considered bold and outrageous at the time, but they truly paved the way for the sterile and aseptic techniques that now are practiced throughout the world.

The activities of the human immune defense mechanisms were recognized about four centuries ago when it became known that some individuals who recovered from a sickness did not get that disease a second time. Edward Jenner is credited with recognizing the concept of immunization when he realized, in the 1790s, that milkmaids who caught cowpox, a mild disease, were protected from the more serious disease of smallpox. He injected the fluid from cowpox pustules into a healthy boy and later injected the boy with fluid from human smallpox lesions. The boy did not get smallpox because the related cowpox gave cross-immunity to smallpox. Placing someone at risk with this type of experimentation is, of course, prohibited today.

Pasteur became known as the "Father of Immunology" for his work in developing immunization techniques against chicken cholera, anthrax in cattle, and rabies in human beings.

The viral diseases of polio, smallpox, and rabies had been described for centuries, but a microbial cause for these and other diseases was not apparent until 1898 when Friedrich Loeffler and Girolamo Fracastorius demonstrated that an agent smaller than bacteria that could not be seen through the microscopes of the day caused foot-and-mouth disease in animals. For the next 40 years or so, a fierce scientific debate raged as to the nature of such small disease agents that were named viruses, the Latin word for poisons. Viruses that infected bacteria were discovered in 1915 and in 1922 were named bacteriophages ("bacteria eaters"). Then, in 1940, the electron microscope was developed, and Wendell Stanley at the Rockefeller Institute in Princeton, New Jersey, published the first pictures of a virus magnified 35,000 times its normal

size. This tobacco mosaic disease virus first was described erroneously as a large protein molecule. Today we know that viruses contain nucleic acids (RNA or DNA), a few molecules of enzymes, structural proteins, and sometimes lipids.

By 1943, viruses were described as the cause of smallpox, chickenpox, rabies, poliomyelitis, yellow fever, mumps, the common cold, hepatitis A, and influenza. Over the next 30 years, several other viruses were first isolated or seen through the electron microscope, including rubella virus, measles virus, Epstein-Barr virus, and other herpesviruses.

In 1967, Alper and Griffith proposed the existence of a new type of infectious agent composed entirely of protein as the cause of a rare degenerative brain disease in humans called Creutzfeldt-Jakob disease. Pruinser coined the term "prion" as a name for this protein in 1982. Today we know that prions are not microorganisms, but are proteins able to induce abnormal folding of normal cellular prion proteins in the brain, leading to brain damage. Prion diseases are usually rapidly progressive and always fatal. Prions also cause brain diseases in animals such as bovine spongiform encephalopathy ("mad cow disease").

Microbe hunters similar to Pasteur and Koch have been active throughout the history of microbiology and infection control. Within the last 40 years or so, new infectious diseases or the causative agents of recognized diseases have been discovered (see Chapter 4). Diseases will continue to emerge as new or renewed opportunities develop for microorganisms to associate with human beings and cause diseases. These diseases might result from closer interactions between the populations of the world and their unique diseases, changes in the disease-producing abilities of microorganisms, unknown factors that may enhance susceptibility of the body to microbial infections, lack of appreciation for maintenance of current vaccine programs and insect control projects, and enhanced complacency concerning personal hygiene and the general cleanliness of objects we contact.

IMPORTANT ACTIVITIES OF MICROORGANISMS

Microorganisms are actually more beneficial than harmful to the human race, but we usually hear about or see only their harmful activities of causing diseases, spoiling food, occluding water lines, or destroying fabrics. Bacteria in the soil convert dead plants, animals, and insects into usable nutrients needed for survival of the live plants. Other soil microorganisms convert atmospheric nitrogen and carbon dioxide into forms that all plants require for growth. Bacteria also form the basis of modern sewage treatment by degrading the organic material in the sewage as it flows over or is mixed with bacterial masses in treatment plants. Also, bacteria are cultured in large vats to make several products, such as vinegar, vitamins, alcohol, organic acids, enzyme cleaners, drain openers, antibiotics, insecticides, and special chemicals used in biomedical research. Microorganisms are used to make rubber products, tobacco, and spices, and are used in processing leather. Some bacteria are used to help clean up oil spills in the oceans because they can degrade the components of crude oil. Special fungi called yeasts make bread dough rise and are used in beer production. Bacteria or fungi are used to pickle cucumbers, to produce cultured dairy products such as yogurt and sour cream, and to make cheeses. Bacteria or yeasts also are used to synthesize special agents such as insulin, other hormones, and hepatitis B vaccines to treat or prevent diseases. Some microbes when administered in adequate amounts can confer a health benefit on a host. Such microbes are called probiotics. Examples of how probiotics are used include as drugs to help treat certain bacterial infections and as food ingredients and dietary supplements for humans and lower animals.

Harmful activities of microorganisms usually result when they are someplace they should not be and when they grow out of control. Microorganisms do not really intend to harm or destroy things; they simply "wish" to survive and grow (increase their numbers). Unfortunately, their growth results in the production of substances that may harm or change their habitat. If their habitat is the human body, disease may occur. If their habitat is food, the food may spoil. If they accumulate in a water line, the water flow is stopped or reduced. Thus harmful activities of microorganisms are actually accidents resulting from their growth.

The first approach to preventing the harmful activities of microorganisms is to attempt to keep them in their proper place by preventing contamination (e.g., infection control or exposure control). If they get someplace where they should not be, they must be removed, killed, or kept from growing to harmful numbers (e.g., by cleaning, sterilization, disinfection, growth inhibition, immunization, or antimicrobial therapy).

SELECTED READINGS

Brock TD: *Milestones in microbiology*, Washington, DC, 1975, American Society for Microbiology.

Gest H: *The world of microbes*, Menlo Park, Calif, 1987, Benjamin Cummings.

Molinari JA: Infection control: its evolution to the current standard precaution, *J Am Dent Assoc* 134:569–574, 2003.

Venugopalan V, Shriner KA, Wong-Beringer A: Regulatory oversight and safety of probiotic use, *Emerg Infect Dis* 16(11):1661–1665, 2010.

REVIEW QUESTIONS

Multiple Choice

1. Mycology is the study of:
   a. bacteria
   b. viruses
   c. fungi
   d. protozoa

2. Infection control is:
   a. sterilizing instruments
   b. disinfecting surfaces
   c. handling sharps carefully
   d. controlling microbial contamination and infection

3. Who became known as the father of oral microbiology?
   a. Willoughby D. Miller
   b. Louis Pasteur
   c. Robert Koch
   d. Ignaz Semmelweis

4. Pasteurization is achieved by which of the following processes?
   a. Cleaning surfaces with a disinfectant
   b. Heating a fluid to 63° C (145.4° F) for 30 minutes
   c. Sterilizing instruments at 49.4° C (121° F) for 20 minutes
   d. Using an alcohol-based hand rub

5. Who first proposed that infection of open wounds was caused by microorganisms in the air?
   a. Louis Pasteur
   b. Oliver Wendell Holmes
   c. Lord Joseph Lister
   d. Chris H. Miller

6. Viruses that infect bacteria are called:
   a. fungi
   b. bacteriophages
   c. prions
   d. protozoa

7. The first microorganisms to be observed under a microscope in 1667 came from:
   a. tooth scrapings and gutter water
   b. lake water and air
   c. rotten meat
   d. a dead possum and the surrounding soil

8. Which of the following statements is true about the activities of microorganisms?
   a. Microorganisms do nothing but cause diseases.
   b. Microorganisms are actually more beneficial than harmful to mankind.

9. When were viruses first seen under the electron microscope?
   a. 1556
   b. 1667
   c. 1940
   d. 1965

10. Who first recognized the importance of handwashing to prevent the spread of disease agents?
    a. Ignaz Semmelweis
    b. Louis Pasteur
    c. Edward Jenner
    d. John Tyndall

11. Which of the following agents cause prion diseases?
    a. Viruses
    b. Bacteria
    c. Special proteins
    d. Yeasts

12. What are probiotics?
    a. Special disinfectants that kill bacterial spores
    b. Antiseptics for open wounds
    c. Microbes administered to confer a health benefit on a host
    d. Antibiotics for lower animals

Please visit http://evolve.elsevier.com/Miller/infectioncontrol/ for additional practice and study support tools.

Characteristics of Microorganisms

OUTLINE

Bacteria
  Bacterial Names and Differentiation
  Cell Morphology and Structure
  Growth and Control

Viruses
  Structure
  Life Cycle

Lytic Cycle
Persistent Infection
Host Cell Transformation
Controlling Virus Replication

Fungi

LEARNING OBJECTIVES

After completing this chapter, the student should be able to do the following:

1. Do the following regarding bacteria:
   • Describe how bacteria are named and differentiated.
   • Describe the general structure of bacteria.
   • Describe what bacteria need for growth.
   • Describe how bacteria are cultured.
   • Describe how bacteria make acids from sugar.

   • Describe how to control the growth of bacteria.
2. Do the following regarding viruses:
   • Describe the general structure and life cycle of viruses.
   • Describe the lytic cycle of viruses.
   • Identify types of persistent viral infections.
   • Describe viral host cell transformation and how to control virus replication.
3. Describe the most important fungus in dentistry.

KEY TERMS

Acidogenic
Aciduric
Antibodies
Bacilli
Bacterial Growth
Bactericidal
Bacteriostatic
Binary Fission
Candidiasis
Capsid
Capsule
Cell Wall
Cocci
Colony-forming Units
Cytoplasm
Cytoplasmic Membrane

Endospore
Endotoxin
Envelope
Enzymes
Facultative Anaerobes
Fimbriae
Flagella
Fungicidal
Genus
Gram-negative
Gram-positive
Lysozyme
Mesophiles
Mesosomes
Metabolism
Microaerophiles

Micrometer
Nucleic Acid Core
Nucleoid
Obligate Aerobes
Obligate Anaerobes
Outer Membrane
Peptidoglycan
Phagocytosis
Pili
Proteases
Psychrophiles
Species
Spirilla
Spore
Thermophiles
Virucidal

Four groups of microorganisms have varying degrees of importance in the field of dentistry and allied dental health. These groups are bacteria, viruses, fungi, and protozoa. Although certain protozoa may occur in the human mouth, this chapter concentrates on bacteria, fungi, and viruses. Although each group has a different life cycle and each group is composed of many different types, the bacteria share two common characteristics: they are too small to be seen by the naked eye, and many members of each group can live on or in the human body, which may result in development of harmful infections.

BACTERIA

Bacterial Names and Differentiation

Bacteria are named like most other life forms, with a first name (genus) and a last name (species). Each genus is composed of one or more species, and some species may be subdivided further into types and strains. For example, the genus *Streptococcus* is composed of approximately 21 different species and the oral species *Streptococcus mutans* is divided into eight subtypes (A to H).

Bacteria have different characteristics and perform different activities that allow them to be distinguished from one another. These include cell morphology (size and shape), staining characteristics, colony characteristics (appearance during growth on agar media), metabolic properties, immunologic properties, and DNA and RNA characteristics.

All sizes and shapes are determined by observation under a microscope that magnifies approximately 1000 times normal size. Because bacteria are difficult to see even under a regular light microscope, procedures for staining the cells with special dyes were developed to aid visualization. A staining procedure developed by Dr. Christian Gram differentiates bacteria into one of two groups. Those bacteria that appear blue or purple are called gram-positive, and those that appear pink or red are called gram-negative. Gram-positive and gram-negative bacteria have other important differences, which are described later. Other staining procedures also aid in identifying bacteria. For example, the Ziehl-Neelsen or Kinyoun acid-fast stain helps visualize acid-fast bacilli and greatly aids in the identification of *Mycobacterium tuberculosis*, the causative agent of tuberculosis.

Another way to visualize bacteria is to place (inoculate) them onto the surface of a semisolid growth medium, called agar, contained in a covered dish, called a Petri plate (described later). If the agar medium contains all the proper nutrients and is incubated at the proper temperature, each bacterium begins to multiply into a small mass of cells (a colony) that can be seen with the naked eye (Figure 2-1). Each visible colony contains hundreds of thousands of bacterial cells and frequently has an appearance (shape, color, size, consistency) different from that of another species. Thus colony morphology is one aspect used to differentiate bacteria.

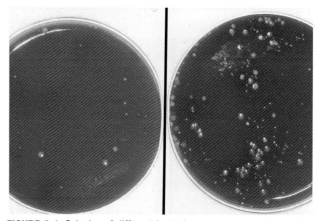

FIGURE 2-1 Colonies of different bacteria on an agar growth medium in Petri plates. Colonies of different bacteria vary in size, shape, color, and texture. **Left,** shows approximately 30 colonies on the plate. **Right,** shows a few hundred colonies. Each colony contains thousands of bacterial cells. Each colony was originally derived from one or a few cells.

Metabolism refers to the physical and chemical changes that occur during bacterial growth (multiplication or increase in numbers of cells). Different bacteria have different metabolic properties, which distinguish one species from another. Detecting these differences may involve performing many tests; for example, determining the nutrients (e.g., sugars and amino acids) used for growth, the requirements for oxygen or carbon dioxide during growth, the waste materials (e.g., acids) produced during growth, and the enzymes (i.e., catalysts that chemically change a substance such as breaking down proteins into amino acids) made during growth.

Table 2-1 assists in understanding the characteristics of microorganisms by describing various macromolecules and their subunits. Bacteria having different chemical substances on their surfaces or that make different extracellular substances (substances that are released from the cell to the outside environment) cause the synthesis of different antibodies (special proteins in serum) when bacteria are placed into animals. These antibodies are part of the immune defense system of human beings and lower animals and are explained further in Chapter 3. Antibodies formed against one bacterium usually will bind only to that bacterium and not to others, and this binding can be visualized in the laboratory by a variety of techniques. Thus, exposing an animal to a known bacterium, allowing the animal to make antibodies to that bacterium, mixing the serum of the animal with unknown bacteria in the laboratory, and looking for a visualized positive reaction can help determine the identity of the unknown bacteria.

All of the properties of bacteria are controlled by specific genes in their DNA. Thus, because different bacteria have different properties, they also have different DNA and RNA. Several techniques can be used to detect differences in these nucleic acids, and these techniques greatly aid in differentiating and identifying bacteria.

TABLE 2-1   Microbial Biochemicals

Macromolecule	Basic Composition	Examples or Occurrence
Protein	Amino acids (e.g., tryptophan, leucine)	Enzymes, viral capsid, cell walls, cytoplasmic membranes, flagella
Polysaccharide	Monosaccharides (e.g., glucose, fructose)	Capsules, storage granules, dextran
Lipid	Fatty acids, glycerol	Cytoplasmic membranes, viral envelopes
Nucleic acid	Adenine, guanine, cytosine, thymine, ribose AGCT	DNA, RNA
Glycoprotein	Polysaccharide, protein	Fimbriae, viral envelope
Lipoprotein	Lipid, protein	Cell wall
Lipopolysaccharide	Lipid, polysaccharide	Endotoxin

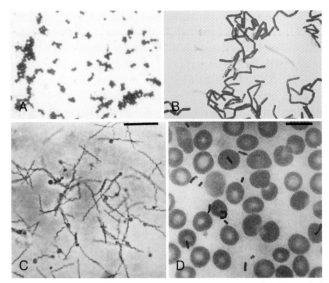

FIGURE 2-2 The common morphologies of prokaryotic cells as revealed by phase-contrast photomicrographs of unstained **(A)** *Staphylococcus aureus* (cocci), **(B)** *Bacillus subtilis* (rods), and **(C)** *Treponema denticola* (spirals) compared with **(D)** human red blood cells. *B. subtilis* has been mixed with the red blood cells in D for size comparison. Bar is 10 μm. (**A,** From VanMeter KC, VanMeter WG, Hubert RJ: *Microbiology for the healthcare professional,* St. Louis, 2010, Mosby. **B,** From Mahon CR, Lehman DC, Manuselis, Jr, G: *Textbook of diagnostic microbiology,* ed 4, St. Louis, 2011, Saunders. **C, D,** From Slots J, Taubman MA: *Contemporary oral microbiology and immunology,* St. Louis, 1992, Mosby.)

Cell Morphology and Structure

Size and Shape

Bacteria are single cells with one of three basic shapes. Spherical cells are called **cocci** (singular coccus); rod-shaped cells are called **bacilli** (singular bacillus); and curved or spiral cells are called **spirilla** (singular spirillum). The cocci and bacilli may exist as single cells, or they may exist in small clusters or in chains (Figure 2-2). The average diameter of a coccus is about 1 **micrometer** (μm). Common bacilli are about 1 μm wide and 5 to 10 μm long.

Spirilla are 0.2 to 1.0 μm wide and up to 30 μm long. A micrometer is 1 millionth of a meter or 1 thousandth of a millimeter, and a millimeter is the smallest division on a metric ruler. Approximately 25,000 cocci laid side by side would create a line just 1 inch long. In comparison, a human red blood cell is about 7 μm in diameter.

Structure

Although bacterial species differ in shape, size, and activity, their structure is similar. Understanding this structure helps explain their role in causing diseases, their resistance to methods of killing, and their activities that are beneficial to the human race. Figure 2-3 shows the structures of a representative bacterial cell; Table 2-2 lists the functions of these structures.

Cytoplasm

The **cytoplasm** is contained within the cytoplasmic membrane and is a viscous material consisting of water, enzymes and other proteins, carbohydrates, lipids, nucleic acids, essential nutrients, oxygen, and waste products. Embedded in the cytoplasm is the bacterial **nucleoid**, which consists of a single, long chromosome of DNA that contains most of the genes (approximately 2500) controlling cell activities. The nucleoid usually is diffused throughout the cytoplasm rather than well defined as in mammalian cells. Some bacteria also have extrachromosomal DNA in small units in the cytoplasm called plasmids. Plasmids frequently carry genes that express special activities such as resistance to chemical and physical agents and antibiotics.

The cytoplasm also contains submicroscopic particles called ribosomes that serve as physical sites for the synthesis of proteins from amino acids. Some bacteria may have granules in the cytoplasm that consist of stored substances such as starch, lipids, or iron.

Cytoplasmic Membrane

The **cytoplasmic membrane** surrounds the cytoplasm and is composed of lipids and protein substances. Its structure is similar to that of mammalian cells, and its functions include regulating the entrance and exit of nutrient materials and waste products, maintaining proper pressure within the cell to keep it from bursting, containing the enzymes responsible for synthesizing the outer cell wall, serving as the physical site for attachment and allocation of newly formed chromosomal DNA during cell division, controlling release of certain extracellular enzymes, and serving as the site of many metabolic reactions through which the cell gains energy for growth.

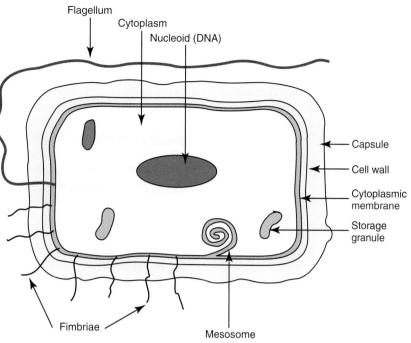

Flagellum
Cytoplasm
Nucleoid (DNA)
Capsule
Cell wall
Cytoplasmic membrane
Storage granule
Fimbriae
Mesosome

FIGURE 2-3 A composite bacterial cell.

TABLE 2-2 Bacterial Structure and Function

Structure	Function/Activity
Cytoplasmic membrane	Transport of nutrients; energy metabolism; secretion of wastes; DNA synthesis; cell wall synthesis
Cell wall	Cell shape; protection from mechanical damage
Outer membrane of gram-negative bacteria	Contains endotoxin; transport of nutrients
Capsule	Protection from drying; antiphagocytic; attachment to surfaces
Flagella	Locomotion
Fimbriae (pili)	Attachment to surfaces; transport of DNA between cells
Nucleoid	DNA control of cell activities
Endospore	Protection against adverse conditions

Mesosomes, present mostly in gram-positive bacteria, are inward foldings of the cytoplasmic membrane. Mesosomes house many hydrolytic enzymes that are released into the extracellular environment and break down macromolecules into their subunits, which are taken into the cell as food.

Antimicrobial agents in many disinfectants, handwashing agents, and mouth rinses kill or inhibit the growth of bacteria by acting on the cytoplasmic membrane. Chlorhexidine gluconate, present in handwashing products and mouth rinses, is thought to affect the cell membrane and interfere with energy metabolism and uptake of nutrients by the cells.

Cell Wall

The bacterial **cell wall** is a rigid structure that gives the cell its characteristic shape (coccus, rod, spirillum) and is not present in mammalian cells. The cell wall is a complex structure in which its basic components (**peptidoglycan**) form a tight-knit "net" over the entire surface of the cell. Peptidoglycan (*peptide*, small protein; *glycan*, polysaccharide) consists of long polysaccharide chains with short side chains of peptides. The peptides of one polysaccharide chain are linked to the peptides of other polysaccharide chains, forming a large continuous macromolecule. Besides giving the cell its characteristic shape, the peptidoglycan also protects the cell from mechanical crushing. Gram-positive bacteria have several layers of peptidoglycan in their cell walls and are much more resistant to external physical forces than gram-negative bacteria, because the latter have only a few layers of peptidoglycan.

The peptidoglycan of the cell wall is the site of action of several antimicrobial agents. **Lysozyme** is an enzyme present in saliva, tears, nasal secretions, and other body secretions and is present inside white blood cells (e.g., phagocytes, which are described later) that destroy bacteria. This enzyme lyses susceptible bacteria by breaking the bond between the subunits of the polysaccharide chain in peptidoglycan. The antibiotic penicillin and its many derivations act by preventing cross-linking of the peptidoglycan units as the cell wall is being synthesized during cell division. Other antibiotics such as vancomycin and the cephalosporins also prevent cell wall synthesis. The action of all of these antimicrobial agents results in "holes" forming in the peptidoglycan that cause a loss of the cytoplasm into the external environment (lysis) and cell death.

Outer Membrane

Gram-negative (but not gram-positive) bacteria have an outer membrane just external to the cell wall. This membrane covers the entire cell surface, and its basic structure and composition are like the cytoplasmic membrane. The outer membrane, however, contains an important component called endotoxin that is composed of lipid, polysaccharide, and protein (lipopolysaccharide–protein complex). When endotoxin is released from bacteria present in the body (after cell death and lysis, or, in some instances, during its synthesis), it can cause damage to nearby body cells and stimulate several reactions in the body, including fever, inflammation, bone destruction, hemorrhage, and vomiting. The action of endotoxin is thought to play a role in many infectious diseases, including periodontal diseases, dysentery, meningitis, typhoid fever, gonorrhea, and cholera.

Capsule

Some gram-positive and gram-negative bacteria contain another structure called the capsule, which also is referred to as a slime layer or glycocalyx. The capsule covers the entire outer surface external to the cell wall in some gram-positive bacteria or external to the outer membrane in some gram-negative bacteria. The capsule is produced by the cytoplasmic membrane and secreted through the cell wall and remains associated with the cell surface in the form of a gelatinous covering. Usually the capsule consists of polysaccharide, but in a few instances it may contain proteins. Some species may have large capsules, such as *Streptococcus pneumoniae* (the cause of lobar pneumonia and middle ear infections); others may have only a thin layer of capsular material, such as *S. mutans* (a cause of dental caries).

Capsules contain a large amount of water (hydrated) and may help bacteria survive in dry environments. The presence of a capsule also influences how bacteria interact with cells and other surfaces in the human body. Surface polysaccharides in the microcapsule of *S. mutans* are involved in sucrose-induced plaque formation on tooth surfaces (see Chapter 5). The presence of capsules also reduces the ability of white blood cells to surround, engulf, and destroy the bacterium through a process called phagocytosis (eating cells) and digestion (see Chapter 3). Thus bacteria with capsules tend to escape these early body-defense mechanisms against bacterial disease agents. Bacteria without capsules are engulfed and destroyed more easily.

Flagella

Some bacteria have long, threadlike appendages called flagella (singular flagellum). These protein structures are attached to the cytoplasmic membrane extending through the cell wall and, if present, the outer membrane and capsule. They have a whiplike motion and allow the bacterium to move through fluids. The number of flagella per bacterial cell may range from one to many, exhibiting different arrangements over the cell surface.

Fimbriae and Pili

Fimbriae and pili are hairlike protein appendages projecting from the cytoplasmic membrane into the external environment. They are much shorter than flagella and have two major functions. Sex pili, found mainly on gram-negative bacteria, serve as a tube through which DNA can be passed directly from a donor cell to a recipient cell during a process called conjugation. This process permits properties expressed by the DNA genes of one cell to be transferred to and expressed by another cell. Fimbriae, also called pili, serve as mechanisms by which cells can attach to other cells or environmental surfaces. The fimbriae act as a bridge between the cell and other surfaces. Attachment fimbriae provide an important virulence property. Almost all bacteria that cause harmful infections on or through mucous membranes must first attach to the epithelial cells of the mucous membrane, or they will be washed away by secretions of the body. Attachment fimbriae provide the mechanisms of attachment in diseases such as "strep throat," scarlet fever, gonorrhea, and diphtheria, and cause some bacteria to attach to each other during the formation of dental plaque.

Endospores

Some bacteria have developed a defense mechanism against death caused by adverse environmental conditions. When available nutrients become depleted, cells of *Bacillus*, *Geobacillus*, and *Clostridium* form a large internal structure that contains the DNA and other substances surrounded by several coats of protein. This dense, thick-walled structure is called a spore or endospore and is one of the most resistant forms of life against heat, drying, and chemicals (Figure 2-4). Once formed, the spore can remain dormant for years and then, when exposed to the proper nutrients and other growth requirements, it can germinate into an actively dividing (vegetative) cell. Only one endospore forms within a bacterial cell, and it germinates into only one vegetative bacterial cell. This is in contrast to fungal spores, in which several spores may form a single cell. Bacterial spores are particularly important in the field of infection control because of their high resistance to heat and antimicrobial chemicals. Spores of *Geobacillus stearothermophilus* and *Bacillus atrophaeus* are used biologically to monitor the use and functioning of heat or ethylene oxide gas sterilizers (see Chapter 12). Also, spores of *B. atrophaeus* and *Clostridium sporogenes* are used to test the antimicrobial effectiveness of liquid sterilants used at room temperature.

Growth and Control

Bacterial growth is defined as an increase in cell numbers; it also is referred to as multiplication. The cells divide by

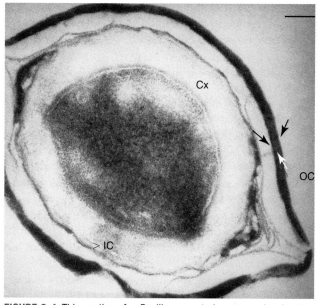

FIGURE 2-4 Thin section of a *Bacillus megaterium* spore showing two spore coats (*IC*, inner coat; *OC*, outer coat). The germ cell wall of the spore coat is seen immediately underlying the thick cortex (*Cx*). Bar is 100 nm. (From Aaronson Al, Fitz-James P: Structure and morphogenesis of the bacterial spore coat, *Bacteriol Rev* 40:360-402, 1976.)

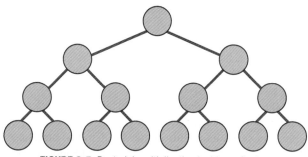

FIGURE 2-5 Bacterial multiplication by binary fission.

a process called **binary fission**, in which each cell divides into two daughter cells (Figure 2-5). In the next generation, each of these daughter cells divides into two similar cells, and this continues until the environmental conditions no longer support growth because of a lack of nutrients; a buildup of toxic products; changes in pH, temperature, and availability of oxygen; or the application of physical or chemical agents that kill the bacteria.

Bacteria have a tremendous ability to multiply, and under optimal growth conditions a population of some bacteria, such as *Escherichia coli*, can double in number (go from one generation to the next) in just 20 minutes. If such growth continues for just 24 hours, one cell can multiply to a mass of cells that is equal to the size of Earth (more than 3 trillion billion cells). This of course can never happen because nutrients soon become depleted and growth stops. To be more realistic, 10 mL of an overnight broth culture of a bacterium seldom achieves a total population of more than 10 billion cells.

Growth Requirements

Bacteria are influenced by a variety of physical and chemical conditions of the environments in which they exist. Each bacterial species requires certain conditions for growth, and, if those conditions do not exist at a given site, the bacterium will not be found at that site. Even subtle differences are important. For example, the differences in the physical and the chemical environments between the buccal surface of a tooth and a periodontal pocket just a few millimeters away are sufficient to result in important differences in the types and numbers of bacteria that are fond at these two sites (see Chapter 5). The greater the differences among environmental sites, the greater the differences in the types and number of bacteria present. Thus the bacteria that survive and grow in the human body can be different from those that survive in the oceans. Conversely, some bacterial species can survive and grow in widely different environments. Five major chemical or physical conditions influence growth of bacteria: temperature, acidity, nutrients, oxygen metabolism, and water.

Temperature

Bacteria can be divided into three groups based on the temperature required for optimal growth. **Thermophiles** grow best at 56° C (132.8° F) with a range of 45° C to 70° C (113° F to 158° F). Such bacteria were found in the hot waters of the "Old Faithful" geyser in Yellowstone National Park. More importantly, the spore-forming thermophilic bacterium *G. stearothermophilus* was selected many years ago to test the use and functioning of heat sterilizers because of its resistance to heat. **Mesophiles** grow at temperatures ranging from 22° C to 45° C (71.6° F to 113° F) with optimal growth at body temperature, 37° C (98.6° F). Most of the bacteria that grow and survive in the human body, including those that cause infectious diseases (such as dental caries, periodontal diseases, tuberculosis, bacterial pneumonia, tetanus, and many others), are mesophiles. **Psychrophiles** grow between temperatures of 1° C and 22° C (33.8° F and 71.6° F), with optimal growth at the typical refrigerator temperature of 7° C (44.6° F). The bacteria present in the oceans, as well as many of those that spoil food stored in a refrigerator, are psychrophiles. Refrigeration has long been used to maintain the freshness of food or extend the storage life of many items that may be contaminated with microorganisms. Refrigeration slows down or prevents the growth of many bacteria and molds, but refrigeration cannot be considered a means of killing microorganisms. If psychrophiles are present, they will continue to grow at normal rates at these low temperatures. If fresh pasteurized milk or high-quality hamburger is purchased at the food market and stored unopened in the refrigerator, it eventually spoils because microorganisms, some of which may be psychrophiles, grow using the nutrients in the milk or meat, producing the physical and chemical changes associated with food spoilage.

Thus if an item or solution becomes contaminated with microorganisms, placing it in the refrigerator or freezer cannot be relied on to kill the microorganisms to make it "safe" for use.

Acidity

pH is a measure of acidity, and the pH scale ranges from 0 (high acidity) to 14 (high alkalinity). Values from 0 to 7 are acidic, and values from 7 to 14 are basic or alkaline. The neutral pH of 7 indicates an equal amount of acid and base or no acid or base present. Examples of acidic solutions are stomach acid (pH 1.5) and orange juice (pH 2.9). Examples of basic or alkaline solutions are household ammonia cleaners (pH 11.9) and human blood (approximately pH 7.4). Pure water has a pH of 7.0.

Most bacteria that survive in the human body grow over a pH range of 5.5 to 8.5, with optimal growth at pH 7.0. Bacteria that produce acids during growth are called acidogenic; those that survive and grow in an acidic environment (usually below pH 5.5) are called aciduric. Acidogenic and aciduric bacteria are important in the initiation and progression of dental caries, as described in Chapter 5.

Nutrients

Bacteria, like mammalian cells, must synthesize all of the macromolecules of protein, polysaccharides, lipids, and nucleic acids (DNA and RNA) needed to grow. These macromolecules are synthesized from the building blocks of amino acids, monosaccharides, fatty acids, and purines/pyrimidines. Bacteria also must use a variety of smaller molecules such as vitamins and inorganic substances (e.g., sodium, potassium, iron, chlorine, manganese, magnesium, sulfur, phosphorus, calcium, and trace elements). If a bacterium cannot synthesize a given building block, such as an amino acid, or a vitamin, such as niacin, these substances must be available from the environment for the bacterium to survive and grow. Just as we require "eight essential vitamins," bacteria also require nutrients for growth.

Different bacteria have different nutritional requirements. For example, *S. mutans* may require six amino acids, five vitamins, all four purines and pyrimidines, and other small molecules, plus an energy source, nitrogen, oxygen, inorganic salts, and trace elements from its environment. Conversely, some types of *E. coli* need only carbon dioxide, a nitrogen source, and trace elements and from this meager "diet" can synthesize all of the macromolecules needed for growth.

Many organic nutrients available for growth may not be in a form that can be used by the bacteria. For example, amino acids are the building blocks for proteins, and many bacteria require certain amino acids to synthesize their own proteins needed for growth. In many instances, proteins rather than the amino acid building blocks are present in the environment, but the entire protein molecules are too large to get into bacterial cells. Thus many bacteria make extracellular proteases, which are enzymes released into the environment that break down proteins into amino acids that can enter the cell. Bacteria also may produce extracellular enzymes that degrade polysaccharides into monosaccharides or lipids into fatty acids, which then can be taken into the cell and be used for growth.

Unfortunately, when these extracellular bacterial enzymes are produced in the human body during a bacterial infection, they may degrade proteins, polysaccharides, or lipids that are important components of body cells, causing damage to these cells. This is one of the mechanisms by which bacteria cause disease.

Oxygen Metabolism

Bacteria are divided into four groups based on their requirement for oxygen:

- **Obligate aerobes** require the presence of oxygen at concentrations of approximately 20% and cannot grow at low oxygen concentrations.
- **Microaerophiles** can tolerate only low concentrations of oxygen of no more than 4%.
- **Obligate anaerobes** cannot tolerate oxygen and grow only in its absence.
- **Facultative anaerobes** can grow in the presence or absence of oxygen.

Almost all bacteria (regardless of their growth requirement for oxygen) have enzymes that produce toxic substances (e.g., superoxide and hydrogen peroxide) from oxygen that can kill the bacteria. These toxic substances also are produced by white blood cells and help these cells kill bacteria after phagocytosis (see Chapter 3). Some bacteria that produce these toxic substances in the presence of oxygen have mechanisms to remove them to prevent death. One mechanism involves the enzyme superoxide dismutase that converts superoxide to hydrogen peroxide and molecular oxygen. Hydrogen peroxide is converted to water and oxygen by the enzyme catalase.

Obligate aerobes, microaerophiles, and facultative anaerobes, all of which can grow in the presence of oxygen, have superoxide dismutase and catalase to detoxify the oxygen metabolites. Obligate anaerobes do not have these enzymes and therefore cannot tolerate the presence of oxygen. Approximately 99% of the bacteria that live in the mouth are obligate anaerobes or facultative anaerobes.

Water

All life forms require water to dissolve nutrients and to permit nutrient entrance or transport into cells. Also, the water molecule is required in several enzymatic reactions to break down (e.g., hydrolyze) certain substances.

Culturing Bacteria

All of the nutritional and physical growth requirements must be met to culture (grow) bacteria in the laboratory. Culture media in the form of a liquid (broth medium) or in a semisolid (JELL-O–like) form (agar medium) provide the nutrients. Agar is a polysaccharide from seaweed that is liquid at boiling temperatures and turns semisolid when it cools to room temperature. Agar is added to a solution of nutrients, brought to a boil, sterilized, and poured into covered dishes (Petri plates) or into tubes to cool and solidify. Samples of bacteria then are placed into sterilized broth media or onto the surface of sterile agar media and incubated under the appropriate atmospheric conditions (anaerobically, without air; aerobically, in air) at the proper temperature.

If bacteria grow in the broth culture, the broth becomes turbid (cloudy). If bacteria grow on the surface of agar media, visible colonies of bacteria appear that may be well separated from each other (see Figure 2-1), or, if a large number of bacteria were originally placed on the agar, a confluent solid mass of growth (lawn) may appear all over the surface.

An agar medium is used primarily to separate bacterial cells physically from each other to obtain a pure culture (growth of only one type of bacterium). Most samples taken from the human body or from nature that are cultured for the presence of bacteria contain many different species. When the sample is spread or streaked (inoculated) over the surface of an agar medium, individual cells or small groups of cells, called colony-forming units (CFUs), are deposited at different sites on the surface. As the agar plate is incubated, each cell or CFU begins to multiply into a pure colony (clone). Thus all of the cells in the colony are derived from the cells or CFUs originally deposited at that site and exist as a pure culture that can be picked off the agar medium and kept separate from all other bacteria. Occasionally, more than one type of bacterial cell can be deposited next to another on the agar surface during inoculation, and both will grow into a mixed, rather than a pure, colony. Such colonies must be picked off and restreaked on a fresh agar plate to separate the types into pure colonies.

Agar plates also provide a means to quantitate the number, or CFUs, of bacterial cells present in a sample. Each single colony that develops on the agar plate after incubation represents 1 CFU present in the original sample.

Most bacteria can survive and grow separately from other cells if the environment is appropriate. Special bacteria can grow only while inside other living cells. Their general structures and mechanisms for growth are the same as those of the free-living bacteria, but they lack some of the metabolic machinery necessary to exist separately. Thus they use the machinery of other cells to grow. Examples of these special bacteria are members of the genera *Rickettsia*, which can cause diseases such as Rocky Mountain spotted fever, typhus, and ehrlichiosis, and *Chlamydia*, which can cause sexually transmitted diseases, pneumonia, and trachoma (disease of the eye).

Metabolic Activities

Metabolism is the sum of chemical reactions that occur in the cell. Metabolism involves the uptake of nutrients into the cell, converting them to substances needed by the cells for survival and multiplication and release of waste products (Figure 2-6). Metabolism includes two phases: catabolism, or the breakdown of nutrients to smaller or more easily usable molecules, and anabolism, or the synthesis of new molecules. Catabolism provides the building blocks or carbon skeletons and the energy needed for anabolism. Anabolism provides the macromolecules needed to make cell components, such as cell walls, DNA, cytoplasmic membranes, fimbriae, flagella, cytoplasmic granules, and capsules. Catabolic and anabolic reactions require biologic catalysts called enzymes.

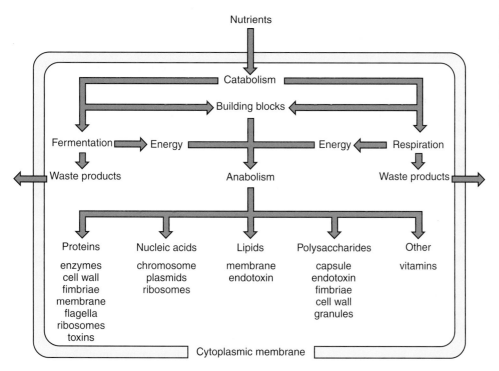

FIGURE 2-6 General bacterial metabolism. Nutrients are taken into the cell and processed through catabolic reactions that generate the building blocks and energy needed to synthesize macromolecules through anabolic reactions. Waste products generated exit the cell.

Enzymes

Metabolism occurs through the action of enzymes, which are catalysts made of protein. Catalysts speed up chemical reactions and are used over and over because they are not changed during the reaction. Action of some enzymes requires small molecules such as magnesium or calcium, called cofactors; other enzymes require organic molecules such as vitamins, called coenzymes. An enzyme (E) molecule binds to a specific molecule referred to as the substrate (S), and the enzyme binds to the part of the substrate molecules that will be changed. This binding causes the breaking of chemical bonds or the formation of new chemical bonds in the substrate molecule, changing the substrate to a new substance called the product (P). This reaction is written as follows:

$$E + S \rightarrow ES \rightarrow E + P$$

A bacterial cell has approximately 1000 different enzymes, and the enzyme names all end with the suffix -*ase* (e.g., protease and hydrolase). Some enzymes break down extracellular substrates into subunits (products) that then can be taken into the cell and used for growth. Other enzyme reactions may change one small molecule into another small molecule. In the example given, pyruvic acid (produced in the cells from the metabolism of sugar) is changed into lactic acid by the enzyme lactate dehydrogenase. Lactic acid produced by streptococci and lactobacilli in dental plaque leaves the cell as a waste product and can cause demineralization of the tooth surface, producing dental caries (see Chapter 5).

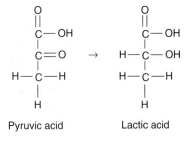

Pyruvic acid   Lactic acid

Catabolism

Bacterial multiplication requires the synthesis of new cell components, and these anabolic reactions require energy. Catabolism provides some of the building blocks for the macromolecules and the energy needed to drive anabolism. All bacteria require nutrients that can serve as sources of energy, and the energy is released from the nutrients as they are processed through catabolic reactions. Two major catabolic pathways that generate energy in bacteria are fermentation and respiration. The pathway used depends on the types of enzymes and metabolic machinery present in the bacterial cell.

Energy Production

A common energy source for many bacteria is glucose. After glucose is transported into the cells, it is processed through one of two major catabolic pathways known as fermentation or respiration (described later). These reactions are associated with the release of energy from the glucose, but the energy cannot be used to drive anabolic reactions unless it is transferred to special molecules such as adenosine triphosphate (ATP). The ATP then participates in the energy-requiring anabolic reactions such as the synthesis of polysaccharides from monosaccharides and proteins from amino acids.

Fermentation

Fermentation is an anaerobic process that usually involves the breakdown of sugars (called glycolysis) with end products of organic acids or alcohols. During fermentation of sugars, hydrogen atoms (also referred to as electrons) are released from the sugar breakdown products. These electrons then bind to organic molecules, changing their structure. In respiration, these electrons bind to oxygen or inorganic substances (as described later). During the fermentation of glucose, pyruvic acid usually accepts the released electrons, changing to lactic acid as a final end product. This is the metabolic pathway that is responsible for dental caries formation, and it is active in caries-conducive oral bacteria such as *S. mutans* and *Lactobacillus* spp. The metabolic machinery present in these oral bacteria gives the cells only one metabolic choice, the generation of building blocks and energy for anabolism through the fermentation of sugar mainly to lactic acid. Other bacteria may produce other products from fermentation, depending on the species and the nutrients available.

Respiration

Respiration by infectious bacteria also involves glycolysis of sugars to pyruvic acid as described for fermentation. The electrons released from the sugar breakdown products, however, are transferred to oxygen in aerobic respiration through a series of molecular processes called the electron transport chain. The pyruvic acid, rather than being changed to an end product lactic acid as in fermentation, is processed further through a series of reactions that yield considerably more energy in the form of ATP.

Controlling Growth

Controlling the growth of bacteria is accomplished by preventing their multiplication or by killing them. Such control is important to prevent damage that they may cause by growing where they should not (e.g., in our bodies, on food, in drinking water).

Preventing Growth

Prevention of growth can be achieved by changing or eliminating a physical or nutritional requirement for growth or by using a chemical agent that interferes with cell division. Agents or conditions that prevent bacterial growth without killing them are called bacteriostatic.

Storing items in the refrigerator stops or slows down bacterial growth, unless the bacteria are psychrophiles. Freezing bacteria stops their growth and, because of formation of ice crystals inside the cell, can rupture the cell membrane. Usually, some cells survive and may begin to grow when thawed.

Eliminating the availability of oxygen prevents the growth of aerobes. Adding oxygen prevents growth of anaerobes. Changing the pH beyond optimal values stops growth except for bacteria that can survive extreme pH values, such as aciduric bacteria in the mouth. Treating bacterial diseases with antibiotics can result in inhibiting growth or in killing the cells, depending on the bacterium and the antibiotic used. Antibiotics are chemicals that interfere with some metabolic activity of the bacterium but usually do not affect the metabolic activity of human body cells. This effect is referred to as selective toxicity. For example, penicillins prevent the formation of the cell wall in certain bacteria, which prevents their growth and usually kills the bacterium. Penicillins do not affect the growth of human body cells because our cells do not have cell walls.

Killing Bacteria

Killing of bacteria is accomplished by physical or chemical means and is an important aspect of disease prevention and infection control. Agents or conditions that kill microorganisms rather than just prevent their growth are called **bactericidal**, **virucidal**, or **fungicidal** agents or conditions. Probably the surest way to kill bacteria (or any other type of microorganism) in the shortest amount of time is to expose them to high temperature, such as that achieved in a steam, dry heat, or unsaturated chemical vapor sterilizer (see Chapter 12). The heat may destroy proteins, break down DNA and RNA, or cause structural damage to the cell membrane.

Several chemicals can kill bacteria and other microorganisms, and the type of chemical used frequently is determined by location of the microorganisms to be killed. Strong chemicals cannot be used to kill microorganisms on or in the body, whereas inanimate objects, such as operatory surfaces, can withstand treatment by such agents. Chemicals kill microorganisms by several mechanisms, depending on the properties of the chemical.

VIRUSES

Viruses cause many different diseases in human beings (e.g., measles, mumps, the common cold, severe acute respiratory syndrome, hepatitis, hemorrhagic fevers, and encephalitis). Viruses can also infect lower animals, plants, fungi, bacteria, algae, and protozoa. Viruses are important in dentistry because they can cause the following:

- Specific oral diseases (e.g., herpes infections and hand-foot-and-mouth disease)
- Diseases elsewhere in the body that may result in lesions occurring in the mouth (e.g., measles)
- Blood-borne diseases (e.g., hepatitis B and acquired immunodeficiency syndrome)
- Other types of diseases that may be transmitted in the dental office without use of proper infection control procedures (e.g., influenza)

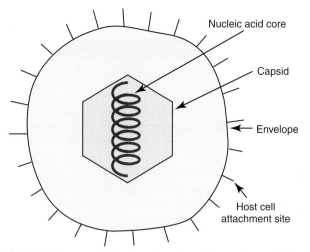

FIGURE 2-7 A representative virus. The shape of the nucleocapsid (capsid plus nucleic acid core) varies. Some viruses do not have an envelope, and the host cell attachment sites are located on the capsid.

Structure

Human viruses are smaller than bacteria, ranging from 0.02 to 0.3 μm. They may have many different shapes, but their general structure consists of a **nucleic acid core** (DNA or RNA) surrounded by a protein coat called a **capsid**. Some viruses also have an outer structure of lipids, proteins, and polysaccharides called the **envelope** (Figure 2-7).

Life Cycle

Unlike most bacteria, viruses are not free-living in that they do not have the metabolic machinery to synthesize new protein coats and nucleic acids. Viruses must use the nutrients and the metabolic machinery of living cells to multiply (replicate themselves). Thus viruses, like the special bacteria *Rickettsia* and *Chlamydia*, are called obligate intracellular parasites and multiply only inside of living cells. Table 2-3 summarizes their life cycle.

To replicate after entering the body, a virus must first adsorb to a surface of a living cell. This attachment is specific for each type of virus, and the virus attaches to certain host cells through special receptors on the capsid or on the envelope. After adsorption, the virus is taken into the cell, and the capsid is removed to release the nucleic acid and a few molecules of enzymes that help initiate replication. At this point in the life cycle, the nucleic acid of the virus (depending on the virus involved) may induce the lytic cycle, a persistent infection, or cell transformation.

Lytic Cycle

In the lytic cycle, the nucleic acid takes over the metabolic machinery of the cell and directs it to produce more virus particles inside the cell. The macromolecules of the host cell are broken down to provide the nutrients needed to synthesize new virus capsids and virus nucleic acids. These

TABLE 2-3 Life Cycle of a Virus

Step	Activity
Adsorption	Virus particle attaches to host cell surface.
Penetration	Virus enters host cell.
Uncoating	Capsid is degraded to release nucleic acid.
Replication*	Host cell machinery is used to synthesize new viral nucleic acid and protein capsid.
Assembly	Capsid is assembled around nucleic acid.
Release	Viral particle migrates to cytoplasmic membrane for budding, or the host cell lyses to release all internal contents.

*Some viruses will incorporate their nucleic acid into the host cell chromosomal DNA, resulting in (1) delay of the viral replication through the lytic cycle or (2) changing of host cell properties through transformation without host cell lysis.

elements then are assembled into new virus particles that are released when the host cell lyses. Each infected host cell may produce thousands of new viruses, each of which can infect a new host cell to produce more viruses. Some viruses are released slowly from their host cells by budding through the host cell cytoplasmic membrane, acquiring a portion of the cell membrane as their envelope.

Persistent Infection

A persistent virus infection may be latent, chronic, or slow. A latent persistent infection may occur if the nucleic acid of the virus is incorporated into the DNA of the host cell chromosomes. This incorporated viral nucleic acid is replicated along with the host cell chromosomes during normal cell division and is carried to each newly formed host cell. The viral nucleic acid may be reactivated later to induce a lytic cycle. This type of latent persistent infection is caused by herpesviruses such as herpes simplex, which causes cold sores. A chronic persistent infection such as hepatitis B is caused by lysis of the infected cells, but the symptoms are often unrecognized. Slow persistent infections are those in which the virus replicates slowly, causing recognizable damage only after several years.

Host Cell Transformation

Some viruses infect host cells and cause changes in the properties of cells without causing lysis of the cell. These new properties may result in uncontrolled cell growth such as the formation of certain tumors such as warts caused by the human papillomavirus.

Controlling Virus Replication

Viruses cause diseases by killing or changing the cells of our body. Artificially controlling the growth of viruses inside the body with chemicals is impossible in most cases. Antimicrobial chemicals (including antibiotics) act by inhibiting the metabolic machinery of the microorganisms. Because viruses use the metabolic machinery of the host cell to replicate, such chemicals would cause damage to the host cells. Thus, because most virus diseases cannot be treated, the approach is to prevent them from occurring through immunization or infection control procedures.

Viruses can be killed when outside of the body by exposure to heat or chemicals as described for bacteria.

FUNGI

Fungi include mushrooms, molds, and yeasts, with certain members of the latter two types capable of causing diseases in human beings. Such diseases may involve the lungs or other organs or tissues (e.g., histoplasmosis, coccidioidomycosis, blastomycosis, cryptococcosis, and phycomycoses) or the skin (e.g., athlete's foot, ringworm, and candidiasis) and infections of the nails, scalp, and hair. In dentistry, the most important fungal infection is oral candidiasis (e.g., thrush or denture stomatitis). The infection is caused by the fungus *Candida albicans*, which may exist as a yeast cell or as a filamentous fungus (mold). This organism also may cause skin infections, vaginal infections, or widespread infection in the body.

C. albicans occurs as a member of the normal oral microbiota in approximately 30% of adults. The fungus is an opportunistic pathogen in that it usually causes harmful infections only when given a special opportunity resulting from depressed body defenses, immature body defenses as in the newborn, changes in the physiology of the body, trauma to tissues (e.g., poor-fitting dentures), debilitating systemic diseases, and long-term antibacterial therapy.

Oral infections with *C. albicans* usually are treated easily with topical antifungal agents, and the yeast cells can be killed outside the body by exposure to heat and to certain chemicals, as described for bacteria and viruses.

SELECTED READINGS

Bagg J, MacFarlane TW, Poxton IR, Smith AJ: *Essentials of microbiology for dental students*, ed. 2, Oxford, 2006, Oxford University Press.

Lamont RJ, Burne RA, Lantz MS, LeBlanc DJ: *Oral microbiology and immunology*, Herdon, PA, 2006, ASM Press.

Sompayrac L: *How pathogenic viruses work*, Boston, 2002, Jones and Bartlett.

REVIEW QUESTIONS

Multiple Choice Questions

1. *Candida albicans* is a:
   a. prion
   b. bacterium
   c. virus
   d. yeast

2. Which of the following microbes do not need to multiply inside of living cells?
   a. DNA viruses ~~virus need host~~
   b. RNA viruses
   c. *Chlamydia* ~~special bacteria~~
   d. Regular bacteria

3. Amino acids are linked together to form:
   a. polysaccharides
   b. DNA and RNA
   c. proteins
   d. fats

4. Which type of bacterium is shaped like a sphere?
   a. Bacillus
   b. Coccus
   c. Spirillum

5. Which is smaller?
   a. Human red blood cell
   b. Bacterium
   c. Virus

6. What bacterial cell structure protects the cell from being crushed?
   a. Cell membrane
   b. Cell wall
   c. Capsule
   d. Fimbriae

7. A special form of bacterium that is dormant and highly resistant to heat and chemicals is a:
   a. vegetative cell
   b. virus
   c. rickettsia
   d. spore

8. Bacteria that make acids are called:
   a. aerobic
   b. anaerobic
   c. aciduric
   d. acidogenic

9. Bacteria that can survive and grow in the presence of acids are called:
   a. aerobic
   b. anaerobic
   c. aciduric
   d. acidogenic

10. Bacteria that die in the presence of oxygen are called:
    a. aerobic *need*
    b. anaerobic
    c. fermentative
    d. acidogenic

11. Structures that allow certain bacteria to attach to surfaces are called:
    a. flagella *movement*
    b. ribosomes
    c. cocci
    d. fimbriae/*pili*

12. What bacterial structure inhibits phagocytosis and allows bacteria to escape death caused by white blood cells?
    a. Nucleus
    b. Capsule
    c. Cytoplasmic membrane
    d. Cell wall

13. What part of the name *Streptococcus mutans* is the species name?
    a. *Streptococcus*
    b. *mutans*

14. Which of the following best describes a psychrophilic bacterium? *crazy cold*
    a. Grows best at cold temperatures such as those in a refrigerator
    b. Produces acids during growth
    c. Is gram-negative
    d. Needs oxygen for growth

15. An antibiotic is a:
    a. chemical substance produced by a microorganism that can inhibit the growth of or destroy some other microorganisms
    b. protein that is produced by the body in response to an antigen and is capable of binding specifically to that antigen
    c. chemical agent used to kill microorganisms on contaminated operatory surfaces
    d. negatively charged ion

Development of Infectious Diseases

OUTLINE

Steps in Disease Development
  Source of the Microorganism
  Escape from the Source
  Spread of Microorganisms to another Person
  Entry into a New Person

Infection
Damage to the Body
Host–Microorganism Interactions
  Pathogenic Properties of Microorganisms
  Host Defense Mechanisms

LEARNING OBJECTIVES

After completing this chapter, the student should be able to do the following:

1. List the steps in the development of an infectious disease, and do the following:
   • Describe the various stages of an infectious disease and describe how each stage is involved in the spread of the disease to others.
   • Differentiate between direct, indirect, droplet, and airborne spread of disease agents.

   • List the ways microbes can enter the body and describe how the route of entry may relate to disease development.
2. List disease-producing properties of microbes.
3. List the four mechanisms by which we defend ourselves against pathogenic microbes.
4. Define immunity, describe how it is involved in protecting against infectious diseases, how it can cause damage to the body, and differentiate between antigens and antibodies.

KEY TERMS

Acquired Defenses
Acute Stage
Anaphylactic Shock
Antibodies
Antigens
Asthma
Asymptomatic Carriers
Body Substance Isolation
Ciliary Escalator
Complement System
Contact Dermatitis

Convalescent Stage
Cytotoxic
Endogenous
Exogenous
Fomites
Hay Fever
Histolytic Enzymes
Incubation Stage
Infection
Infectious Diseases
Innate Defenses

Interferon
Lymphokines
Macrophages
Malaise
Neutrophils
Opportunistic Pathogens
Pathogens
Prodromal Stage
Standard Precautions
Toxigenic Diseases
Universal Precautions

Diseases in the body have several causes. Some causes are associated with microorganisms, but others result from malfunctioning of an organ (e.g., hyperthyroidism and diabetes), a nutritional deficiency (e.g., rickets and scurvy), an allergic reaction (e.g., hay fever, asthma, and poison ivy), and abnormal growth of cells (e.g., cancer and tumors).

An **infectious disease** occurs when a microorganism in the body multiplies and causes damage to the tissues. The microorganisms that cause infectious diseases are called **pathogens**.

Two types of infectious diseases are **endogenous** and **exogenous**. These terms refer to the source of the microorganism. Endogenous diseases are caused by microorganisms that are normally present on or in the body without causing harm, but something happens that allows them to express their disease-producing potential. Examples of oral endogenous infectious diseases caused by members of the normal oral flora are dental caries, pulpitis, periodontal diseases, and cervicofacial actinomycosis. The causative agents of these diseases are called **opportunistic pathogens**. These agents cause diseases only when given a special opportunity to enter deeper tissues of the body or to accumulate to levels that can harm the body.

An exogenous disease is caused by microorganisms that are not normally present on or in the body but contaminate the body from the outside. Most infectious diseases are exogenous diseases (e.g., hepatitis B, "strep throat," acquired immunodeficiency syndrome [AIDS], measles, chickenpox, the common cold, and influenza).

Some exogenous microorganisms also can cause disease without entering and multiplying in the body. These are called **toxigenic diseases** and occur after eating food in which microorganisms have multiplied and produced toxins or poisons (e.g., *Staphylococcus* food poisoning and botulism).

STEPS IN DISEASE DEVELOPMENT

Box 3-1 lists the steps for development of exogenous infectious diseases. Exogenous infectious diseases develop through six basic steps, each of which may be modified slightly, depending on the specific microorganism involved and the related environmental conditions. The basic steps are described next as related to disease development in a dental office environment. Prevention of disease development occurs by interfering with one of the basic steps as described in Part 2: Infection Control (see Chapters 6 to 29).

Source of the Microorganism

The major sources of disease agents in the dental office are the mouths of the patients. Although microorganisms can be present almost anywhere in the office (surfaces, dust, water, air, and the dental team), microorganisms of greatest concern are in the mouths of patients. These microorganisms are

---

BOX 3-1

Steps in the Development of an Infectious Disease

1. Source of microorganism
2. Escape of microorganism from the source
3. Spread of microorganism to a new person
4. Entry of microorganism into the person
5. Infection (survival and growth of microorganism)
6. Damage to the body

From Miller CH, Cottone JC: The basic principles of infectious diseases as related to dental practice, *Dent Clin North Am* 37:1-20, 1993.

---

described more fully in Chapters 5 and 7 and include those that may be present in saliva, respiratory secretions, and blood that may escape from the mouth during dental care. Members of the dental team also may harbor pathogenic microorganisms, but the chances for the spread of these agents in the office are much lower than for those involving microorganisms in patients. Nevertheless, spread of microorganisms from the dental team to patients is an important concern and is described in Chapter 8.

Although the patient's mouth is in general the most important source of pathogens in the dental office, accurate detection of which patients may indeed be harboring these pathogens is not possible. Therefore, to successfully prevent the spread of pathogens in the office, the dental team must apply infection control procedures during the care of all patients using the concept of **standard precautions**. Standard precautions combines the concept of **universal precautions** (the need to treat blood and other body fluids from all patients as potentially infectious) with **body substance isolation** (designed to reduce the risk of transmission of pathogens from moist body surfaces) into one set of standards. Thus standard precautions mean to consider blood, all body fluids, including secretions and excretions (except sweat), nonintact skin, and mucous membranes as potentially infectious in all patients. The importance of standard precautions is based on an understanding of **asymptomatic carriers** of disease agents and an analysis of the four stages of the infectious disease process in the body as related to spread of disease agents to others.

Asymptomatic Carrier

Persons who have disease agents on or in their bodies but have no recognizable symptoms of the diseases are called asymptomatic carriers. These persons are probably the most important source for spread of disease agents because they may spread pathogens to others and not even be aware that they are infected. Also, the dental team will not be aware of the potentially infectious nature of patients because carrier patients may look normal, with no recognizable symptoms.

An asymptomatic carrier state may occur at different stages during an infectious disease.

Stages of an Infectious Disease

The four stages of an infectious disease are incubation, pro-dromal, acute, and convalescent. Pathogens may be spread to others during each of these stages.

Incubation Stage

The incubation stage of an infectious disease is the period from the initial entrance of the infectious agent into the body to the time when the first symptoms of the disease appear. During this time, the disease agent simply is surviving in the body or is multiplying and producing harmful products that ultimately damage the body. This incubation period may range from a few hours to years, depending on the disease-producing potential of the microorganism, the number of microorganisms that enter the body, and the resistance of the body to the microorganism. All infectious diseases have an incubation stage, because we seldom, if ever, are exposed to a sufficient number of microorganisms to cause immediate symptoms. The entering microorganisms must multiply to sufficient numbers that overwhelm local or bodywide defense systems before enough damage occurs to result in a recognizable symptom (e.g., fever, swelling, skin discoloration, ulceration, pain, bleeding, watery eyes, and runny nose). The length of the incubation stage varies. For influenza, incubation is usually 2 to 3 days, whereas for hepatitis B, incubation is usually several weeks. Persons infected with the human immunodeficiency virus serotype 1 (HIV-1) may be free of recognizable symptoms for 10 years or longer after the virus initially enters the body.

Prodromal Stage

The prodromal ("running before") stage of a disease involves the appearance of early symptoms. The microorganism multiplies to numbers just large enough to cause the first symptoms commonly called malaise (not feeling well). These symptoms may include slight fever, headache, and upset stomach.

Acute Stage

The acute stage is when the symptoms of the disease are maximal and the person is obviously ill. Although this person certainly has a potential to spread disease agents, the person may not be the most important source in the dental office. The acutely ill are not likely to come to the dental office for care except in an emergency. Their presence in the office also may depend on the severity of their symptoms and the nature of the disease.

Convalescent Stage

The convalescent stage of a disease is the recovery phase. The number of microorganisms may be declining, or the harmful microbial products are being destroyed rapidly as the body defenses successfully combat the disease. Nevertheless, infectious agents are present and may be spread during this stage. Although the patient is aware of the disease, the declining symptoms may not be recognizable by others.

Some persons may never recover fully from an infectious disease. The symptoms may occur over a long period or may occur intermittently. The chronic (long-term) stages may occur in diseases such as hepatitis B and tuberculosis, in which the disease agent may be retained in the body for long periods. As more fully described in Chapter 6, some persons may be infected with the hepatitis B virus and not experience any symptoms until 25 or more years later, with development of severe liver damage. Yet the virus was present in their bodies all of this time and may have been spread to others.

Normal Patient

A normal patient in this context is one who has no infectious diseases and is not a carrier of obvious pathogens. Normal and asymptomatic patients appear the same with no recognizable symptoms, however. This fact substantiates the need for standard precautions because one cannot always differentiate between normal patients and those capable of spreading harmful microorganisms.

Even normal patients have opportunistic pathogens in their mouths, as more fully described in Chapter 5.

Escape from the Source

Step 2 in the development of an infectious disease is the escape of microorganisms from the source. Microorganisms escape from the mouth during natural mechanisms such as coughing, sneezing, and talking. These modes are indeed how respiratory diseases, such as the common cold, measles, chickenpox, and influenza, normally are spread. Providing dental care results in several artificial mechanisms by which microorganisms can escape from the patient's mouth.

Anything that is removed from a patient's mouth is contaminated (hands, instruments, handpieces, x-ray film, cotton products, needles, teeth, saliva, tissue, appliances, and temporaries). In addition, microorganisms can escape from the mouth in spatter droplets and aerosol particles generated by use of the handpiece, ultrasonic scaler, and air/water syringe. Spatter droplets are the larger droplets that may contain several microorganisms and can hit the skin, eyes, nostrils, lips, and mouth of the dental team. These droplets settle rapidly from the air and can contaminate nearby surfaces. Aerosol particles are mostly invisible but contain a few microorganisms that may be inhaled or remain airborne for some time, depending on their size and on the air currents in the office.

Spread of Microorganisms to another Person

Microorganisms that have escaped from a patient's mouth may be spread to others by four basic modes of disease transmission: *direct contact, indirect contact, droplet infection, and airborne infection* (Table 3-1).

Direct Contact

Touching soft tissue or teeth in the patient's mouth results in direct contact with microorganisms with immediate

TABLE 3-1 **Modes of Disease Transmission**

Mode	Example
Direct contact	Contact with microorganisms at the source such as in the patient's mouth
Indirect contact	Contact with items contaminated with a patient's microorganisms such as surfaces, hands, contaminated sharps
Droplet infection	Contact with the larger droplets in sprays, splashes, or spatter-containing microorganisms
Airborne infection	Contact with the smaller droplet nuclei (aerosol particles) containing microorganisms

TABLE 3-2 **Routes of Entry of Microorganisms into the Body**

Route	Examples
Inhalation	Breathing aerosol particles generated from use of prophylaxis angle
Ingestion	Swallowing droplets of saliva/blood spattered into the mouth
Mucous membranes	Droplets of saliva/blood spattered into the eyes, nose, or mouth
Breaks in the skin	Directly touching microorganisms or being spattered with saliva/blood onto skin with cuts or abrasions; punctures with contaminated sharps

spread from the source. The mere presence of microorganisms on the skin gives them an opportunity to penetrate the body through small breaks or cuts in the skin and around the fingernails of ungloved hands. Transference may involve diseases such as herpes infections of the fingers, other skin diseases, and sexually transmitted diseases.

Indirect Contact

A second mode of spread, called indirect contact, can result from injuries with contaminated sharps (e.g., needlesticks) and contact with contaminated instruments, equipment, surfaces, and hands. The inanimate surfaces are referred to as fomites. These items and tissues can carry a variety of pathogens such as hepatitis B and C viruses, usually because of the presence of blood, saliva, or other secretions from a previous patient. Skin infection and the common cold also are spread by this mode.

Droplet Infection

A third mode of spread is droplet infection. This mode encompasses large-particle droplet spatter (larger than 5 μm) that is transmitted by close contact. Spatter generated during dental care may contact unprotected broken skin or mucous membranes of the eyes, noses, and mouths of members of the dental team. This contact delivers microorganisms directly to the body. Regular surgical masks, eyeglasses, and face shields interrupt this mode of transmission, which can involve the influenza, mumps, and rubella viruses, and herpesviruses.

Airborne Infection

A fourth mode of spread is airborne infection that involves small particles (sometimes referred to as droplet nuclei or aerosol particles) of a size smaller than 5 μm. These particles can remain airborne for hours and can be inhaled. Tuberculosis, chickenpox, and measles are spread by this mode, and surgical masks are not designed to protect against airborne spread. A particulate respirator (e.g., N-95 respirator) would be needed to afford such protection.

Entry into a New Person

Microorganisms that are spread to a new person frequently cause no damage unless they actually enter the body. The four basic routes of entry have been mentioned already (Table 3-2).

Microorganisms at the surface of the skin can enter through small cuts or abrasions that often are unnoticed. Injuries with contaminated sharp items cause direct penetration through the skin into the body. Also, microorganisms in spatter or aerosols may contact and enter the body through mucous membranes of the eye, nose, and mouth, or they may be inhaled. Ingestion is another route of entry.

Infection

Infection is the multiplication and survival of microorganisms on or in the body. An infection does not always indicate disease, but disease seldom results without infection (the exception is toxigenic diseases). Our bodies are infected constantly with large numbers of bacteria multiplying and surviving in our mouths, nose, eyes, intestines, and skin on a normal basis.

Damage to the Body

As mentioned previously, infecting microorganisms usually must multiply to a harmful level for disease to occur. Thus harmful infection is the final step in development of an infectious disease. The final two steps of infection and damage are complex and involve a battle between the infecting microorganism and the defenses of the body, as described in the next section.

HOST–MICROORGANISM INTERACTIONS

Microorganisms present on or in the body multiply if the conditions are appropriate. Bacteria and fungi take in available nutrients, metabolize, multiply, and produce extracellular products that may damage the body. Viruses invade appropriate host cells, replicate, and damage the host cells during the process. The body attempts to restrict microbial invasion and multiplication and to counteract harmful microbial products. The result of these interactions is health or disease.

Pathogenic Properties of Microorganisms

Pathogenic properties of microorganisms are properties that facilitate development of disease and are categorized as those that enhance infection, interfere with host defenses, and cause direct damage to the body (Table 3-3).

Enhancement of Infection

Properties that enhance the initial survival and multiplication of microorganisms in the body are the surface fimbriae on bacteria and host cell attachment sites on viral envelopes or capsids. These features allow the microorganism to attach to host cells or other surfaces; for viruses, this attachment is required before the viruses can multiply.

Attachment to host surfaces is also necessary for infection by many bacteria, especially if they are to establish themselves on mucosal surfaces such as in the mouth. Bacteria that do not attach to or are not mechanically trapped in oral sites are washed off surfaces by saliva and swallowed. The accumulation of dental plaque is an example of the result of bacterial attachment to host surfaces, in this case leading

TABLE 3-3   Pathogenic Activities and Properties of Microorganisms

Activity	Property	Examples
Enhances infection	Attaches to host cells	
	bacterial fimbriae	*Streptococcus pyogenes*
	bacterial surface polymers	*Streptococcus mutans*
	viral envelope or capsid	All viruses
	Multiplies at body site	
	utilizes available nutrients	Most pathogens
	resists acids	*Lactobacillus acidophilus*
Interferes with host defenses	Destroys phagocytes	
	leukocidin	*Aggregatibacter actinomycetemcomitans*
	exotoxin A	
	Inhibits phagocyte attraction	*Pseudomonas aeruginosa*
	extracellular products	*Capnocytophaga* sp.
	Avoids phagocyte engulfment	
	bacterial capsule	*Streptococcus pneumoniae*
	bacterial fimbriae	*Streptococcus pyogenes*
	Resists phagocytic digestion	
	resistant bacterial surfaces	*Mycobacterium tuberculosis*
	products inhibit killing	*Legionella pneumophila*
	Suppresses or avoids immune system	
	kills lymphocytes	Human immunodeficiency virus (HIV)
	changes surface antigens	Influenza viruses
	destroys antibodies	*Streptococcus sanguis*
	avoids contact with antibodies	Herpes simplex viruses
Damages cells or tissues	Produces histolytic enzymes	
	collagenase	*Porphyromonas gingivalis*
	hyaluronidase	*Staphylococcus aureus*
	Contains endotoxin	Gram-negative bacteria
	Produces exotoxins	
	tetanus toxin	*Clostridium tetani*
	botulinum toxin	*Clostridium botulinum*
	enterotoxins	*Staphylococcus aureus*
	Produces cytotoxic chemicals	
	hydrogen sulfide	*Fusobacterium nucleatum*
	ammonia	*Bacteroides* sp.
	acids	
	Induces damage by the immune system	*Streptococcus mutans*
	causes persistent, localized infections	Periodontopathogens
	causes chronic infections	Hepatitis B virus

to dental caries. Other examples of diseases requiring initial attachment by bacteria are streptococcal pharyngitis, genitourinary gonorrhea, gonococcal pharyngitis, conjunctivitis, *Salmonella* gastroenteritis, and shigellosis.

Bacteria that attach to specific body sites must be able to multiply in the environment of that site to become established and eventually cause damage. Thus their nutritional requirements must be compatible with the specific host site. For this reason, only specific bacteria can survive at and damage specific sites in the body. For example, lactobacilli and many strains of *Streptococcus mutans* can survive in an environment high in acid (they are aciduric) such as within a carious lesion. Thus, although many other oral bacteria cannot multiply under these conditions, these aciduric species continue to thrive in the lesion and contribute to the progression of caries.

Interference with Host Defenses

Many microorganisms are pathogenic because they interfere with host defense mechanisms. Bacteria with capsules, such as *Streptococcus pneumoniae*, which causes lobar pneumonia, resist phagocytic engulfment, whereas other bacteria, such as *Mycobacterium tuberculosis*, which causes tuberculosis, may be engulfed but resist phagocytic digestion. Such bacteria gain a foothold during infection because they evade destruction by phagocytes, one of the early lines of defense.

The same is true for bacteria such as *Aggregatibacter actinomycetemcomitans*, an important periodontal pathogen that produces a toxin (leukocidin) that kills certain phagocytes. Other microorganisms interfere with the latter stages of host defense, cell-mediated and antibody-mediated immunity. For example, HIV-1 can destroy certain T lymphocytes that are involved in regulating the immune response. Also, some streptococci can produce protease enzymes that destroy antibody molecules.

Direct Damage to the Body

As bacteria or fungi multiply in the body, they produce extracellular enzymes that can degrade macromolecules. If these macromolecules are parts of host cell surfaces or are tissue components, this process can kill cells or damage the tissue. Examples of such histolytic enzymes are the collagenase produced by the bacterial species of *Porphyromonas*, *Bacteroides*, and *Clostridium*; hyaluronidase produced by some streptococci; and a variety of proteolytic enzymes produced by many bacteria.

Bacteria also produce waste products, many of which are cytotoxic, such as ammonia, acids, and hydrogen sulfide, or cause demineralization of enamel and dentin, such as lactic acid and other organic acids. Gram-negative bacteria contain endotoxin that, when released, affects phagocytes and blood platelets and can induce an inflammatory response. Other bacteria may produce exotoxins that interfere with cell or body functions, such as food poisoning toxins and tetanus toxins.

Viruses cause damage by killing or interfering with the normal functions of the host cells they invade, and all

types of microorganisms contain or produce substances that stimulate an inflammatory response or an immune response. These host responses are protective, but, if they are stimulated continually by persistence of the microorganism, these responses may produce more damage than protection. One example is the damage that occurs in periodontal disease with the long-term presence of plaque and its antigens in periodontal pockets.

Host Defense Mechanisms

Host defense against harmful infections are grouped into two categories: **innate defenses** that are always active and **acquired defenses** that must be stimulated to become active.

Innate Host Defenses

Innate host defenses consist of four groups of properties or activities of the body that guard against infection by contaminating microorganisms (Table 3-4). Although these defenses are formidable, they do not prevent all diseases.

Physical Barriers

The unbroken skin serves as an excellent barrier and prevents microorganisms from penetrating to deeper tissues where multiplication and spread to other body sites may occur. The mucous membranes of the eyes, nose, mouth, respiratory tree, vagina, and intestinal tract also provide resistance to penetration by microorganisms. The architecture of the skin with its many layers and the arrangement of cells of mucous membranes serve as the mechanisms that resist penetration.

TABLE 3-4   Innate Host Defense Mechanisms

Mechanism	Examples
Physical barriers	Skin
	Mucous membranes
	Architecture of respiratory tree
Mechanical barriers	Washing action of secretions and excretions
	Sticky nature of mucus
	Ciliary escalator
	Desquamation of skin and mucous membrane cells
	Coughing and sneezing
	Hair in the nose
Antimicrobial chemicals	Hydrochloric acid in stomach
	Organic acids on skin and in vagina
	Lysozyme
	Phagocytic killing systems
	Interferon
	Complement fragments
	Microbial products
Cellular barriers	Phagocytes

Adapted from Miller CH, Cottone JC: The basic principles of infectious diseases as related to dental practice, *Dent Clin North Am* 37:1-20, 1993.

Another physical barrier is the architecture of the respiratory tree, which prevents particles of 5 μm and greater in size from reaching the alveoli (air sacs) of the lung. This restricts entrance of many microorganisms that may be present in large droplets or dust particles that are inhaled.

Mechanical Barriers

Mechanical barriers include the cleansing action of secretions such as saliva and tears and excretions such as urine that wash away microorganisms present at these respective body sites. Innate protection of the respiratory tree also includes the secretion of "sticky" mucus that tends to trap inhaled particles that then are moved up and away from the lungs by the ciliary escalator (movement of the hairlike cilia on the surface of mucosal epithelial cells that moves the mucus toward the throat). The natural reflexes of coughing and sneezing also expel particles from the respiratory tree.

Another mechanical barrier involves the desquamation (shedding) of skin cells and mucous membrane cells. As these outer surface cells are lost, microorganisms attached to these cells also are removed from the body.

Antimicrobial Chemicals

A variety of antimicrobial chemicals are present in the body that kill or inhibit the multiplication of microorganisms. Hydrochloric acid in the stomach and organic acids on the skin and in the vagina can prevent bacterial multiplication. The enzyme lysozyme can lyse and kill some bacteria and is present in saliva, tears, nasal secretions, intestinal secretions, colostrum, and inside phagocytes. Other antimicrobial mechanisms of phagocytes involve oxygen products, peroxidase, and lactoferrin. When infected with a virus, many of our body cells produce a substance called interferon. Interferon is released from infected cells and makes nearby cells resistant to virus replication.

A special group of proteins called the complement system is present in blood and tissue fluids and can participate in antimicrobial activities by working in concert with the immune response (it "complements" the immune system). The complement system provides a very early defense mechanism and can attract phagocytes to a site of infection, enhance phagocytosis of microorganisms, lyse certain gram-negative bacteria, and destroy the envelope of some viruses.

Cellular Barriers

As previously described, certain white blood cells such as neutrophils and macrophages can destroy microorganisms through the process of phagocytosis. These phagocytes first engulf (swallow up) microorganisms and then kill and digest them using enzymes that degrade the microbial structures. Phagocytes provide an important defense system and are present throughout the body in connective tissue, tissue and lymphatic fluid, lymph nodes, blood, and many organs.

Acquired Immunity

Immunity is a state of being resistant to the harmful effects of specific microorganisms. If a microorganism invades the body, it usually activates a special host defense system directed specifically against that invading microorganism. After this system is activated, it attempts to prevent serious harm from that microorganism and may provide protection against subsequent invasion of the body by that same microorganism. This defense system is called acquired immunity because this system is always ready to respond to microbial infections but does not actually do so until after an infection has occurred. In contrast, the innate body defenses are always active, even before infection has occurred.

Activation of the Immune Response

The immune response is activated by antigens (sometimes referred to as immunogens). Examples of antigens are bacteria, viruses, fungi, protozoa, extracellular macromolecules produced by these microorganisms, and other macromolecules or cells that are normally not present in the body. During an infection, while the innate body defenses are trying to kill or limit the spread of the invading microorganism, the body recognizes the microorganism and its macromolecular products (antigens) as being foreign to the body. This recognition is accomplished by special macrophages distributed throughout the body that process antigens through phagocytosis and then interact with the cells of the immune system: B lymphocytes and T lymphocytes. This interaction causes these lymphocytes to multiply and yield large numbers of cells that can recognize the specific invading antigens. These lymphocytes then begin a series of activities that can destroy the microorganism or interfere with its pathogenic properties. These activities are grouped into two categories: cell-mediated response and antibody-mediated response.

Cell-Mediated Response

The activated T lymphocytes develop into several different types of T lymphocytes that can (1) regulate the antibody-mediated response, (2) destroy virus-infected host cells in an attempt to stop further multiplication of the virus in the body, (3) produce chemicals called lymphokines that in general activate other types of cells (e.g., phagocytes) to be more active in killing the invading microorganism, and (4) destroy certain nonmicrobial cells in the body that have changed and become recognized as foreign to the body (e.g., cancer cells).

Antibody-Mediated Response

The activated B lymphocytes develop into different types of B lymphocytes that produce lymphokines (that act like those produced from T lymphocytes) and into plasma cells that produce antibodies. Antibodies are protein molecules that can bind to the specific antigens that originally stimulated their formation. When the antibodies bind to these antigens, the antigens (e.g., microorganisms or their harmful products)

TABLE 3-5   **Protective Activities of Antibodies**

Activity	Examples
Enhance phagocytosis to destroy microorganisms	Binding to the bacterial capsule, eliminating its antiphagocytic activity Binding to a microorganism and attaching the microorganisms to the surface of a phagocyte that promotes engulfment Activating the complement system that in turn activates phagocytes
Interfere with microorganism attachment to host cells to prevent infection	Binding to bacterial fimbriae or to viral capsid and envelope before the microorganism attaches to host cells Binding to microorganism surfaces and causing several cells or viral particles to clump
Inactivate toxins to prevent damage to the body	Binding to bacterial leukocidin molecules, preventing damage to neutrophils
Inactivate histolytic enzymes to prevent damage to the body	Binding to the collagenase molecule, preventing destruction of collagen
Lysis of gram-negative bacteria or enveloped viruses	Binding to the surface of microorganisms and activating the complement system that destroys the outer membrane or viral envelope
Lysis of virus-infected cells	Binding to virus-infected cells and attaching the cell to a macrophage that then kills the virus-infected cells

are destroyed, inactivated, or more easily removed from the body, depending on the nature of the antigen (Table 3-5).

Long-Term Immunity

The initial immune response to an invading microorganism usually results in an increased number of lymphocytes that can respond to that microorganism if it attempts to invade the body again. During subsequent invasions, the body "remembers" that microorganism and, because of the large number of specific lymphocytes now present, can respond rapidly to destroy the microorganism before it can damage the body. Thus, once we have had an infectious disease, we frequently do not get that same disease again. Notable exceptions include dental caries, periodontal disease, and gonorrhea. Also, in some instances, different microorganisms can cause the same disease. For example, more than 100 viruses can cause the common cold, and an immune response to one microorganism seldom protects against another microorganism.

Artificial Immunity

Artificial immunity involves being immunized or vaccinated against a specific disease. We are inoculated with an antigen (e.g., a dead microorganism, a weakened microorganism, the antigenic part of a microorganism, or an inactivated toxin) that will not cause disease or damage to the body but will stimulate the immune system. On receiving the vaccine, the body is deceived and, reacting as if the infection were real, mounts an immune response for protection. In most instances, this protection lasts for many years (e.g., hepatitis B vaccination), but in some cases booster inoculations are needed periodically to maintain protection

(e.g., tetanus vaccinations). Chapter 9 describes diseases for which vaccines are available in the United States, including hepatitis B.

Damage by the Immune System

Activation of the immune system by certain antigens can cause damage to the body. Approximately 10% of the population is allergic to substances that either can serve directly as an antigen or are changed into antigens after they enter the body. The immune response to the antigen (in these cases called an allergen) results in damage to the body, usually occurring at the body site exposed to the allergen. For example, some persons who breathe in pollens have antibody-mediated allergic reactions in the nose and eyes, called hay fever, or in the respiratory tree, called asthma. Allergies to foods (e.g., chocolate) are usually expressed as hives on the skin. Allergy to a substance that is distributed throughout the body (e.g., penicillin inoculation) may result in a widespread reaction affecting the blood system, lungs, and heart, and is called systemic anaphylactic shock.

Cell-mediated allergic reactions also occur in some persons with chronic infections such as may occur in hepatitis B, syphilis, and tuberculosis. Oils from the poison ivy plant, nickel from jewelry, and chemicals in latex gloves also may cause cell-mediated allergic reactions, called contact dermatitis.

Skin testing is used to determine which specific allergens are causing problems. In many instances, an allergic person outgrows the allergy, but some persons remain allergic for life and must take special precautions to avoid contact with the allergens.

SELECTED READINGS

Abbas AK: *Cellular and molecular immunology*, ed 6, Philadelphia, 2007, Elsevier.

Bagg J, MacFarlane TW, Poxton IR, Miller CH: *Essentials of microbiology for dental students*, Oxford, 1999, Oxford University Press.

Miller CH, Cottone JC: The basic principles of infectious diseases as related to dental practice, *Dent Clin North Am* 37:1–20, 1993.

Sompayrac L: *How pathogenic viruses work*, Boston, 2002, Jones and Bartlett.

REVIEW QUESTIONS

Multiple Choice

1. The most important source of potentially infectious microbes in the dental office is:
   a. water
   b. air
   c. insects
   d. the patients' mouths

2. Microbes spreading from a patient's mouth to your hand and then to another patient's mouth represents what type of spread from patient to patient?
   a. Indirect contact
   b. Direct contact
   c. Droplet infection
   d. Airborne infection

3. The best definition of an asymptomatic carrier is a patient who is infected with a microorganism and:
   a. has no obvious symptoms
   b. dies
   c. is obviously sick
   d. later is completely cured

4. During the development of an infectious disease, what has to happen before the step "spread to a new host"?
   a. Damage to the new host
   b. Infection
   c. Entry into the new host
   d. Escape from the source

5. Antibodies are best defined as:
   a. the active ingredients in antimicrobial handwashing products
   b. microbes that can enter the body and stimulate an immune response
   c. different types of chemicals such as penicillin that can kill microbes
   d. proteins made in the body that bind to and destroy microbes and other antigens

6. Allergies are best defined as:
   a. infectious diseases caused by harmful infections with viruses
   b. reactions to harsh chemicals that directly damage tissues
   c. immune responses that cause damage to the body

7. The incubation stage of an infectious disease occurs:
   a. after contamination and before symptoms
   b. during the height of the symptoms
   c. after the symptoms have subsided

8. Infection is best defined as the:
   a. occurrence of severe symptoms of a disease
   b. entrance of microbes into the body
   c. growth and survival of microbes on or in the body

9. The difference between droplet and airborne infections is that:
   a. airborne infections are caused by smaller infectious particles
   b. droplet infections are caused by smaller infectious particles
   c. airborne infections are caused by larger infectious particles

10. Destruction of collagen in periodontal tissue by collagenase from *Porphyromonas gingivalis* is an example of what type of bacterial pathogenic property?
    a. Enhancement of infection
    b. Interference of host defenses
    c. Direct damage to the body

11. Mucous membranes of the mouth represent what type of innate host defense barrier of the human body?
    a. Physical
    b. Mechanical
    c. Antimicrobial
    d. Chemical

12. The material in a vaccine that stimulates an immune response is called an:
    a. antibody
    b. antigen
    c. antibiotic
    d. acidogen

13. Which of the following is an infectious disease?
    a. The hereditary malfunctioning of an organ
    b. The abnormal growth of body cells
    c. An allergic reaction
    d. Tissue damage caused by a microorganism

14. Hay fever and asthma are examples of:
    a. endogenous infectious diseases
    b. allergic reactions
    c. artificial immunity
    d. mechanical barriers

15. Dental caries is what type of infectious disease?
    a. Endogenous
    b. Exogenous
    c. Toxigenic

Please visit http://evolve.elsevier.com/Miller/infectioncontrol/ for additional practice and study support tools.

4 Emerging Diseases

OUTLINE

Ecological Changes

Changes in Human Demographics or Behaviors

International Travel and Commerce

Technology

Microbial Changes

Breakdown in Public Health Measures

Unexplained Emergence

LEARNING OBJECTIVES

After completing this chapter, the student should be able to do the following:

1. Define an emerging disease.
2. List some of the infectious diseases that have appeared since 1970.
3. List the six ways infectious diseases may emerge and give an example with each, and describe the unexplained emergence of Ebola hemorrhagic fever.

KEY TERMS

Emerging Diseases
Zoonotic

Overall, infectious diseases remain the third leading cause of death in the United States and the second leading cause of death worldwide. Of the 15 million deaths that occur worldwide each year, 3.75 million (25%) are directly caused by infectious diseases. This is surpassed only by deaths from cardiovascular diseases at 29%. Emerging diseases are new infectious diseases that have not been recognized before as well as known infectious diseases with changing patterns. Infectious diseases can be expected to emerge continually, and the number of these diseases, as listed in Table 4-1, will continue to grow. Diseases emerge because conditions change that bring microorganisms and human beings together in new ways. These changing conditions can be grouped into six categories, as listed in Table 4-2.

ECOLOGICAL CHANGES

Ecological changes that result in disease emergence usually involve zoonotic diseases (diseases involving animals) or insect-borne diseases. Such changes involve bringing human beings into close contact with animals or insect vectors, resulting in the spread of microorganisms from animals to human beings. One example is the emergence of Korean hemorrhagic fever, a disease of human beings that involves high fever and internal bleeding, which is caused by the Hantaan virus from rodents. When rice fields are created, field mice flourish because of the new source of food. Harvesting the rice brings human beings into close contact with these infected mice, resulting in spread of the virus.

In 1993, an unusually mild and wet summer in the southwestern United States likely enhanced contact between human beings and rodents carrying a previously unrecognized hantavirus now named Sin Nombre virus. The rodent population flourished, and human beings probably entered the wilds more frequently as a result of the favorable weather. This likely caused the initial cluster of 24 human cases of hantavirus pulmonary syndrome in this area. This syndrome produces symptoms of fever, muscle aches, nausea, vomiting, headache, and, ultimately, severe respiratory distress with death in approximately half of those infected. Although the initial outbreak occurred in the Four Corners region of the United States (Arizona, New Mexico, Colorado, Utah), more than 300 cases now have been confirmed in the United States. The deer mouse (which is distributed widely in North America) is found to be the most common host for the Sin Nombre virus. The disease also is associated with cotton rats, rice rats, and the white-footed mouse, and has now been detected in several other countries, including Argentina, Brazil, Canada, Chile, Paraguay, and Uruguay.

Other rodent viruses cause human diseases, including the Machupo virus that causes Bolivian hemorrhagic fever, the Argentine hemorrhagic fever virus, and the Lassa fever virus. The exact mode of spread of microorganisms from rodents to human beings is not always known but may involve contact with rodent feces or aerosolized urine.

TABLE 4-1   **Some Recently Recognized Disease/Microorganism Associations**

Year*	Microorganism	Disease
1970	Coxsackievirus	Hand-foot-and-mouth disease
1972	Norwalk virus	Gastroenteritis
1973	Rotavirus	Infantile diarrhea
1975	Astrovirus	Gastroenteritis
1975	Parvovirus B19	Fifth disease; aplastic crises–chronic hemolytic anemia
1976†	Ebola virus	Ebola hemorrhagic fever
1977	*Cryptosporidium parvum*	Acute enterocolitis
1977	Enteric adenovirus	Gastroenteritis
1977	Hantaan virus	Hemorrhagic fever with renal syndrome
1977	Hepatitis D virus	Hepatitis D (bloodborne)
1977	*Legionella pneumophila*	Legionnaires disease
1981	*Staphylococcus aureus*	Toxic shock syndrome associated with tampons
1982	*Escherichia coli* O157:H7	Hemorrhagic colitis; hemolytic uremic syndrome
1983	*Helicobacter pylori*	Gastric ulcers
1983	HIV type 1	HIV disease; HIV infection and AIDS‡
1987	Hepatitis E virus	Hepatitis E (waterborne, food-borne)
1987	Rift Valley fever virus	Hemorrhagic fever
1988	Human herpesvirus 6	Roseola (actual disease known since 1910)
1989	*Ehrlichia chaffeensis*	Human ehrlichiosis
1989	Hepatitis C virus	Hepatitis C (bloodborne)
1990	Barmah forest virus	Polyarthritis in West Australia
1990	*Haemophilus influenzae*	Brazilian purpuric fever (new strain: aegyptius)
1991	*Guanarito* virus	Venezuelan hemorrhagic fever
1991	Hepatitis F virus	Hepatitis
1992	*Bartonella henselae*	Cat-scratch disease
1992	*Vibrio cholerae* O139	Epidemic cholera (new strain)
1993	Sin nombre virus	Hantavirus pulmonary syndrome
1994	Sabia virus	Brazilian hemorrhagic fever
1995	Hepatitis G virus	Hepatitis G
1995	Human herpesvirus 8	Associated with Kaposi sarcoma
1995	Alkhurma virus	Hemorrhagic fever
1996	Australian bat lyssavirus	Paralysis, delirium, convulsions
1998	Hendra virus	Respiratory disease
1998	Menangle virus	Respiratory disease
1998	Nipah virus	Meningitis, encephalitis
1999	West Nile virus	Encephalitis
2003	Coronavirus	Severe acute respiratory syndrome (SARS)
2003	Monkeypox virus	Skin infection
2004	Torque teno virus	Acute respiratory disease
2005	Chikungunya virus	Polyarthralgia
2009	Saffold virus	Infects the myocardium and central nervous system
2009	SFTS bunyavirus	Thrombocytopenia and fever
2012	Novel coronavirus	Respiratory syndrome with renal failure

*Year microorganism was isolated, identified, or first associated with disease.

†Subsequent outbreaks have occurred in 1979, 1994, 1995, 1996, 2001, and 2007.

‡HIV, human immunodeficiency virus; AIDS, acquired immunodeficiency syndrome.

TABLE 4-2 **Causes and Examples of Disease Emergence**

Cause	Disease Examples
Ecological changes	Argentine hemorrhagic fever Bolivian hemorrhagic fever Hantavirus pulmonary syndrome Korean hemorrhagic fever Lassa fever Lyme disease Rift Valley fever West Nile fever in the United States
Changes in human demographics or behaviors	Hepatitis B and C Human immunodeficiency virus (HIV) disease Tuberculosis
International travel and commerce	Cholera Encephalitis Severe acute respiratory syndrome
Technology	*Escherichia coli* hemolytic uremic syndrome Hepatitides B and C HIV disease Legionnaires disease *Salmonella* food poisoning
Microbial changes	Infections with antibiotic-resistant strains Influenza
Breakdown in public health measures	Cryptosporidiosis Diphtheria

Another ecological change resulted in disease emergence in 1987 along the Senegal River in Mauritania, Africa. Building dams in the river valley facilitated irrigation as planned but also greatly increased the water breeding grounds for the mosquitoes that carry viruses. This caused the emergence of Rift Valley fever, a viral disease caused by a mosquito vector that results in high fever and sometimes retinitis and, rarely, fulminant hepatitis with hemorrhage. This disease also became visible again in Kenya in 1997, after that part of East Africa received torrential rains, yielding a "bumper crop" of mosquitoes. In 2000, outbreaks were seen for the first time outside of Africa, in Saudi Arabia and Yemen. In 2003, this disease reemerged in Mauritania.

Lyme disease initially was recognized in the United States in 1975 in a group of children who lived in Lyme, Connecticut. Lyme disease is caused by the bacterial spirochete *Borrelia burgdorferi*, which is transmitted to human beings through the bite of ticks. The disease results in a rash (associated with the tick bite) and starts with flulike symptoms. Weeks later, the subject may develop cardiac or neurologic problems, muscle aches and pains, or intermittent attacks of arthritis. The emergence of this disease likely was caused by ecological changes in forests near populated sites that increased the population of the deer and the deer tick, the vector of Lyme disease in human beings. Situations that encourage human beings to venture near and into forests also contribute to this emergence, and affected individuals may include campers, hunters, hikers, bird watchers, and even golfers. Today, approximately 16,000 cases of Lyme disease are reported annually throughout the United States, with most cases occurring in the northeastern states.

CHANGES IN HUMAN DEMOGRAPHICS OR BEHAVIORS

Human population movements or changes in how human beings associate with each other can create new conditions that favor disease spread. Movement and crowding of persons into cities in poor countries result in numerous infectious disease problems such as the spread of dengue virus from mosquitoes breeding in open water containers, causing dengue hemorrhagic fever. Crowding also leads to transference of other mosquito-borne diseases such as yellow fever and several forms of viral encephalitis. The movement of persons infected with human immunodeficiency virus (HIV) from the villages of Africa to large cities introduced the infection to larger susceptible populations. The movement of more than 500,000 starving Rwandans into Zaire (now the Democratic Republic of the Congo) in 1994 resulted in more than 50,000 deaths in the refugee camps from cholera and *Shigella* dysentery.

Human demographics also play a role in disease spread in the United States. Increased population densities, as may occur with the homeless or with institutionalized persons (e.g., prisoners), have contributed to the increase in the numbers of tuberculosis cases in the United States in recent years. Bringing children together in some day care centers has contributed to the spread of disease agents such as cytomegalovirus. Human behavior also influences disease spread and emergence. Unprotected sexual contact among members of various populations and an increase in injection drug abuse facilitate the sharing of human body fluids among individuals. If the body fluids are infected with microorganisms, the microorganisms rapidly reach new hosts. These behaviors are the primary reasons for the emergence and spread of HIV and the continued occurrence of most cases of hepatitides B and C.

The behaviors of misuse and overuse of antibiotics lead to conditions that select for antibiotic-resistant strains of bacteria; for example, antibiotics prescribed when not necessary and antibiotics used for prevention of infections. Such practices have resulted in the emergence and occurrence of harmful infections by antibiotic-resistant strains that are much more difficult to treat. Such conditions are described more fully under Microbial Changes below.

INTERNATIONAL TRAVEL AND COMMERCE

In a few hours, or a few days at the most, just about anyone can travel just about anywhere. We carry our microorganisms with us when we travel and can spread them easily to others in faraway lands. Also, microorganisms that contaminate water, foods, plants, animals, insects, and goods literally can be shipped throughout the world. A recent example of this is the emergence of cholera in South and Central America. Cholera is an intestinal bacterial disease spread by contaminated water or food that results in severe diarrhea and dehydration. A new strain of the cholera causative agent (*Vibrio cholerae* O139 Bengal) emerged in 1992 in southern Asia, where cholera is endemic. Within a year, this new strain was detected in South and Central America, where, along with *V. cholerae* O139, it has caused more than a million cases of cholera and resulted in approximately 10,000 deaths. This was the first epidemic of cholera in South and Central America in the twentieth century. The exact mode of spread of strain O139 from Asia to South and Central America is not known, but transmission possibly involved the water on and in cargo ships. *V. cholerae* has been isolated from the ballast, bilge, and sewage waters of cargo ships.

As evidence that *V. cholerae* O139, originally detected in Indonesia, has reached U.S. shores, this strain was isolated from oysters and oyster-eating fish in Mobile Bay, Alabama, in 1992. However, an associated epidemic or even a large outbreak of cholera has not occurred in the United States. During the period when a million cases of cholera developed in South and Central America (1991 to 1994), only 158 cases were reported in the United States. This difference likely involves better import controls and sanitation in the United States.

Another example of shipping industry involvement in disease emergence is viral encephalitis spread by the Asian tiger mosquito. Encephalitis involves infection of the central nervous system that may cause fever, headache, vomiting, nausea, lethargy, paralysis, or convulsions. Tiger mosquitoes originally were found in Asia, but they now have been detected (along with the encephalitis) in the United States, Brazil, and Africa. Apparently these mosquitoes were transported from Asia in water that collected in used automobile tires on the decks of cargo ships. Since coming to the United States in 1982, the Asian tiger mosquito has established itself in at least 21 states and is involved in causing eastern equine encephalomyelitis.

An interesting incident involving foreign commerce occurred in Reston, Virginia, in 1989. Monkeys from the Philippines were shipped to an animal care facility in Reston. The monkeys were infected with an Ebola virus (referred to as the Ebola-Reston strain) that caused a hemorrhagic fever, and the virus was spread to other monkeys in the facility. The fear was that this deadly virus might escape the facility and cause an epidemic in human beings. Fortunately, the Reston virus was different from the African strains of the Ebola virus (see the following discussion) and did not cause disease in human beings.

West Nile virus was discovered first in Uganda in 1937. The virus usually causes mild encephalitis but can produce a severe and fatal disease. This virus was first recognized in the western hemisphere in an outbreak in New York in 1999. By the end of 2006, 4269 cases had been reported in the United States, with 177 deaths. The disease is transmitted by ornithophilic (bird-loving) mosquitoes and also occurs in horses, many types of birds, and some other animals. The virus apparently is not spread directly from person to person or animal to person. At the same time the human outbreak in New York was detected, large die-offs of wild and captive birds were noticed in the Bronx Zoo and other parts of New York. Human cases occurred at sites near wetlands where migratory birds, ornithophilic mosquitoes, and human beings were concentrated. These events, along with the history of European cases, suggest that zoo, pet, wild, or domestic birds were responsible for introduction of this virus into the United States through normal migration or importation.

In early 2003, a disease emerged in China and the cities of Hong Kong, Hanoi, and Singapore called severe acute respiratory syndrome (SARS). The syndrome is a pneumonia-like disease caused by a previously unrecognized coronavirus from domesticated animals (possibly cats) that is spread by droplet infection or by indirect or direct contact. The first cases detected in other countries and in Canada and the United States were in individuals who recently had traveled from China or Vietnam. Approximately 8500 cases of SARS have been identified.

TECHNOLOGY

Technological advancements involving the development of new devices and processes are important to many aspects of life. However, sometimes this new technology creates new ways to bring microorganisms and human beings together. For example, mass food processing combines large amounts of raw materials for widespread distribution. Unfortunately, a small amount of contaminated raw material can taint a large amount of processed food. Apparently this happened in 1993, when a pathogenic strain of *Escherichia coli* (O157:H7) contaminated meat used to make hamburger for a fast-food chain. The *E. coli* was distributed to restaurants over a four-state area in the northwest United States, infecting approximately 700 persons and causing two deaths. Another important point is that undercooking of the meat allowed the *E. coli* to survive and cause problems. This strain of *E. coli* was first recognized in 1983 and causes hemorrhagic colitis involving bloody diarrhea and abdominal cramps. A life-threatening complication called hemolytic uremic syndrome may develop, and this was the cause of the two deaths in the 1993 outbreak. Hemolytic uremic syndrome involves malfunction of the kidneys and lysis of red blood cells. Fifteen additional outbreaks with the O157:H7 strain were reported in 1993, resulting in more than 100 outbreaks now reported in the United States. Most outbreaks resulted from consumption of contaminated, undercooked ground beef, which has resulted in the FDA-ordered destruction or recall of millions of pounds of hamburger. Other outbreaks have involved contaminated fruits, yogurt, water, apple juice, coleslaw, and dried salami. *E. coli* O157:H7 also has been spread to others in swimming pools and daycare centers.

In 1994, approximately 4000 cases of *Salmonella* food poisoning occurred in 36 states because of contamination of a batch of ice cream mix processed by a large food company. The mix was prepared and pasteurized (heated to 71.7° C [161° F] for 15 seconds to kill disease-producing bacteria) and transported to the packaging and distribution plant. Unfortunately, the mix was transported in a truck that had been previously used to transport raw eggs. Eggs are the leading source of *Salmonella* food poisoning in the United States. Apparently the truck had not been disinfected properly before transporting the ice cream mix, which was not repasteurized before freezing, packaging, and distribution.

The life-saving technology of concentrating special blood products to administer to hemophiliacs and others is important. Unfortunately, such technology also has created an efficient way to transmit bloodborne viruses (e.g., HIV and hepatitis B and C viruses) to those who receive these blood products. Blood transfusion with contaminated blood presents a similar mode of spread. The Centers for Disease Control and Prevention (CDC) estimates that through 2009 there have been 1,142,714 cases of acquired immunodeficiency syndrome (AIDS) diagnosed in the United States. A small percent of these had occurred in those with hemophilia and other coagulation disorders, and in transfusion recipients. Today, blood can be tested for the presence of HIV, hepatitis C, and hepatitis B and no longer serves as a significant mode of spread for these agents.

The development of water-handling devices certainly has made our lives easier, but it has led to new sites that harbor potential pathogens. For example, legionnaires disease (a pneumonia caused by the bacterium *Legionella pneumophila*; see Chapter 7) was first recognized in 1976 among attendees at an American Legion convention in Philadelphia. A few hundred staying at a particular hotel became infected with *L. pneumophila* through the hotel water system or the air-conditioning system and became ill. Since then, *L. pneumophila* has been found to exist in our natural waters and to accumulate on surfaces of water-handling devices (e.g., cooling fins of air-conditioning units, in humidifiers, grocery store vegetable sprayer nozzles, shower heads, therapeutic whirlpools, and dental unit water lines). Inhalation of contaminated water aerosols or aspiration of oral fluids colonized with this opportunistic bacterium may lead to disease, mainly if a person's immune system is compromised and particularly susceptible to respiratory diseases.

MICROBIAL CHANGES

Most mutations in the microbial world are probably lethal because the change destroys some mechanism necessary for multiplication. However, some mutations do not cause death and occasionally even make the microorganism more virulent or more difficult to kill. Two such examples have been mentioned already: *V. cholerae* O139 and *E. coli* O157:H7.

Another well-known example of microbial change is the influenza virus, which changes constantly. Nearly every year, everyone becomes susceptible to the influenza virus regardless

of past bouts with it. The immune system of those who have had influenza usually does not recognize the new virus and offers little or no protection. Likewise, last year's vaccine usually does not work against this year's new strain of virus, so annual flu shots are necessary to achieve the maximum protection.

Another major cause of disease emergence is the development of drug resistance (resistance to antibiotics) among several bacteria. Some of the changes that occur in bacteria involve the development of resistance to one or more antibiotics. For example, if resistance to penicillin has developed in a bacterium causing an infection, and penicillin (which has always taken care of the infection in the past) is administered to the infected patient, the bacterium not only will continue to make the person sick but also will continue to multiply in higher numbers, enhancing its chances of spreading to others. As this continues with subsequent patients, the resistant bacterium reaches more and more persons, causing the same disease, which can no longer be treated with the original antibiotic. With time, a large percentage of those susceptible to this bacterium become infected with the antibiotic-resistant strain. Such infection usually causes delays in effective therapy, giving the bacterium a sometimes dangerous foothold in the early stages of disease.

Several pathogenic antibiotic-resistant bacteria have emerged, including drug-resistant *Streptococcus pneumoniae*, vancomycin-resistant enterococci, methicillin-resistant *Staphylococcus aureus*, and multiple drug-resistant *Mycobacterium tuberculosis*, all of which are important in dentistry and are described further in Chapter 7.

BREAKDOWN IN PUBLIC HEALTH MEASURES

Countless public health measures to protect against the spread of infectious diseases have been instituted in the United States, but they must be maintained to remain effective. One measure is the production of safe drinking water (referred to as potable water). The breakdown of a water treatment process in the city of Milwaukee in 1993 resulted in approximately 400,000 cases of an intestinal infection caused by the protozoon *Cryptosporidium parvum*. This protozoon exists in the intestines of animals and thus ends up in groundwater that empties into the streams that serve as the source of the drinking water of the nation. If water treatment plants do not effectively remove this protozoon (and many other microorganisms) from the drinking water, problems can occur. Other municipal waterborne outbreaks of cryptosporidiosis have occurred in Texas, Georgia, and Oregon.

Many major cities periodically issue "boil water" notices indicating that persons should boil tap water before consuming it or using it in cooking. These notices usually result from a temporary problem at the water treatment plant or with the lines that distribute the water from the plant to homes and workplaces. Commonly, a notice will be generated if a water main (a large water distribution pipeline) breaks as a result of below-freezing temperatures, earthquakes, settling of the ground, or age of the water distribution system. These events can allow potentially contaminated groundwater into the drinking water that flows downstream from the break.

With the formation of the new independent states from the former Soviet Union, some public health vaccination programs were relaxed, which resulted in the development of 45,000 new cases of diphtheria in 1994, with a prediction of 200,000 cases in the following year unless action was taken. Strengthening of the vaccination programs resulted in "only" 60,000 cases in 1995. Diphtheria in the United States is rare because of our effective vaccination program involving DPT inoculations (D stands for diphtheria; P stands for pertussis, the bacterium that causes whooping cough; and T stands for tetanus). Approximately five cases a year have been reported since 1980, and since 1988 all the cases in the United States have been imported. However, if the United States were to relax its vaccination program as occurred in the former Soviet Union, we would experience similar problems because the bacterium (*Corynebacterium diphtheriae*) is still present, living in the throats of asymptomatic carriers.

UNEXPLAINED EMERGENCE

Ebola hemorrhagic fever was first recognized in 1976 in two outbreaks (one in northern Zaire and one in southern Sudan) that involved 602 persons in Africa. This rapidly progressing viral disease causes a high fever with bleeding from multiple sites and the ultimate shutdown of the major organs. The Ebola-Zaire strain of the virus was fatal in 88% of the cases, and the Ebola-Sudan strain was fatal in 53% of the cases. The third outbreak of Ebola hemorrhagic fever was in Sudan in 1979 and involved 34 persons. Another outbreak in 1994 in a Gabon mining camp killed 29 of the 49 persons infected. An outbreak in 1995 involving 315 cases spread through families and a hospital in and around Kikwit, Zaire, resulting in 255 deaths, which is a case fatality rate of 81%. Kikwit has a population of approximately 400,000 and is approximately 1000 km (621 miles) south of the site of the original outbreak in 1976 in the small village of Yambuku, Zaire. The Ebola viruses involved in the Kikwit and Yambuku outbreaks (even though the outbreaks occurred 19 years apart) have been shown to be almost identical. In 1996, 91 persons became infected in Gabon, and these cases may have been associated with eating an infected chimpanzee. In 2000 to 2001, an outbreak occurred in Uganda that involved 425 cases and 225 deaths, and another outbreak occurred in Gabon and the Democratic Republic of the Congo with 96 deaths among the 122 cases. Disease spread was associated with family and health care provider contacts with infected persons.

Great fear exists that Ebola hemorrhagic fever will break out in a small village and that those infected will carry the virus to a site of a larger population, causing a major epidemic and even a pandemic. In the 1995 outbreak, the fear was that the disease would spread from Kikwit to the capital of Zaire, Kinshasa, about 240 miles to the east. Maybe the reason this did not occur is that the disease progresses so rapidly that the victims die in a matter of days, which limits their contact with others. In the 1976, 1995, and 2001 outbreaks, person-to-person spread occurred through close personal contact with infected blood and other body fluids. Those infected included family members and health care providers, although the exact modes of spread still need to be better defined. An obvious problem in these outbreaks is the lack of modern medical facilities and barrier products that could have better protected health care workers from exposure to their infected patients. Additional outbreaks have occurred in the Democratic Republic of the Congo in 2001, 2002, and 2003. In 2004 an outbreak occurred in Sudan. All totaled, approximately 2000 cases of Ebola hemorrhagic fever have occurred, most of which have been fatal.

The natural reservoir (source) where the Ebola virus strains "hide out" between outbreaks is unknown, but attempts to identify the source are being made by culturing samples from local animals, insects, and the environment. The index patient in the 1995 outbreak is thought to have been a charcoal maker who worked in the forest near Kikwit, so this area was being analyzed very carefully. However, the cause of Ebola emergences is still unknown.

SELECTED READINGS

Centers for Disease Control and Prevention: Diphtheria epidemic—new independent states of the former Soviet Union, 1990-1994, *MMWR Morb Mortal Wkly Rep* 44:177–181, 1995.

Centers for Disease Control and Prevention: Hantavirus pulmonary syndrome–United States, 1993, *MMWR Morb Mortal Wkly Rep* 43:45–48, 1994.

Centers for Disease Control and Prevention: *Infectious disease information: emerging infectious diseases*, http://www.cdc.gov/ncidod/diseases/eid/index.htm. Accessed November, 2007.

Centers for Disease Control and Prevention: *MRSA in healthcare setting*. Available at http://www.cdc.gov/ncidod/dhqp/ar_MRSA_spotlight_2006.html. Accessed November 2006.

Centers for Disease Control and Prevention: Update: *Vibrio cholerae* O1-Western hemisphere, 1991-1994, and *V. cholerae* O139–Asia, 1994, *MMWR Morb Mortal Wkly Rep* 44:215–219, 1995.

Corso PS, Kramer MH, Blair KA, et al: Cost of illness in the 1993 waterborne *Cryptosporidium* outbreak, Milwaukee, Wisconsin, *Emerg Infect Dis* 9:426–431, 2003.

Huang C, Slater B, Rudd R, et al: First isolation of West Nile virus from a patient with encephalitis in the United States, *Emerg Infect Dis* 8:1367–1371, 2002.

Kurashina K, Horda T: Nosocomial transmission of methicillin-resistant *Staphylococcus aureus* via the surfaces of the dental operatory, *Br Dent J* 201:297–300, 2006.

Morse SS: Factors in the emergence of infectious diseases, *Emerg Infect Dis* 1:7–15, 1995.

Nielson ACY, Bottiger B, Banner J, et al: Serious invasive scaffold virus infections in children, 2009, *Emerg Infect Dis* 18:7–12, 2012.

Stratton CW: Dead bugs don't mutate: susceptibility issues in the emergence of bacterial resistance, *Emerg Infect Dis* 9:10–16, 2003.

Wilson ME: Travel and the emergence of infectious diseases, *Emerg Infect Dis* 1:39–46, 1995.

Xue-Jie Y, Mi-Fang L, Shou-Yin Z, et al: Fever with thrombocytopenia associated with a novel bunyavirus, *N Engl J Med* 364:1523–1532, 2011.

REVIEW QUESTIONS

Multiple Choice

1. An emerging disease is a disease that:
   a. has not been recognized before
   b. has been known to occur for more than 20 years
   c. is caused by an unknown virus
   d. occurs only in women

2. Hand-foot-and-mouth disease caused by a coxsackievirus was first recognized in:
   a. 2003
   b. 1990
   c. 1970
   d. 1942

3. What caused hantavirus pulmonary syndrome to emerge?
   a. Ecological changes
   b. International travel
   c. Development of new technologies
   d. Breakdown of public health measures

4. What caused legionnaires disease to emerge?
   a. Ecological changes
   b. International travel
   c. Development of new technologies
   d. Breakdown of public health measures

5. Severe acute respiratory syndrome is caused by:
   a. *Escherichia coli*
   b. a coronavirus
   c. *Streptococcus mutans*
   d. a human herpesvirus

Please visit http://evolve.elsevier.com/Miller/infectioncontrol/ for additional practice and study support tools.

Oral Microbiology and Plaque-associated Diseases

OUTLINE

LEARNING OBJECTIVES

After completing this chapter, the student should be able to do the following:

1. Describe the general nature of the normal oral microbiota.
2. Describe the mechanism of dental caries formation, and do the following:
   - List the types of dental caries.
   - Define biofilm and describe how it forms on teeth.
   - List the microbes most important in causing dental caries.
3. Do the following regarding periodontal diseases:
   - Describe the mechanism of periodontal diseases.
   - Differentiate the types of periodontal diseases.
   - List the microbes most important in causing periodontal diseases.
4. List the general approaches to preventing plaque-associated diseases.
5. Describe how other harmful infections may develop from normal oral flora.

KEY TERMS

Biofilm
Calculus
Cellulitis
Chronic Periodontitis
Demineralization
Dental Caries
Dental Plaque
Gingivitis

Glucosyltransferases
Juvenile Periodontitis
Mutans Streptococci
Necrotizing Ulcerative Gingivitis
Non–self-cleansing Areas
Pellicle
Periapical Infection
Periodontitis

Prepubertal Periodontitis
Pulpitis
Rapidly Progressive Periodontitis
Subacute Bacterial Endocarditis
Sucrose
Transient Bacteremia

The mouth contains the normal oral microbiota that have colonized and continually are maintained on the teeth and soft tissues and in saliva. These microorganisms usually cause no harm except when they are allowed to accumulate in the form of dental plaque or are displaced from the mouth to deeper tissues such as the tooth pulp or to other body sites such as the bloodstream.

NORMAL ORAL MICROBIOTA

The human mouth usually is first exposed to microorganisms at birth during passage through the birth canal. Most of the mother's vaginal bacteria that enter the child's mouth are transient (short-lived) and do not establish themselves as regular members of the oral microbiota. With time, the child is exposed to microorganisms from the environment, and the main sources of microorganisms that colonize the child's mouth appear to be the mouths of other persons, particularly the mother and other close family members.

For microorganisms to become established members of the oral microbiota, they must attach to oral surfaces and be able to multiply in the oral environment. Eruption of the primary teeth results in a major change in this environment, now providing tooth surfaces, gingival crevices, and more opportunity for bleeding into the mouth. New bacteria, such as *Streptococcus mutans*, appear that can survive only on the teeth. Anaerobes increase in number because of the added anaerobic sites around the teeth. Thus different sites in the mouth (tongue, buccal epithelium, supragingival tooth surfaces, subgingival tooth surfaces, and crevicular epithelial surfaces) support different combinations of microorganisms. As one grows older, more and more microorganisms colonize the mouth, and, in general, the composition stabilizes by the early teen years.

The normal oral microbiota consists mostly of bacteria, although about one-third of the population also has the yeast *Candida albicans* in their mouth. The oral microbiota is complex with at least 42 known genera of bacteria represented (Box 5-1), although not every person has all of these genera present all of the time. Each genus may be represented by several species, resulting in a complex group of gram-positive and gram-negative bacteria. It is estimated that we can grow only about one-half to two-thirds of the bacteria present in the mouth, and this growth is important in identifying bacteria. Thus there are still many unknown species of bacteria in the human mouth. A gram of dental plaque (about one-quarter of a teaspoonful) contains almost 200 billion bacteria, and saliva contains 10 million to 100 million bacteria per milliliter.

MICROBIOLOGY OF CARIES

Dental caries is an infectious disease and is caused by a demineralization of tooth structure by acids produced during metabolism of dietary sugars by bacteria associated with the tooth surfaces (Figure 5-1). Different types of caries occur depending upon the tooth site affected (e.g., occlusal caries, smooth surfaces caries, interproximal caries, root caries). As with any infectious disease, four factors are necessary for caries to occur: susceptible host, microorganisms, substrate, and time.

Susceptible Host

Not all individuals are susceptible to all infectious diseases. Resistance may be attributable to many factors (other than specific immunity) that are not well understood. In the case of caries-free persons, resistance has not been explained clearly, but may involve characteristics of saliva, anatomic differences in the teeth, or the nature of the oral microbiota. Nevertheless, for caries to occur, the person must be susceptible to the disease.

BOX 5-1

Some Bacterial Genera in the Mouth

Gram-negative
Aggregatibacter
Bacteroides
Campylobacter
Capnocytophaga
Catonella
Cardiobacterium
Centipeda
Dialister
Eikenella
Fusobacterium
Haemophilus
Lautropia
Leptotrichia
Mitsuokella
Moraxella
Neisseria
Parvimonas
Porphyromonas
Prevotella
Selenomonas
Synergistetes
Tannerella
Treponema
Veillonella

Gram-positive
Actinomyces
Arachnia
Atopobium
Bifidobacterium
Corynebacterium
Eubacterium
Filifactor
Gemella
Granulicatella
Lactobacillus
Micrococcus
Mogibacterium
Peptostreptococcus
Propionibacterium
Rothia
Solobacterium
Stomatococcus
Streptococcus
Wolinella

Microorganisms

Bacteria capable of causing caries must be present in the mouth and must be associated closely with the teeth. This association may be in the form of dental plaque, a microbial

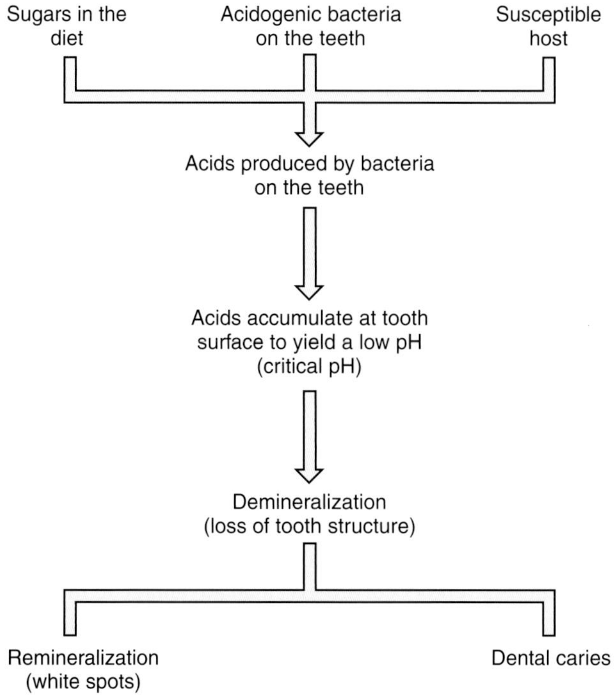

Sugars in the diet   Acidogenic bacteria on the teeth   Susceptible host

↓

Acids produced by bacteria on the teeth

↓

Acids accumulate at tooth surface to yield a low pH (critical pH)

↓

Demineralization (loss of tooth structure)

Remineralization (white spots)   Dental caries

FIGURE 5-1 Formation of dental caries. In a person susceptible to dental caries, the acidogenic bacteria on the teeth ferment sugars in the diet to acids (mainly lactic acid). The acids accumulate on the tooth surface, lowering the pH to a critical level of approximately 5.2. At this pH, the minerals in the tooth start to dissolve, causing loss of tooth structure (demineralization). A natural body defense mechanism called remineralization attempts to restore the lost calcium and phosphate in the tooth, which will appear as a white spot on the tooth. If remineralization occurs more slowly than demineralization, dental caries occurs.

mass that accumulates on the teeth in the absence of oral hygiene, or may result from an impaction of bacteria and food in the non–self-cleansing areas of the dentition (pits and fissures, interproximal sites, gingival crevices).

Dental Plaque (Biofilm)

Plaque is a biofilm composed of bacterial cells embedded in an intercellular matrix (Figure 5-2). The matrix contains macromolecules and small molecules that (1) are produced by the multiplying bacteria, (2) may enter the mouth in the diet, and (3) originate from mammalian cells, saliva, or blood.

Plaque begins to reform within seconds after the teeth are cleaned. Glycoproteins from saliva are first absorbed onto the tooth surface to a thin proteinaceous layer called the pellicle that coats all tooth surfaces exposed to saliva. Next, the bacteria attach to the pellicle, and these serve as an initial "layer" to which other bacterial cells attach. These other cells may come from saliva, or they may be the daughter cells formed from previously attached cells that are multiplying. Plaque accumulates most rapidly in the non–self-cleansing areas of the dentition where the tip of the tongue, the musculature of the cheeks, and the occlusion of the teeth cannot remove the accumulating bacteria.

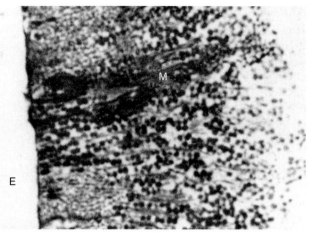

FIGURE 5-2 Relatively thin predominantly coccal flora (plaque) on the enamel surface associated with nondisease gingival tissue. E, Enamel; M, columnar microcolony. (From Listgarten MA: Structure of surface coatings of teeth, *J Periodontol* 47:3, 1976.)

As the plaque accumulates in the absence of oral hygiene, potentially harmful products from the multiplying bacteria accumulate and may cause damage to the teeth (caries) or to the nearby periodontal tissues (gingivitis or periodontitis). In some persons, plaque can mineralize (accumulate calcium) forming a hardened material referred to as calculus or tarter.

Many are the mechanisms by which bacteria attach to tooth surfaces or to each other during plaque formation. Some mechanisms involve interactions of the bacteria with glycoproteins or calcium from saliva or the pellicle, some involve fimbriae or special receptors on the surfaces of the bacteria, and others involve extracellular macromolecules produced by the bacteria that then can bind to cell surfaces. One approach to prevention of plaque-associated diseases (caries, periodontal diseases) other than brushing and flossing is to develop special mouth rinses that interfere with bacterial attachment to the teeth to prevent plaque from accumulating.

Caries-conducive Bacteria

Although dental plaque contains many different species of bacteria, some are more important than others in directly contributing to the initiation or progression of dental caries (Table 5-1).

A group of closely related streptococci called the mutans streptococci consist of the most caries-conducive bacteria in the mouth. Members of this group that are most commonly present in the human mouth are *S. mutans* and *Streptococcus sobrinus*. Other species in this group occur in the mouth less frequently. The *mutans* streptococci have all three pathogenic properties important for caries formation:

- Production of acids from carbohydrates (being acidogenic)
- Survival at low pH (being aciduric)
- Accumulation on teeth

The *mutans* streptococci are thought to be the most important oral bacteria in initiating caries, particularly on smooth tooth surfaces (buccal and lingual) where plaque that can resist the cleansing action of the tongue and cheeks "rubbing" against the teeth is needed for caries to develop. *Mutans* streptococci are important plaque formers and can accumulate rapidly in plaque in the presence of sucrose (table sugar). The *mutans* streptococci have special enzymes (glucosyltransferases) that split sucrose, linking together the glucose units of the sucrose molecules to form polysaccharides called glucans (Figure 5-3). The remaining fructose part of sucrose is taken into the cell and processed through catabolic fermentation reactions to produce energy with mainly lactic acid as a waste product (see Chapter 2). The glucans bind to the cells and act as bridges that bind to other cells. This binding permits new daughter cells to attach to the cell mass and accumulate in the developing dental plaque. The *mutans* streptococci not only produce acids (are acidogenic) from sugar metabolism but also are capable of surviving and metabolizing in the presence of these acids at a low pH (are aciduric), whereas most bacteria die at a low pH.

Lactobacillus species such as *Lactobacillus acidophilus* and *Lactobacillus casei* are thought to be more important in the progression of a carious lesion after other bacteria (mainly *mutans* streptococci) have initiated the tooth destruction. Although lactobacilli are highly acidogenic and aciduric, they do not have effective attachment mechanisms to allow them to accumulate in plaque that develops over noncarious teeth. Thus the other bacteria present in plaque (e.g., *mutans* streptococci) are more important than lactobacilli in the initial attack on the tooth. Low numbers of lactobacilli, however, are accidentally "trapped" in plaque as it develops and may be present in saliva. If the plaque bacteria produce acids, causing demineralization of the tooth, the aciduric bacteria such as lactobacilli and *mutans* streptococci are given an advantage to multiply more rapidly. The nonaciduric bacteria begin to die, leaving more nutrients available for the aciduric bacteria. The best place for lactobacilli to thrive is within the highly acidic carious lesion itself. As the lactobacilli thrive, they and the *mutans* streptococci produce even more acids, if sugars are present, causing the lesion to progress.

Actinomyces naeslundii is a good plaque former and can accumulate to high numbers in plaque. The bacteria is not as conducive to caries as the *mutans* streptococci, likely because they are only slightly acidogenic and not aciduric. However, *A. naeslundii* is important in root caries formation but the mechanisms of its involvement have not been defined clearly.

TABLE 5-1	Important Caries-conducive Bacteria in Human Beings	
Bacterium	**Pathogenic Properties**

Mutans streptococci
  Streptococcus mutans
  Streptococcus sobrinus
	Acidogenic; aciduric; accumulate on teeth

Lactobacillus species	Acidogenic; aciduric
Actinomyces naeslundii	Accumulates on teeth; slightly acidogenic

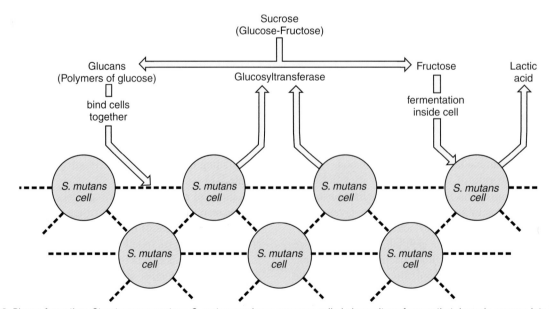

FIGURE 5-3 Plaque formation: *Streptococcus mutans*. *S. mutans* produces enzymes called glucosyltransferases that degrade sucrose into free fructose and polymers of glucose called glucans. The glucans bind to the surfaces of the *S. mutans* cells, linking them together into a mass in the plaque. The cells take in the fructose and metabolize it through fermentation with production of energy for multiplication and lactic acid as a waste product. Dashed lines indicate glucans.

Substrate

The third factor needed for caries development is a dietary substrate that oral bacteria metabolize through catabolic fermentation to produce acids. Sucrose is the most caries-conducive component of our diet, but other sugars such as fructose, glucose, lactose, and starch also can be fermented by bacteria and can contribute to the disease.

Time

As with any infectious disease, time is needed for the disease to become recognized. This time can be called the incubation time, as described in Chapter 3. Dental checkups are scheduled frequently at 6-month intervals because this approximates the usual incubation time for clinically detectable caries.

MICROBIOLOGY OF PERIODONTAL DISEASES

Like dental caries, periodontal diseases are also infectious diseases caused by members of the normal oral microbiota that have been allowed to accumulate in gingival sulcus plaque (Figure 5-4). As the bacteria multiply, they produce histolytic enzymes, toxic metabolites, exotoxins, endotoxins, and immunosuppressive and antiphagocytic factors (which are described in Chapter 3). The accumulation of these bacteria and their potentially harmful products and antigens then produce periodontal diseases by the following mechanisms:

- Direct damage to the tissue
- Inflammation
- Interference with some host defense mechanisms
- Stimulation of the immune response in the periodontal tissues, which can cause damage

Types of Periodontal Diseases

If the disease process affects only the gingival tissue, resulting in an inflammatory response, including swelling, redness, and maybe spontaneous bleeding, the disease is called simple or acute gingivitis. This disease is reversible. When the plaque (and its tissue damaging products) is removed, the gingival tissue returns to normal. Another gingivitis, called necrotizing ulcerative gingivitis or trench mouth, is associated with plaque accumulation and predisposing factors such as stress. This gingivitis also is reversible if the predisposing factors are eliminated and plaque accumulation is controlled.

If the disease process affects the bone in which the teeth are set, the disease is called periodontitis. The disease involves the development of periodontal pockets around the teeth where the gingival tissue has separated from the teeth. These pockets are filled with plaque bacteria and limit access to cleaning. Some of the plaque products directly or indirectly destroy the periodontal tissues and the alveolar bone, which can result in a loosening or loss of the teeth involved. Periodontitis is not reversible. Removal and subsequent control of the plaque, however, can stop further progress of the disease in many instances.

The type of periodontal disease that develops from the accumulation of plaque is influenced by the specific types of bacteria present in the plaque and by how the body responds to the infection. For example, the continuous presence of plaque in persons with normal body defense mechanisms likely leads to chronic periodontitis, a slowly progressing destruction of the bone in which the teeth are set that occurs over a period of years. This is the most common form of periodontitis that usually occurs in persons older than age 35 years.

In those persons with some defect in body defenses (usually decreased phagocytosis), the bone destruction that occurs in periodontitis may occur rapidly, within months or weeks, as in rapidly progressive periodontitis (most commonly seen in those younger than age 35 years), juvenile periodontitis (most common during the early teen years), or prepubertal periodontitis (occurring in those with primary teeth). Immunosuppression resulting from human immunodeficiency virus infection also may predispose individuals to a rapidly progressing periodontitis.

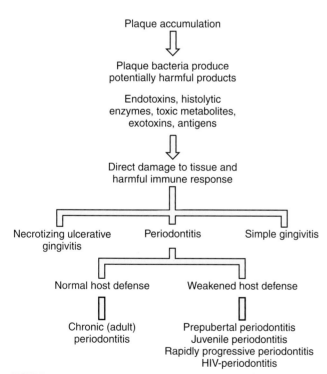

FIGURE 5-4 Development of plaque-associated periodontal diseases. As plaque accumulates in the gingival crevice, the bacteria multiply and produce harmful products that can cause direct damage to the periodontal tissues and that continually stimulate the immune system, resulting in tissue damage. The types of bacteria in the plaque and the nature of the body defense mechanisms combating the infection determine which form of periodontal disease may result.

Microorganisms in Periodontal Diseases

Subgingival plaque associated with all forms of periodontal disease contains many bacteria that possess a wide variety of pathogenic properties. Thus many species can contribute to the disease processes, but some appear to be more important than others and often are called periodontopathogens (Box 5-2). Although caries-conducive bacteria are gram-positive, most of the periodontopathogens are gram-negative; the exceptions include *Peptostreptococcus*, *Streptococcus*, and *Actinomyces*. The latter two genera are associated mostly with gingivitis rather than with periodontitis. Although some research has discovered strong associations of specific species with specific types of periodontitis (e.g., *Aggregatibacter actinomycetemcomitans* with juvenile periodontitis and *Porphyromonas gingivalis* with chronic periodontitis), this is not always true in every case of the diseases.

PREVENTION OF PLAQUE-ASSOCIATED DISEASES

Regular brushing and flossing have long been used for preventing plaque-associated diseases. Fluoride and pit and fissure sealants also are effective against caries. Fluoride has three principal topical mechanisms of action: inhibiting bacterial metabolism after diffusing into the bacteria as hydrogen fluoride; inhibiting demineralization when present at the crystal surfaces of teeth during an acid challenge; and enhancing remineralization. Caries and periodontal diseases still occur, however, and other preventive approaches are being used or studied. A current approach involving microbiology is the use of antimicrobial mouth rinses. Other approaches still under investigation include more effective means of delivering antimicrobial agents to sites of infection, development of new antimicrobial agents, replacement of oral pathogens with nonpathogenic strains, and use of vaccines or other chemical agents that may prevent bacterial attachment or disrupt preformed plaque.

ACUTE DENTAL INFECTIONS

As untreated carious lesions progress and approach the tooth pulp, microbial by-products may enter the pulp and cause inflammation called **pulpitis**. As the disease continues, the bacteria enter the pulp chamber, enhancing the inflammation and destroying the pulp tissue. Further progression may extend the infection through the tooth apex, causing a **periapical infection**. Depending on the host response and probably the types of bacteria involved, the surrounding facial tissues may become infected, producing a **cellulitis**. In general, endodontic treatment involves removing necrotic (dead) pulp tissue, killing and removing the remaining bacteria in the root canals, and filling the canals with inert material to prevent further access of bacteria to the periapical tissues. Treatment with antibiotics also may be necessary to slow down bacterial growth involved with periapical infections and cellulitis. Thus the normal oral bacteria present in carious lesions that extend to the pulp tissues become the causative agents of these acute dental infections.

OTHER INFECTIONS

Members of the normal oral flora may be involved in other harmful infections if given the opportunity to invade tissues, as in pulpitis. For example, *Actinomyces israelii*, a gram-positive anaerobic, rod-shaped bacterium, or other *Actinomyces* species found in plaque may cause a harmful infection in the jaw and neck area called cervicofacial actinomycosis. This disease is rare, resulting from entrance of these bacteria into oral tissues as a result of tooth extractions or some other trauma. Actinomycosis of the lung is another rare disease that results from aspiration (breathing in) of *Actinomyces* species into the lung from the mouth.

The slightest trauma in the mouth that results in bleeding (e.g., toothbrushing, biting the cheek, and dental procedures) may permit members of the normal oral microbiota to enter the bloodstream, causing a **transient bacteremia**. Normally, the phagocytes in the blood rapidly destroy these bacteria before they have a chance to cause problems. If a person has had previous damage to the heart valves, however, such as in rheumatic heart disease, certain oral bacteria in the blood may induce further damage to these valves or cause **subacute bacterial endocarditis** (inflammation of the inside of the heart). For this reason, some dental patients with previous heart damage must be given antibiotics prophylactically (for prevention) when they receive dental care. When bacteria do enter the bloodstream and cause damage to tissues, the condition is referred to as septicemia rather than bacteremia.

Other harmful infections caused by oral microorganisms are those resulting from a bite or a puncture or cut with a contaminated dental instrument. Several microorganisms are implanted through the skin in these instances, which can lead to a harmful infection that sometimes needs antibiotic treatment. Thus many members of the normal oral microbiota have pathogenic potential if they are allowed to gain entrance to deeper tissues or if they gain entrance to the bodies of others.

SELECTED READINGS

Bagg J, MacFarlane TW, Poxton IR, Miller CH: *Essentials of microbiology for dental students,* Oxford, 1999, Oxford University Press.

Centers for Disease Control and Prevention: Recommendations for using fluoride to prevent and control dental caries in the United States, *MMWR Recomm Rep* 50(RR-14):1–42, 2001.

Featherstone JDB: The science and practice of caries prevention, *J Am Dent Assoc* 131:887–899, 2000.

Lamont RJ, Burne RA, Lantz MS, LeBlanc DJ, editors: *Oral microbiology and immunology,* Herndon, PA, 2006, ASM Press.

REVIEW QUESTIONS

Multiple Choice

1. The most important bacterium in causing dental caries is:
   a. *Streptococcus pyogenes*
   b. *Bacillus subtilis*
   c. *Staphylococcus aureus*
   d. *Streptococcus mutans*

2. Dental plaque is:
   a. a microbial mass
   b. composed of pieces of food that have stuck to the teeth
   c. mineralized proteins
   d. dried saliva

3. Which of the following dietary components are most important in the cause of dental caries?
   a. Proteins
   b. Fats
   c. Cholesterol
   d. Sugars

4. Which is true about periodontal diseases?
   a. Gingivitis involves the bone in which the teeth are set.
   b. The same bacteria that cause dental caries also cause periodontal diseases.
   c. Plaque causes periodontal diseases.
   d. Periodontitis occurs only in older adults.

5. Which is true about the normal oral microbiota?
   a. Dental plaque has about 200 billion bacteria per gram.
   b. Usually only four different species of bacteria can exist in the human mouth.
   c. All the bacteria in the mouth are cocci.
   d. The oral microbiota are not involved in causing dental caries or periodontal diseases.

6. Which of the following bacteria is the most important in causing the progression of a carious lesion after the lesion has been initiated?
   a. *Streptococcus sanguis*
   b. *Lactobacillus acidophilus*
   c. *Porphyromonas gingivalis*
   d. *Prevotella intermedia*

7. Which of the following bacteria is most important in causing periodontal diseases?
   a. *Streptococcus mutans*
   b. *Porphyromonas gingivalis*
   c. *Lactobacillus acidophilus*
   d. *Streptococcus sanguis*

8. Sucrose is converted to what polysaccharide that causes bridging between cells of *Streptococcus mutans* during plaque formation?
   a. Starch
   b. Fructan
   c. Glycogen
   d. Glucan

9. Which of the following periodontal diseases is not related to weakened host defenses?
   a. Chronic adult periodontitis
   b. Rapidly progressive periodontitis
   c. Juvenile periodontitis
   d. Prepubertal periodontitis

10. Inflammation of the tissue in the root canal of a tooth is called:
    a. pulpitis
    b. dental caries
    c. cellulitis
    d. periapical infection

PART TWO

Infection Control

Bloodborne Pathogens

OUTLINE

LEARNING OBJECTIVES

After completing this chapter, the student should be able to do the following:

1. Define bloodborne diseases and pathogens and explain why an understanding of these diseases is important to the practice of dentistry.
2. Compare the five major types of viral hepatitis and describe the relative infectivity of viral hepatitis after an occupational exposure.
3. Describe the antigens and antibodies related to the different types of hepatitis.
4. Describe the relative infectivity of HIV after an occupational exposure, and list ways to prevent the spread of HIV.

KEY TERMS

Acquired Immunodeficiency
   Syndrome (AIDS)
Acute Retroviral Syndrome
Bloodborne Diseases
Bloodborne Pathogens
Carrier State
HBcAg
HBeAg

HBsAg
Hepatitis
Hepatitis A Virus
Hepatitis B Vaccine
Hepatitis B Virus
Hepatitis C Virus
Hepatitis D Virus
Hepatitis E Virus

HIV Disease
Human Immunodeficiency Virus (HIV)
Lymphocytes
Percutaneous
Retroviruses
Seroconversion
Viral Hepatitis

As described in Chapter 3, the patient's oral cavity is the single most important source of potentially pathogenic microorganisms. Pathogenic agents may be present in the mouth as a result of four basic processes: bloodborne diseases, oral diseases, systemic diseases with oral lesions, and respiratory diseases. Bloodborne diseases are discussed in this chapter; oral and respiratory diseases are presented in Chapter 7.

Bloodborne pathogens may infect different blood cells or other tissues of the body, but during infection the pathogens exist in or are released into the blood or other body fluids, which may include semen, vaginal secretion, intestinal secretions, tears, mother's milk, synovial (joint) fluid, pericardial (around the heart) fluid, amniotic fluids (surround the developing fetus), and saliva. Because blood or other body fluids may contain these pathogens, the disease may be spread from one person to another by contact with the fluids. Thus the diseases are called bloodborne diseases. Bloodborne pathogens may enter the mouth during dental procedures that induce bleeding. Thus contact with saliva during such procedures may result in exposure to these pathogens if they are present. Because determining whether blood is actually present in saliva is difficult, saliva from all dental patients should be considered potentially infectious.

VIRAL HEPATITIS

Five common hepatitis viruses cause clinically similar diseases: hepatitides A, B, C, D, and E (Table 6-1). Hepatitis A virus and hepatitis E virus are transmitted mainly through contaminated food and water (fecal–oral routes of spread), whereas hepatitis B virus (HBV), hepatitis C virus (HCV), and hepatitis D virus (HDV) are bloodborne diseases usually transmitted by direct or indirect contact with infected body fluids.

Hepatitis means an inflammation of the liver. Often the inflammation is virally related; however, hepatitis also may be caused by excessive alcohol consumption, exposure to some hazardous chemicals, and as a complication of other infections.

Hepatitis B

Hepatitis B is a major health problem in the United States and worldwide. Hepatitis B is endemic (occurs regularly) in many parts of the world. The number of new infections per year in the United States has declined from an estimated 260,000 in the 1980s to approximately 38,000 in 2009. Approximately 8000 persons with acute infections will require hospitalization. Approximately 180 persons will die of fulminant hepatitis (an overwhelming and rapidly destructive form of the disease), whereas more than 3700 persons will become chronic carriers of the virus. Approximately 3000 persons with chronic hepatitis B die each year. Current estimates by the Centers for Disease Control and Prevention (CDC) suggest that there are almost a million HBV carriers in the United States. Each person has some potential to spread the virus to others. More than 200 million persons are

TABLE 6-1   **Comparison of Hepatitis Viruses**

Feature	Hepatitis A	Hepatitis B	Hepatitis C	Hepatitis D	Hepatitis E
Family characteristics	Picornavirus Nonenveloped single-stranded RNA	Hepadnavirus Double-stranded DNA	Flavivirus Enveloped single-stranded RNA	Satellite/defective Nonenveloped single-stranded RNA	Calicivirus Nonenveloped single-stranded RNA
Incubation period	15-40 days	45-180 days	1-5 months	21-90 days	15-60 days
Nature of onset	Usually acute	Usually insidious	Usually insidious	Usually acute	Usually acute
Transmission	Fecal–oral Poor hygiene Contaminated food or drink	Parenteral Permucosal Sexual contact Prenatal Other	Usually parenteral Permucosal Sexual contact Idiopathic Other	Usually parenteral Permucosal Sexual contact Other	Fecal–oral Waterborne
Carrier states	None	Yes (5%-10%)	Yes (75%-85%)	Yes	None
Chronic infections	No	Yes	Yes	Yes	No
Possible sequelae	None reported	Hepatocellular carcinoma Cirrhosis	Hepatocellular carcinoma Cirrhosis	Hepatocellular carcinoma Cirrhosis	None reported
Mortality from acute infection	Rare	1%-2% (higher if older than age 40 years)	1%-2%	2%-30%	1%-3% 15%-25% if pregnant
Immunity	Anti-HAV	Anti-HBsAg Anti-HBcAg	Anti-HCV (less effective)	Anti-HBsAg	Anti-HEV
Immunization	Yes	Yes	No	Yes via HBV vaccination	No
Serologic screening	Yes	Yes	Yes	Yes via HBV	No
Occupational hazard for dentistry	No	Yes	Yes, but lower than HBV	Yes	No

Abbreviations: HAV, Hepatitis A virus; HBcAg, hepatitis B core antigen; HBsAg, hepatitis B surface antigen; HBV, hepatitis B virus; HCV, hepatitis C virus; HEV, hepatitis E virus.
Modified from Palenik CJ: Hepatitis C virus and dental personnel, *Dent Today* 23:56-59, 2004.

estimated to be carriers worldwide. HBV accounts for 34% of all types of acute viral hepatitis.

Hepatitis B Virus

The HBV is an enveloped DNA virus that infects and multiplies in human liver cells. During the course of an infection, the virus and cells containing the virus are released in high numbers into the bloodstream and other body fluids, explaining its description as a bloodborne disease agent. A milliliter of blood from an infected person may contain as many as 100 million virus particles, meaning that only small amounts of blood or other body fluids are necessary to transmit the disease to others. The virus has three components that are important antigens; some components are on its surface (hepatitis B surface antigen, or HBsAg), and two are inside the virus (hepatitis B core antigen [HBcAg] and hepatitis Be antigen [HBeAg]) (Table 6-2). The hepatitis B vaccines consist of the HBsAg that is synthesized using yeast cells in a laboratory by genetic engineering techniques.

Hepatitis B virus has been shown to remain viable at room temperature for at least 1 month. The virus can be killed or inactivated by commonly used methods of sterilization and disinfection, including the steam autoclave, or a 10-minute exposure to 1:100 diluted bleach, 1:16 diluted phenolic glutaraldehyde, 75 parts per million (ppm) iodophor, or 70% isopropyl alcohol. Thus HBV is easy to kill when outside the

TABLE 6-2 **Hepatitis Terminology**

	Abbreviation	Term	Definitions/Comments
Hepatitis A	HAV	Hepatitis A virus	Etiologic agent of "infectious" hepatitis; a picornavirus; single serotype
	Anti-HAV	Antibody to HAV	Detectable at onset of symptoms; lifetime persistence
	IgM anti-HAV	Immunoglobulin M (IgM) class antibody to HAV	Indicates recent infection with hepatitis A; detectable for 4 to 6 months after infection
Hepatitis B	HBV	Hepatitis B virus	Etiologic agent of "serum" hepatitis; also known as Dane particle
	HBsAg	Hepatitis B surface antigen	Surface antigen(s) of HBV detectable in large quantities in serum; several serotypes identified
	HBeAg	Hepatitis e antigen	Soluble antigen; correlates with HBV replication; high titer HBV in serum and infectivity of serum
	HBcAg	Hepatitis B core antigen	No commercial test available
	Anti-HBs	Antibody to HBsAg	Indicates past infection with and immunity to HBV, passive antibody from hepatitis B immune globulin or immune response from hepatitis B vaccine
	Anti-HBe	Antibody to HBeAg	Presence in serum and HBsAg carrier indicates lower titer of HBV
	Anti-HBc	Antibody to HBcAg	Indicates prior infection with HBV at some undefined time
	IgM anti-HBc	IgM class antibody to HBcAg	Indicates recent infection with HBV; detectable for 4 to 6 months after infection
Hepatitis C	HCV	Hepatitis C virus	Causative agent of hepatitis C, the most common chronic bloodborne pathogen disease
	Anti-HCV	Antibody to HCV	Anti-HCV can be detected in 97% of infected persons, but antibody does not tell whether the infection is new (acute), chronic (long-term), or no longer present
Hepatitis D	HDV	Hepatitis D virus	Etiologic agent of delta hepatitis; can cause infection only in the presence of HBV
	sHDAg	Small hepatitis D antigen	Detectable in early acute delta infection
	lHDAg	Large hepatitis D antigen	Detectable in early acute delta infection
	Anti-HDV	Antibody to delta antigen	Indicates present or past infection with delta virus
Hepatitis E	HEV	Hepatitis E virus	Diagnosis by exclusion; no serologic tests to diagnose HEV infection are commercially available in the United States
Immune globulin	IG	Immune globulin	Antibodies to HAV and lesser amounts to HBV
	HBIG	Hepatitis B immune globulin	Contains high titers to HBV

body, provided the killing agent comes into direct contact with the virus. Hepatitis B virus is more easily killed than *Mycobacterium tuberculosis* and bacterial spores.

Disease States

Human beings are the only known natural hosts of HBV. Approximately 90% of those infected with HBV undergo complete recovery without developing a **carrier state** (Figure 6-1). Approximately 2% to 10% become carriers of the virus, with approximately half eliminating the virus from their bodies within 5 years. The other half become chronic carriers, and approximately 25% of these will develop chronic active hepatitis. Persons who have chronic active hepatitis have a 200 to 300 times greater chance of later developing liver cancer (hepatocellular carcinoma). Premature mortality from chronic liver disease occurs in approximately 15% to 25% of the chronically infected.

The carrier state is defined as being HBsAg-positive on at least two occasions when tested at least 2 months apart or being HBsAg-positive and immunoglobulin M anti–HBc-negative at a single test. Anyone who is positive for HBsAg has a potential to spread the disease to others. Those who are also HBeAg-positive have high concentrations of the virus in their blood and therefore are considered as being highly infectious.

Transmission

HBV is spread percutaneously (through the skin) or permucosally (through mucous membranes) by contact with infected body fluids, for example, at birth, during sexual activities, or with contaminated needles or other sharp objects. Perinatal transmission of the virus to infants at birth is efficient. If the mother is positive for HBsAg and HBeAg, the infant has a 70% to 90% chance of being infected. If the mother is only HBsAg-positive, the risk to the infant drops to 20%. Up to 90% of infected infants become chronic carriers. When infection occurs between 1 and 5 years of age, 30% of children become chronic carriers. Above the age of 5 years the rate drops to approximately 6%.

The virus also may be spread in environments involving frequent close contact with an infected person, as in households or institutions for developmentally disabled children. This latter route of spread likely involves unnoticed contact of infected body fluids with skin lesions or mucosal surfaces.

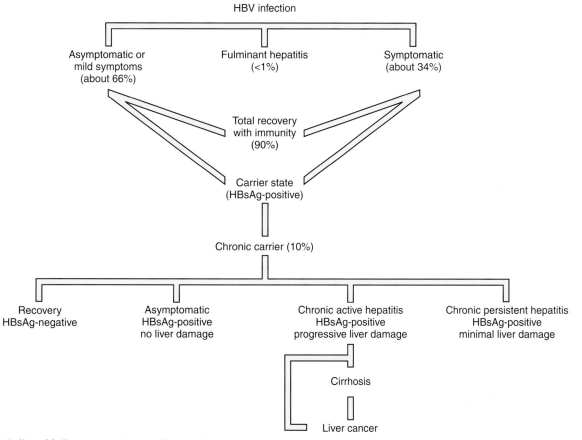

FIGURE 6-1 Hepatitis B outcomes. Hepatitis B virus infection may result in clinical symptoms in approximately one third of the cases and no symptoms or unrecognized symptoms in approximately two thirds of the cases. A rapidly progressive fulminant disease leading to death occurs in less than 1% of the cases. Approximately 90% of all infected persons recover. The remaining 10% develop chronic infection and may carry the virus for up to 6 months and then have complete recovery. Others remain as chronic carriers, being asymptomatic, having chronic active hepatitis or having chronic persistent hepatitis.

Infection occurs when blood or body fluids from an infected person enter the body of a person who is not immune to HBV. High-risk behaviors for acquiring hepatitis B include the following:

- Sharing of contaminated needles during intravenous drug abuse
- Sexual intercourse with an infected person without using a condom
- Becoming pregnant while infected with HBV; may lead to perinatal infection

Spread of HBV through transfused blood or blood products is now rare because of routine testing of blood for HBsAg and donor screening. A fecal–oral route of transmission does not occur commonly. No transmission appears to occur through tears, sweat, stool, urine, or droplet infection.

Symptoms

If symptoms develop after infection, they begin to appear 45 to 180 days (average of 60 to 90 days) after exposure. Roughly one third of those infected (see Figure 6-1) exhibit the more easily recognizable symptoms of yellowing of the skin (jaundice) and whites of the eyes, light-colored stools, dark urine, joint pain, fever, rash, and itching. Clinical illness is more common among infected individuals older than 5 years of age. Approximately another one third of those infected develop less descriptive mild symptoms that may include malaise ("not feeling good"), loss of appetite, nausea, and abdominal pain. The remaining one third develop no symptoms at all. Thus two thirds of all those infected develop no symptoms or mild nondescript symptoms that often are unrecognized as being related to hepatitis. Yet symptomatic and asymptomatic carriers can spread the virus to others. This unrecognizable infection with HBV and with other viruses (such as human immunodeficiency virus [HIV], described later) serves as the basis for universal and standard precautions—applying infection control procedures during care for all patients, not just those who are considered infectious.

Development of a hepatitis B chronic carrier state may occur more commonly in those who are asymptomatic and is more likely to occur in the young. Women who are pregnant should seek the advice of their personal physician about being tested for HBV, so that, if infected, proper procedures can be instituted to protect the newborn. One could be infected unknowingly with HBV, not develop any recognizable symptoms, become a chronic carrier, unknowingly spread the virus to others, and die years later of HBV liver damage. Hepatitis B is obviously an insidious disease.

Risk for the Dental Team

Several blood-testing surveys of dental workers conducted between 1975 and 1982 attempted to determine how many of the different types of dental workers had been infected with HBV. Although some of the studies involved only small groups of workers, the results suggested that approximately 13% of dental assistants, 17% of dental hygienists, 14% of dental laboratory technicians, and 9% to 25% of dentists had been infected. At that time, approximately 5% of the general population was estimated to have been infected. Thus unvaccinated members of the dental team are at least 2 to 5 times more likely to become infected with HBV than the general population.

In the early to mid-1980s, 10,000 to 12,000 cases of HBV infection (approximately 4% of all cases) occurred annually in persons who had an occupational risk for exposure to body fluids. In 1994, this number dropped to approximately 1000 cases, showing about a 90% decrease in HBV among health care workers. This decrease can be related to the development of a protective vaccine and the increased application of better engineering and work practice controls and personal protective equipment. However, exposure still can occur readily through injuries with contaminated sharp instruments and needles. Consequently, hepatitis B remains the most important occupationally acquired disease for dental professionals.

The greatest dental occupational risks for exposure are the following:

- Injuries from contaminated sharps (needlesticks, instrument punctures, cuts, bur lacerations)
- Blood and saliva contamination of cuts and cracks on the skin or ungloved hands or hands with torn gloves
- Spraying of blood and saliva onto open lesions on the skin or onto mucous membranes

Dentist-to-Patient Spread of Hepatitis B

The chances of a patient acquiring any disease in a dental office are low. In the past, HBV has been spread from dentists to patients, as documented in 11 separate instances. In each instance, the dentist was highly infectious (HBeAg-positive) and apparently did not wear gloves routinely. These instances occurred between 1974 and 1987, with none, as yet, being reported since. The drop in the spread of HBV from dentists to patients coincides with the time (around 1984) when infection control in dentistry was reemphasized as a result of the advent of **acquired immunodeficiency syndrome (AIDS)**.

Patient-to-Patient Spread of Hepatitis B

After a lull of 14 years, HBV raised its ugly head again in 2001 as the cause of an infection in a dental patient, as reported by Redd et al in May 2007. Hepatitis B was spread from one patient to another patient on the same day in 2001 in an oral surgery practice. The source patient was a 36-year-old chronic carrier positive for HBsAg and HBeAg, the latter indicating high communicability. She had some teeth extracted on the day of the incident but did not tell anyone in the office that she was an HBV carrier. A little over 2.5 hours after her teeth were extracted, the same oral surgeon and staff extracted seven teeth from a 61-year-old woman who later developed hepatitis B, but recovered. Molecular epidemiologic techniques determined that the same virus caused hepatitis B in both women. Fourteen of the 15 employees in the practice were tested and showed evidence of HBV vaccination, and none showed any evidence of previous HBV infection. Testing of 25 of the 27 patients seen after the source patient that week in the practice revealed that 19 of them were immune to hepatitis B. This included three of the five patients seen after the source patient on the same day. CDC investigators visited the practice after the incident and determined that the office was clean, that standard precautions were being practiced, and that appropriate infection control procedures were in place at that time.

Since no clear-cut mode of viral spread was identified in this case, the CDC investigators could only speculate on the mechanism of transmission involved. One possibility mentioned was the spread of the virus from a contaminated environmental surface. HBV is known to survive for several days in dried blood, and maybe a contaminated surface was not properly managed after treatment of the source patient.

This case alerts us to the continued importance of the potential spread of HBV in dentistry and the importance of HBV vaccination. The spread of this virus in this case was likely limited by the high incidence of HBV immunity in the staff and patients.

Hepatitis B Vaccine

The availability of safe and effective vaccines for hepatitis B is fortunate. Because no successful medical treatment exists to cure this disease, prevention is of paramount importance. Chapter 9 presents details on the vaccines and the vaccination series. The vaccines are strongly recommended for all members of the dental team. The Occupational Safety and Health Administration of the U.S. Department of Labor actually requires dentist-employers to offer the hepatitis B vaccine series free of charge to office staff who may have any potential for exposure to blood or saliva. The requirement applies to employers in all health care and other professions in which body fluid exposure is possible. Also, in late 1991 the CDC recommended hepatitis B vaccination for all newborns, and in 1995 the CDC recommended vaccination for 12-year-olds who were not vaccinated previously. In 2006, CDC recommended vaccination for all unvaccinated adults at risk for HBV infection and for all adults requesting protection from HBV infection. They also stated that acknowledgment of a specific risk factor should not be a requirement for vaccination. Because no vaccine is 100% effective, the CDC does recommend testing for immunity (anti-HBsAg antibody) 1 to 2 months after one receives the third inoculation of the vaccine series.

Hepatitis C

Hepatitis C virus (HCV) previously was called parenterally transmitted non-A, non-B hepatitis (see Table 6-2). HCV is thought to cause approximately 30% of acute viral hepatitis cases in the United States and is a bloodborne disease. Approximately 16,000 persons in the United States are estimated to become infected with HCV every year, but only approximately 20% of those infected have any (generally mild) recognizable symptoms.

Approximately 50% of hepatitis C cases are associated with intravenous drug abuse, 15% to 25% are associated with sexual exposure, 3% with blood transfusions, and 1% with occupational exposure in health care workers. The remaining cases have unidentified routes of transmission. HCV has been transmitted to medical health care workers through needlestick injuries. However, as long as Standard Precautions and other infection control procedures are used, dental and medical procedures in the United States generally do not pose a risk for spread of HCV.

An alarming fact about hepatitis C is that 75% to 85% of those infected apparently become chronic carriers, and 20% develop chronic liver disease. An estimated 3.2 million persons have chronic infection with HCV, and deaths from cirrhosis may occur in 1% to 5% of all those infected.

Until recently, HCV was diagnosed by indirect means showing that the patient did not have type A or type B hepatitis. The causative virus was first isolated in 1989, and a blood test for antibodies to HCV was designed in 1991. This test aids in diagnosing the disease, identifying those who are or have been infected, and in screening potential blood donors. As yet, no vaccine is available for hepatitis C, but development of the badly needed test for HCV is leading to firmer information on modes of spread of this virus. Those at the highest risk are injection-drug users and recipients of clotting factors made before 1987. Those at intermediate risk include hemodialysis patients, recipients of blood and/or solid organs before 1992, people with undiagnosed liver problems, and infants born to infected mothers. Those with low risk include health care and public safety workers, people having sex with multiple partners, and people having sex with an infected steady partner. Neither the hepatitis A nor the hepatitis B vaccine provides any protection against hepatitis C.

Hepatitis D

Infection with hepatitis D virus (HDV), previously known as the delta agent, is regarded as a complication of hepatitis B (see Table 6-1). This bloodborne virus may cause infection only in the presence of an active HBV infection. HDV is a defective virus that needs a part of the HBV to complete its life cycle.

Infection with HDV may occur as a coinfection with HBV (HDV and HBV infect simultaneously) or as a superinfection of HDV in an HBV carrier. Both instances usually result in clinical acute hepatitis, and coinfection usually resolves, whereas superinfection frequently causes chronic HDV infection and chronic active hepatitis. Routes similar to those of HBV transmit the HDV. Outbreaks of hepatitis D have been reported in the United States. Thus, those who are susceptible to HBV infection, occupationally or otherwise, are also susceptible to HDV infection. Successful vaccination against hepatitis B also should prevent hepatitis D.

Hepatitides A and E

Hepatitis A does not pose a particular occupational risk to dental workers or patients, because this form of hepatitis is spread primarily by the fecal–oral route involving consumption of contaminated food or water (see Table 6-1). A vaccine is available for hepatitis A; vaccination is recommended for persons who may travel to countries with poor sanitation systems. Isolated instances of hepatitis A spread by contact with body fluids other than feces have been reported.

Hepatitis E is a liver disease that is usually self-limiting with no chronic state. Like the hepatitis A virus, the hepatitis E virus is spread by contaminated food or water, and only a handful of cases have been reported in the United States. In contrast, hepatitis E is a problem in Asia, Middle Eastern countries, Africa, and Central America, and is usually spread by fecal-contaminated drinking water.

HUMAN IMMUNODEFICIENCY VIRUS DISEASE

The human immunodeficiency virus (HIV) causes HIV disease, which involves HIV infection and progresses to a final phase called acquired immunodeficiency syndrome. In the summer of 1981, AIDS was reported as a new clinical disease, and the CDC now estimates that approximately 1.25 million persons in the United States have been infected with HIV. Worldwide, HIV is thought to have infected approximately 42 million persons. At the end of 2003, an estimated 1,039,000 to 1,185,000 persons in the United States were living with HIV/AIDS, with 24% to 27% undiagnosed and unaware of their HIV infection. In 2006, 35,314 new cases of HIV/AIDS in adults, adolescents, and children were diagnosed in the 33 states with long-term, confidential name–based HIV reporting. In 2010 the CDC estimated that 47,129 people were diagnosed with HIV infection in 46 states. Since the epidemic began, an estimated 1,129,127 people have been diagnosed with AIDS in the United States and 619,400 have died.

Human immunodeficiency virus disease involves destruction of the immune system of the body, making an individual susceptible to life-threatening opportunistic infections and cancers. Progression from the initial phase of the disease (HIV infection) to the terminal phase of the disease (AIDS) has been lengthened significantly through the combined use of antiviral drugs. Effective therapy in the United States has made HIV disease a manageable affliction. Life after infection now can be expected to approach 25 years.

Human Immunodeficiency Virus

HIV is a member of a group of single-stranded RNA viruses called retroviruses. HIV type 1 (HIV or HIV-1) is the most common worldwide cause of HIV disease. HIV type 2 causes another less aggressive immunodeficiency syndrome, especially in Western Africa. Infection with HIV-2 in the United States is uncommon, with most cases occurring in immigrants from Africa and among injection-drug abusers.

HIV primarily infects T4 lymphocytes but also can infect macrophages and a few other cell types. These special lymphocytes are the cells that regulate the immune response. HIV selectively attaches to and enters T4 lymphocytes (also called CD4 lymphocytes). The viral RNA is converted quickly into viral DNA, which then is incorporated as viral genes into the chromosomes of the host lymphocyte. Thus the lymphocyte and its succeeding generations of cells are infected permanently with the HIV-1 genes. These genes may remain latent (delayed) for prolonged periods, but they induce the production of new virus particles within the lymphocytes. This virus production occurs throughout HIV disease but at widely different rates in different patients.

Virus production destroys lymphocytes and yields more viruses that can infect and destroy even more lymphocytes. This process eventually depletes the body of T4 cells. Thus HIV produces a seemingly latent infection in which the infected person usually remains asymptomatic until the level of T4 lymphocytes becomes critically low.

HIV undergoes mutations that produce several different genetic forms as the virus replicates inside lymphocytes and other cells. This genetic variation may explain the difference in the course of HIV disease in different individuals, with some strains of HIV being more virulent than others. This genetic variation also is one reason why a vaccine for prevention has not yet been developed. A vaccine made against one HIV strain may not protect against other strains.

Although an approach to kill HIV after it is in the body is not known, HIV can be killed easily when outside the body. All forms of heat and gas sterilization readily kill it. The virus also is killed by commonly used liquid sterilants and surface disinfectants, provided the killing agent comes into direct contact with the virus. HIV is killed much more easily on instruments and surfaces than *M. tuberculosis* and bacterial spores.

Disease States and Symptoms

Human Immunodeficiency Virus Infection

Approximately 4 weeks after the initial infection with HIV, many persons experience a sore throat, fever, swollen glands, diarrhea, joint pain, and fatigue. This condition is called acute retroviral syndrome, which signifies an acute HIV infection. This process commonly occurs soon after many viral infections. Symptoms may be slight or even may go unnoticed. Antibodies to HIV usually develop within 6 to 12 weeks after initial infection, and, by 6 months, 95% of those infected have developed antibodies (seroconverted). Unfortunately, these antibodies do not protect against the disease; however, they do provide a means to diagnose HIV disease. A person with antibodies to HIV is referred to as being "HIV-positive," indicating that the person is infected with the virus.

After acute HIV infection has occurred, most persons have no further clinical symptoms until months or years later, when the killing of T4 lymphocytes or other cells becomes prominent. Nevertheless, persons with asymptomatic HIV infection still can transmit the virus to others. Some HIV-positive persons experience persistent swollen glands under the arms and in the groin but are otherwise asymptomatic. The condition is referred to as generalized lymphadenopathy.

Acquired Immunodeficiency Syndrome

Replication of HIV in T4 lymphocytes kills the lymphocytes, and, as an increasing number of cells are killed, the immune system becomes progressively weaker. This immunodeficiency results in increased susceptibility to opportunistic infections that normally do not cause infections or cause less-severe infections in those with healthy immune systems. When an HIV-positive patient experiences one or more of these indicator opportunistic infections or a cancer, the patient is diagnosed as having AIDS. The symptoms experienced depend on the type of infection or cancer that occurs. Eventually, one of these diseases causes death. The infectious diseases may be caused by bacterial, viral, fungal, or protozoal agents. The leading cause of death in an AIDS patient is *Pneumocystis jiroveci* pneumonia, a fungal infection.

Highly active antiretroviral therapy can suppress HIV replication in some for decades, allowing patients to enjoy longer and healthier lives and making them less infectious to others.

Oral Manifestations of Acquired Immunodeficiency Syndrome

In many instances, early manifestations of AIDS occur as oral lesions. Oral manifestations include fungal diseases such as candidiasis (thrush), histoplasmosis, geotrichosis, or cryptococcosis; viral diseases such as warts, hairy leukoplakia, or human herpesvirus type 1 (herpes simplex) infection; bacterial diseases such as rapidly progressing periodontitis or gingivitis; and cancerous diseases such as Kaposi sarcoma (recently associated with human herpesvirus type 8) and non-Hodgkin lymphoma.

Transmission

HIV is transmitted primarily from an infected person through the following routes:
- Intimate sexual contact (vaginal, anal, oral) involving contact or exchange of semen or vaginal secretions
- Exposure to blood, blood-contaminated body fluids, or blood products (e.g., sharing intravenous drug paraphernalia)
- Perinatal contact (from infected mother to child)

Other exposures resulting in HIV-infection are variations of these three basic modes of transmission. HIV infection is not spread by casual contact. Table 6-3 lists risk factors for acquiring AIDS. Note the overall increase in percent of heterosexual contacts involving an infected partner as a risk factor.

TABLE 6-3 Estimated AIDS Cases by Exposure Category in the United States: Through 1993, 2001, 2006, and 2009

Exposure Category	TOTAL AIDS CASES (%)			
	1993*	2001†	2006#	2009‡
ADULTS/ADOLESCENTS				
Men who have sex with men	56	46	48	48
Injection-drug abusers	23	25	25	25
Men who have sex with men who are injection-drug abusers	6	6	7	7
Heterosexual contact	7	11	18	18
Other‡	8	2	2	2
CHILDREN (<13 YEARS OLD)				
Mother with/at risk for HIV infection	87	91	93	91
Other‡	13	9	7	9

*Based on 289,320 cases of AIDS. Centers for Disease Control and Prevention: *HIV/AIDS Surveillance Report* 5:1-19, 1993.

†Based on 816,149 cases of AIDS. Centers for Disease Control and: Prevention: *HIV/AIDS Surveillance Report* 13(2):1-48, 2001.

#Based on 1,099,161 cases of AIDS. Centers for Disease Control and Prevention. *HIV/AIDS statistics and surveillance: basis statistics.* http://www.cdc.gov/hiv/topics/surveillance/basic.htm. Accessed April 2012.

‡Includes hemophilia/coagulation disorder, transfusion, and risk not reported or identified.

Sexual Contact

Nationwide, unprotected sex has resulted in the greatest number of AIDS cases. The risk of exposure to HIV is present when unprotected genital or anal intercourse is performed with individuals whose HIV status is not known, be it homosexual, bisexual, or heterosexual contact. Having multiple sex partners of unknown HIV status increases this risk even further. Clearly, HIV disease is a sexually transmitted disease, as are genital herpes, gonorrhea, syphilis, nongonococcal urethritis, genital warts, and several other conditions. The presence of a sexually transmitted disease, particularly herpes, syphilis, or chancroid, increases the chance of acquiring HIV infection 100 to 200 times if one is exposed.

As of 2009, 48% of AIDS cases involved men who had sex with men, whereas heterosexual contact accounted for 18% of cases. The latter is an increase of 7% since 2001 (see Table 6-3).

Exposure to Blood

Intravenous drug abuse is a high-risk behavior when users share injection needles, allowing the transfer of blood remaining in the used needles from one person to another. Twenty-five percent of cases involve injecting-drug use.

Men who have sex with men who inject drugs have been associated with 7% of AIDS cases in the United States (see Table 6-3).

Injection of infected blood directly into the bloodstream is an efficient route of transmission. Percutaneous (through the skin) injuries with contaminated needles or other sharp objects and contamination of skin or mucous membranes containing small cuts or abrasions or dermatitis are variations of this "shared needles" mode of transmission.

Administration of infected blood products (e.g., to those with bleeding disorders such as hemophilia) or transfusions with infected blood have caused approximately 3% of the total reported cases of AIDS. In 1985, tests were developed that detected HIV-infected blood, and since then these modes of transmission essentially have been eliminated.

HIV has been isolated from numerous body fluids, including blood, semen, vaginal and cervical secretions, cerebrospinal fluid, synovial fluid, amniotic fluid, pericardial fluid, saliva, tears, breast milk, and urine.

Although HIV has been isolated from saliva, so far this route in casual or household contacts has not resulted in any documented cases of transmission. Transmission also was shown not to occur in a 2.5-year follow-up study of 198 health care workers, 30 of whom were bitten or scratched by an HIV-infected patient. The low risk for transmission through saliva may be attributable to the low concentration of the virus in the saliva of infected persons. A proteinaceous factor in human saliva also has been shown to interfere with the HIV infection process. Nevertheless, "saliva in dentistry" still is considered potentially infectious because of the intimate contact with the patient's mouth during dental care and because most dental procedures result in varying degrees of bleeding into the mouth. Some natural bleeding also may occur in the mouths of dental patients who have gingivitis or other oral soft-tissue lesions. Thus "saliva in dentistry" commonly contains blood.

Mother to Child

Many infants who have HIV-positive mothers are infected before birth by passage of the virus across the placenta, at the time of birth by contact with mother's blood during delivery, or, less commonly, through breast milk. Effective drug therapy during pregnancy can reduce the chances of mother-to-child transmission by close to 90%. Approximately 0.9% of all reported AIDS cases in the United States have occurred in children younger than age 13 years (pediatric AIDS cases), and 93% of these occurred by spread from infected mothers, with the remainder involving hemophilia, transfusion, or unidentified risks (see Table 6-3).

Risk for the Dental Team

The risk of HIV disease transmission from dental patients to members of the dental team is low; nevertheless, some small potential exists for this to occur. Through 2010, the CDC received reports of 57 health care workers in the United

TABLE 6-4   Occupational Risk of HIV Infection for Health Care Workers 1981-2010*

Occupation	NUMBER OF OCCUPATIONALLY ACQUIRED HIV INFECTIONS	
	Documented	Possible
Nurse	24 (42%)	36 (25%)
Laboratory worker, clinical	16 (28%)	17 (12%)
Physician, nonsurgical	6 (11%)	13(9%)
Laboratory worker, nonclinical	3 (5%)	0
Housekeeper/maintenance worker	2 (4%)	14 (10%)
Technician, surgical	2 (4%)	2 (1%)
Embalmer/morgue technician	1 (2%)	2 (1%)
Health aide/attendant	1 (2%)	15 (11%)
Respiratory therapist	1 (2%)	2 (1%)
Technician, dialysis	1 (2%)	3 (2%)
Dental workers[†]	0	6 (4%)
Emergency medical technician/paramedic	0	12 (9%)
Physician, surgical	0	6 (4%)
Technician/therapist, other	0	9 (7%)
Other health care occupations	0	6 (3%)
Total	57	143

*CDC. *Surveillance of occupationally acquired HIV/AIDS in healthcare personnel, as of December 2010.* http://www.cdc.gov/HAI/organisms/hiv/Surveillance-Occupationally-Acquired-HIV-AIDS.html. Accessed April 2012.
[†]Three dentists, one oral surgeon, and two dental assistants.

States with documented, occupationally acquired HIV infections (Table 6-4). The routes of exposure resulting in these cases were:

- 48 percutaneous (puncture/cut injury)
- 5 mucocutaneous (mucous membrane or skin)
- 2 both percutaneous and mucocutaneous
- 2 unknown route

Forty-nine of the 57 healthcare personnel were exposed to HIV-infected blood; one to visibly bloody fluid; three to concentrated virus in the laboratory; and four to an unspecified fluid. In addition to these 57 cases, 143 cases with possible occupationally acquired HIV infections have been reported (see Table 6-4). Since 2003, no new documented cases and five new cases of possible occupational transmission have been reported. No documented cases of occupationally related HIV transmission have occurred among dental personnel. However, six possible cases have been noted (three dentists, one oral surgeon, two dental assistants).

A "documented" case involves seroconversion (HIV-negative at the time of exposure, later becoming

HIV-positive) following a percutaneous or mucocutaneous (mucous membrane and skin) occupational exposure to blood, body fluids, or tissues. A "possible" case involves persons with no determined behavioral or transfusion risks who reported past percutaneous or mucocutaneous occupational exposure to blood, other body fluids, or tissues but did not have a documented seroconversion. This means that they became HIV-positive; but, because they did not get tested at the time of exposure, it is possible that they were already positive at that time.

Risk of transmission increases when hollow bore needles are involved, especially if the needles are obviously soiled with blood, have been inserted into an artery or vein, or have caused a deep tissue injury. Another important factor is whether the source patient dies within 2 months of the exposure. Generally, the greatest concentration of HIV in blood (viral load) occurs soon after infection (acute retroviral syndrome) and during the AIDS stage of HIV disease.

Risk for Dental Patients

The risk for a dental patient of acquiring HIV disease in the office from a member of the dental team must be low. Although the bloodborne HBV has been spread in rare instances from dentist to patient, spread of HIV is suggested in only one instance in dentistry. Apparently, a dentist with HIV infected six of his patients being treated in his Florida dental office during the years 1987 to 1990. The investigation of this case involved a comparison of the HIV from the dentist with the viruses isolated from the infected patients, and this demonstrated significant similarity in the viruses. Unfortunately, the investigation did not discover the mode of virus spread from the dentist to the six patients, but the final conclusion by the investigators from the CDC and the Florida Department of Health suggested that direct spread from the dentist to the patients was most likely, rather than spread from contaminated instruments, equipment, or surfaces.

Until recently, this Florida dentist case was the only known instance in all of dentistry and medicine of possible spread of HIV disease from a health care worker to patients. The case still remains the only known instance in dentistry, but in February 1997 the French government reported that a woman patient contracted HIV disease from a physician in France in 1992. All of the details are not available, but evidence released so far supporting this transmission (comparing the viruses from the patient and the physician) is compelling. The available information suggests that the physician (an orthopedic surgeon) may have contracted the disease from a patient in 1983 but was not tested for HIV status until 1994. The physician performed an orthopedic procedure of some 10 hours in length on the woman patient in 1993; this is the time when the transmission is assumed to have occurred. To date, 968 of this physician's surgery patients have been tested and only the one woman has been found to be HIV-positive. Further attempts have been made to identify and define the low risk of spread from health care workers to patients by performing HIV testing on patients who have been cared for by other HIV-positive health care workers. Of about 28,000 medical and dental patients tested so far, none has shown to have acquired HIV diseases from any of the 63 infected dentists or physicians involved. Nevertheless, maintenance of proper infection control during care for all patients is important.

Prevention

Sexual Contact

Recommendations for preventing the spread of HIV through sexual contact include abstinence or limiting sexual activities to one partner who is not infected and who does not have any other sex partners. A lesser level of protection is offered by safer sex practices such as the use of condoms to eliminate or minimize contact of each partner with body fluids that may contain HIV.

Blood Contact

Injection-drug abusers must not use blood-contaminated needles. Continued screening for HIV-infectivity of blood for transfusion and of blood products began in June 1985 and must continue. All members of the dental team and other health care workers must protect themselves from exposure to blood, saliva in dentistry, and other potentially infectious body fluids. Contaminated sharps must be handled and disposed of properly. Gloves, mask, and protective eyewear and clothing must be used during the care of all patients and in other instances to prevent direct or indirect contact with body fluids. All health care workers also must prevent their blood or body fluids from coming into contact with the patients being treated, and instruments and equipment used on more than one patient must be decontaminated properly before reuse. The infection control procedures involved in these approaches to disease prevention are described in Chapter 8 and in Chapters 10 to 18.

Perinatal

Monotherapy or combined drug treatment has been shown to reduce perinatal transmission of HIV significantly. Side effects of treatment commonly develop in the mothers. The overall safety of the combination therapy still is being investigated. The rate of congenital abnormalities appears to be similar between groups of infected women who did and did not receive drug therapy while pregnant.

SELECTED READINGS

Centers for Disease Control and Prevention: *A comprehensive immunization strategy to eliminate transmission of hepatitis B virus infection in the United States,* http://www.cdc.gov/mmwr/preview/mmwrhtml/rr5516a1.htm?s_cid=rr5516a1_e. Accessed April 2012.

Centers for Disease Control and Prevention: *Surveillance of occupationally acquired HIV/AIDS in healthcare personnel, as of December 2010* http://www.cdc.gov/HAI/-organisms/hiv/Surveillance-Occupationally-Acquired-HIV-AIDS.html. Accessed April 2012.

Centers for Disease Control and Prevention: National Institute for Occupational Safety and Health: Alert: preventing needlestick injuries in health care settings, Cincinnati, 1999, US Department of Health and Human Services, Public Health Services. CDC, DHHS (NIOSH) Pub No 2000–198.

Centers for Disease Control and Prevention: Recommendations for prevention and control of hepatitis C virus (HCV) infection and HCV-related chronic disease, *MMWR Recomm Rep* 47(RR-19):1–38, 1998.

Centers for Disease Control and Prevention: Recommended infection control practices for dentistry, 2003, *MMWR Recomm Rep* 52(RR-17):1–66, 2003.

Centers for Disease Control and Prevention: Revised recommendations for HIV testing of adults, adolescents, and pregnant women in healthcare settings, *MMWR Recomm Rep* 55(RR-14):1–24, 2006.

Centers for Disease Control and Prevention: Updated US Public Health Service guidelines for the management of occupational exposures to HBV, HCV and HIV and recommendations for postexposure prophylaxis, *MMWR Recomm Rep* 50(RR-11):1–43, 2001.

Centers for Disease Control and Prevention: Viral Hepatitis. http://www.cdc.gov/ncidod/diseases/hepatitis. Accessed April 2012.

Cottone JA, Puttaiah R: Hepatitis B virus infection: current status in dentistry, *Dent Clin North Am* 40:293–307, 1996.

Glick M: The role of the dentist in the era of AIDS,, *Dent Clin North Am* 40:343–357, 1996.

Palenik CJ: Protection from infectious diseases–hepatitis, *Dent Asep Rev* 32(2):1–2, 2011.

Redd JT, Baumbach J, Kohn W, et al: Patient-to-patient transmission of hepatitis B virus associated with oral surgery, *J Infect Dis* 195:1311–1314, 2007.

Wasley A, Grytdal S, Gallagher K: Centers for Disease Control and Prevention: Surveillance for acute viral hepatitis—United States 2006, *MMWR Surveill Summ* 57(SS-2):1–28, 2008.

REVIEW QUESTIONS

Multiple Choice

1. Which is a correct statement about hepatitis B?
   a. Only about one third of those infected have recognizable symptoms.
   b. Most dental assistants who have been working for more than 5 years get hepatitis B.
   c. Most persons who get hepatitis B die.
   d. Hepatitis B is usually spread through drinking contaminated water.

2. How does HIV cause AIDS?
   a. It destroys the liver.
   b. It destroys the body's defenses against diseases.
   c. It destroys the ability to control muscle action.
   d. It paralyzes the body.

3. The vaccine for hepatitis B protects against:
   a. hepatitides A, B, C, and D
   b. hepatitis B and may prevent type D
   c. hepatitides B, C, and D
   d. hepatitis D

4. The risk of getting AIDS as a dental assistant is:
   a. very high
   b. high
   c. moderate
   d. very low

5. About how many persons in the world have been infected with HIV?
   a. 4000
   b. 400,000
   c. 4 million
   d. 42 million
   e. 400 million

6. All of the following types of viral hepatitis are bloodborne except hepatitis
   a. A
   b. B
   c. C
   d. D

7. Occupationally acquired hepatitis B in health care workers is most commonly contracted:
   a. by ingesting contaminated water
   b. through sharps injuries
   c. through inhalation of respiratory aerosols

8. The best way for one to avoid contracting a bloodborne disease in the office is:
   a. not to shake hands with the patients
   b. to wear a mask all day long even between patients
   c. to handle sharps carefully

9. A hepatitis B carrier is:
   a. HBsAg-positive
   b. anti–HBsAg-positive
   c. HIV-positive

10. Which of the following is not a mode of spread of HIV disease?
    a. Percutaneous
    b. Inhalation
    c. Sexual activities
    d. From infected mother to child at birth

11. Most persons who develop HIV disease become HIV-positive within _____ after exposure.
    a. 1 to 2 weeks
    b. 6 to 12 weeks
    c. 5 to 6 years
    d. 9 to 10 years

12. About what percent of persons infected with hepatitis C virus become chronic carriers of the disease?
    a. 5
    b. 25
    c. 55
    d. 80
    e. 99

Please visit http://evolve.elsevier.com/Miller/infectioncontrol/ for additional practice and study support tools.

Oral and Respiratory Diseases

OUTLINE

Oral Diseases
Human Herpesviruses Types 1 and 2
Oral Candidiasis
Oral Syphilis and Gonorrhea
Herpangina and Hand-Foot-and-Mouth Disease
Systemic Diseases with Oral Lesions
Secondary Syphilis
Chickenpox
Infectious Mononucleosis
Respiratory Diseases
Streptococcal Pharyngitis
Tuberculosis

Streptococcus Pneumoniae
Human Herpesvirus Type 5
Human Herpesviruses Types 6, 7, and 8
Influenza
Other Respiratory Diseases
Waterborne Disease Agents
Legionnaires Disease
Pseudomonas **Infection**
Methicillin-Resistant *Staphylococcus Aureus*

LEARNING OBJECTIVES

After completing this chapter, the student should be able to do the following:
1. List infectious diseases that occur in the mouth.
2. List systemic diseases that may produce oral lesions.
3. List respiratory infectious diseases that may be spread in the dental office, including the known

herpesviruses spread by respiratory droplets and the diseases they cause.
4. List waterborne disease agents that may be spread through contaminated dental unit water.
5. Discuss how to prevent the spread of methicillin-resistant Staphylococcus aureus (MRSA) in the dental office.

KEY TERMS

Chickenpox
Denture Stomatitis
Hand-Foot-and-Mouth Disease
Herpangina
Herpes Labialis
Herpetic Whitlow

Human Herpesviruses
Infectious Mononucleosis
Influenza
Legionnaires Disease
Opportunistic Pathogen
Oral Candidiasis

Purified Protein Derivative
Shingles
Streptococcal Pharyngitis
Thrush
Tuberculosis

ORAL DISEASES

Chapter 5 discussed the plaque-associated diseases of caries and periodontal diseases. This chapter presents information on other oral diseases and respiratory diseases that may be spread in a dental office (Table 7-1). A key aspect of the potential for spread of respiratory diseases in the dental office is that dental patients (and many other persons) are asymptomatic carriers of a variety of pathogens present in their oral or respiratory fluids (Table 7-2).

Human Herpesviruses Types 1 and 2

Human herpesviruses cause several diseases (Table 7-3). Human herpesvirus type 1 (herpes simplex virus 1) may cause infections of the mouth, skin, eyes, and genitals, and those who have depressed immune systems (who are immunocompromised) may have a widespread (systemic) infection.

Approximately 90% of adults have been infected with human herpesvirus 1. Only 10% of infected persons (usually children) experience the typical symptoms of oral herpes

---

TABLE 7-1   Important Infectious Diseases and Pathogens Associated with the Mouth

Disease	Pathogen
ORAL DISEASES	
Bacterial	
Gonococcal pharyngitis	*Neisseria gonorrhoeae*
Streptococcal pharyngitis and scarlet fever	*Streptococcus pyogenes*
Syphilis	*Treponema pallidum*
Viral	
Primary herpetic gingivostomatitis	Human herpesvirus 1 or 2
Recurrent herpes (e.g., herpes labialis)	Human herpesvirus 1 or 2
Hand-foot-and-mouth disease	Coxsackievirus
Herpangina	Coxsackievirus
Hairy leukoplakia	Human herpesvirus type 4
Fungal	
Candidiasis (thrush)	*Candida albicans*
Denture stomatitis	*Candida albicans*
SYSTEMIC DISEASES WITH ORAL LESIONS	
Bacterial	
Secondary syphilis	*Treponema pallidum*
Viral	
Chickenpox	Human herpesvirus type 3 (varicella-zoster virus)
Infectious mononucleosis	Human herpesvirus type 4 (Epstein-Barr virus)
OTHER DISEASES SPREAD BY RESPIRATORY/ORAL FLUIDS	
Bacterial	
Tuberculosis	*Mycobacterium tuberculosis*
Diphtheria	*Corynebacterium diphtheriae*
Pneumonia	*Streptococcus pneumoniae, Staphylococcus aureus, Mycoplasma pneumoniae, Chlamydia pneumoniae, Moraxella catarrhalis, Haemophilus influenzae*
Meningitis, sinusitis, conjunctivitis	*Haemophilus influenzae* type b
Meningitis	*Neisseria meningitidis*
Bronchitis	*Haemophilus influenzae, Moraxella catarrhalis*

continued

TABLE 7-1 **Important Infectious Diseases and Pathogens Associated with the Mouth—cont'd**

Disease	Pathogen
Viral	
Common cold	Rhinoviruses and several others
Influenza	Influenza viruses
Bronchitis	Influenza A, parainfluenza virus, coronavirus
Pneumonia	Influenza virus, adenovirus, respiratory syncytial virus
CMV disease	Cytomegalovirus
Infectious mononucleosis	Human herpesvirus type 4 (Epstein-Barr virus)
Erythema infectiosum (fifth disease)	Human parvovirus B19
Measles	Rubeola (measles) virus
Rubella	Rubella virus
Mumps	Mumps virus

TABLE 7-2 **Estimated Asymptomatic Rates for Some Pathogens Present in Oral or Respiratory Fluids**

Microorganisms	Disease	Carrier Rate
Streptococcus pneumoniae	Pneumonia, middle ear infection, meningitis, sinusitis	Preschoolers (33%) Adults (5%-70%)
Streptococcus pyogenes	"Strep throat," scarlet fever, skin infections	Children (0%-20%) Adults (0%-5%)
Staphylococcus aureus	Skin infections, secondary pneumonia	Adults (20%-40%)
Haemophilus influenzae type b	Meningitis, middle ear infection, sinusitis, conjunctivitis	Population (3%-5%)
Neisseria meningitidis	Meningitis	Adults (3%-30%)
Corynebacterium diphtheriae	Diphtheria	Population (0%-5%)
Human herpesvirus type 4	Infectious mononucleosis	Adults (10%-20%)
Human herpesvirus type 1	Oral, ocular herpes	Adults (0.5%-15%)
Candida albicans	Thrush, denture stomatitis	Adults (33%)

TABLE 7-3 **Human Herpesviruses (HHV)**

Type	Other Name	Disease
HHV 1	Herpes simplex type 1 (HSV-1)	Oral, ocular, and some genital herpes
HHV 2	Herpes simplex type 2 (HSV-2)	Genital herpes, some oral herpes
HHV 3	Varicella-zoster virus (VZV)	Chickenpox, shingles
HHV 4	Epstein-Barr virus (EBV)	Infectious mononucleosis, hairy leukoplakia of tongue
HHV 5	Cytomegalovirus (CMV)	CMV disease, retinitis
HHV 6	None	Roseola
HHV 7	None	Not yet known
HHV 8	None	Kaposi sarcoma

(primary herpetic gingivostomatitis). In this disease, vesicle-type lesions occur in the mouth. Most (if not all) herpesviruses cause recurrent diseases (periodic recurrence of the disease). An example is herpes labialis, sometimes called fever blisters, with lesions periodically appearing on the lips (Figure 7-1). During active human herpesvirus 1 infections, vesicles at any site of the body contain the virus, which may be spread to others by direct contact with these lesions. The human herpesvirus 1 also may be present in saliva in those with oral or lip lesions and in a small percentage of those who are infected but have no active lesions (see Table 7-2). In such instances, direct contact with lesions may cause infection of the skin, or sprays or aerosols of the saliva may result in spread of the virus to unprotected eyes of the dental team. Entrance of the virus through breaks in the skin on unprotected hands and fingers can lead to vesicle development at these sites called herpetic whitlow. Chapters 10 and 11 describe a vivid example of how the human herpesvirus 1 may be spread from a lip lesion of one patient to the mouths of other dental patients via the ungloved hands of a dental hygienist. Human herpesvirus 1 causes approximately 10% of genital herpes cases.

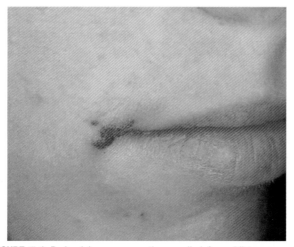

FIGURE 7-1 Perioral herpes, sometimes called fever blisters or cold sores. (From Ibsen OAC, Phelan JA: *Oral pathology for dental hygienists*, 5th ed, St. Louis, 2009, Saunders.)

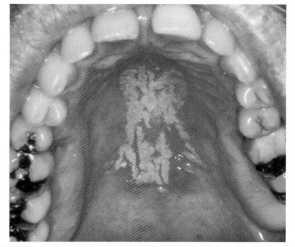

FIGURE 7-2 Oral candidiasis. (From Ibsen OAC, Phelan JA: *Oral pathology for dental hygienists*, 5th ed, St. Louis, 2009, Saunders.)

Human herpesvirus type 2 (herpes simplex virus 2) causes approximately 90% of genital herpes infections but occasionally causes oral infections. Although most infections are asymptomatic, human herpesvirus 2 can cause vesicle-type lesions in the mouth, or on the skin in the male and female genital and anal areas, or internally in the female. As with other herpesvirus infections, these vesicles may recur periodically. The vesicles contain the virus and are contagious on contact, but the virus also can be spread in the absence of symptoms. Genital herpes is one of the most common sexually transmitted diseases.

Treatment of herpesvirus infections with acyclovir usually reduces the severity and duration of the disease but does not prevent the recurrence of the disease. Acyclovir is structurally similar to guanosine triphosphate, which is a building block for DNA. When acyclovir is incorporated into the viral DNA being synthesized inside of body cells infected with the virus, that DNA becomes nonfunctional, and the virus does not survive.

Oral Candidiasis

Candida albicans is yeast that occurs in the mouth asymptomatically in approximately one third of adults. The yeast is an **opportunistic pathogen** usually causing a harmful infection only under special circumstances that give it an advantage to multiply to harmful levels. Such harmful infections are referred to as **oral candidiasis** (Figure 7-2) and appear as whitish lesions (called **thrush**) or reddish areas (**denture stomatitis**). Circumstances that may result in oral disease might include the following:

- Conditions that disturb body defense mechanisms such as the systemic diseases of human immunodeficiency virus (HIV) infection and leukemia
- Long-term broad-spectrum antibacterial therapy that gives the unaffected yeast a better chance to grow

- Trauma to the mouth from poorly fitting dentures causing *C. albicans* to produce denture stomatitis
- Poor resistance in the mouth of newborns orally contaminated with the yeast during passage through the mother's infected birth canal

Yeast infections with *C. albicans* may occur at other sites of the body, including the skin and the vagina. Infections in the vagina are the cause of "yeast infections" in females.

Spread of *C. albicans* from a patient's mouth to the dental team is theoretically possible through direct contact with lesions or sprays or aerosols of infected saliva. However, unless the contaminated member of the dental team has lowered body defenses, the contamination likely will not lead to a harmful infection.

Oral candidiasis can be treated with one of several antifungal agents, which include nystatin, ketoconazole, and clotrimazole.

Oral Syphilis and Gonorrhea

Other important oral disease-causing agents that may have some potential for spread to the dental team are *Treponema pallidum* and *Neisseria gonorrhoeae*.

T. pallidum is a spirochete bacterium and is the causative agent of syphilis. Approximately 5% to 10% of the cases of syphilis first occur in the mouth in the form of a lesion called a primary chancre, an open ulcer frequently on the tongue or lip (Figure 7-3). These lesions contain the live spirochetes, which may be spread by direct contact. The possibility of the spirochete entering small cuts or breaks in the skin of unprotected hands of the dental team exists and has been documented, in one instance causing syphilis of the finger.

N. gonorrhoeae causes another sexually transmitted disease, gonorrhea, which is an infection through the mucous membranes inside the penis or vagina. This gram-negative bacterium may be spread to the mouth during certain sex practices with an infected person, and the bacterium might

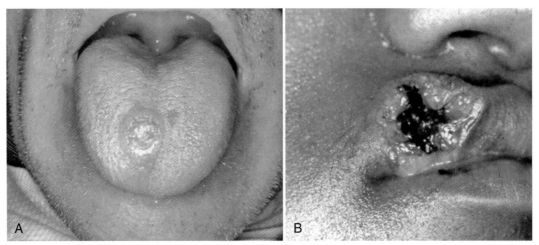

FIGURE 7-3 Oral/peri-oral syphilis. A, Tongue lesion. B, Lip lesion. (From Ibsen OAC, Phelan JA: *Oral pathology for dental hygienists*, 5th ed, St. Louis, 2009, Saunders.)

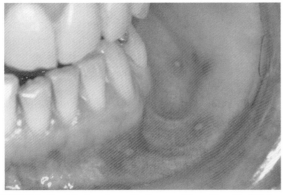

FIGURE 7-4 Hand-foot-and-mouth disease. (From Newville BW, Damm DD, Allen C, Bouquot JE: *Oral and maxillofacial pathology*, 3rd ed, St. Louis, 2009, Mosby.)

cause an inflammation of the throat area. Although spread of *N. gonorrhoeae* from a patient with oral gonorrhea to a member of the dental team has never been documented, some potential may exist for this to occur during generation of dental aerosols. *N. gonorrhoeae* can cause eye infections.

Herpangina and Hand-Foot-and-Mouth Disease

Herpangina appears as vesicles on the soft palate or elsewhere in the posterior part of the mouth that break down to ulcers that last for about a week. Seldom do the vesicles appear on the gingiva, buccal mucosa, or tongue, which differentiates this disease from intraoral herpes infections. Fever, sore throat, and headache frequently accompany the vesicular stage. The lesions are caused by specific types of coxsackievirus (usually group A types 1 to 6, 8, 10, and 22). Coxsackievirus (usually type A16) also may cause a vesicular type of disease, with vesicles occurring in the mouth, on the hands, and on the feet (hand-foot-and-mouth disease) (Figure 7-4). In this instance, the oral vesicles occur primarily on the cheek mucosa and tongue, but sometimes on the hard palate and anywhere else in the mouth. Usually children and young adults are affected; no specific treatment is available that attacks the virus.

SYSTEMIC DISEASES WITH ORAL LESIONS

Secondary Syphilis

In untreated syphilis, a secondary phase of the disease may appear 2 to 10 weeks after the initial lesion occurs and has subsided. This secondary phase results from spread of the *T. pallidum* bacteria from the initial lesion through the blood and may involve the appearance of mucous patches on mucous membranes in the mouth. The lesions contain the live spirochetes and may be spread to others by direct contact. Syphilis usually responds to penicillin therapy.

Chickenpox

Human herpesvirus type 3 (varicella-zoster virus) causes chickenpox (Figure 7-5) as the primary disease (usually in the young) and shingles (Figure 7-6) as the recurrent disease (usually in those older than age 50 years). Although chickenpox commonly produces skin lesions, this disease is classified as a respiratory disease. Human herpesvirus 3 enters the body by droplet infection, invades the respiratory tract, and is spread through the bloodstream to the skin and other organs. After approximately 2 weeks, vesicles frequently occur in the mouth in addition to those typically present on the skin. The virus is spread through saliva and nasal secretions in addition to contact with skin lesions.

The disease is highly contagious through droplet infection and is usually mild in children but can be more severe in teenagers and adults. Occasionally an adult who escaped the primary infection as a child develops chickenpox, which is usually more severe and has a higher mortality rate because of an increased incidence of encephalitis. A vaccine for chickenpox was cleared by the U.S. Food and Drug Administration in 1996 and is described further in Chapter 9.

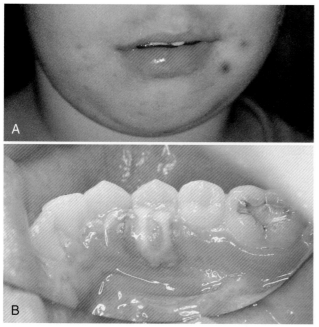

FIGURE 7-5 Chickenpox. A, Skin lesions. B, Gingival lesions. (From Ibsen OAC, Phelan JA: *Oral pathology for dental hygienists*, 5th ed, St. Louis, 2009, Saunders.)

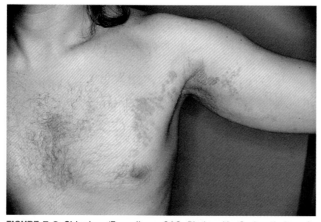

FIGURE 7-6 Shingles. (From Ibsen OAC, Phelan JA: *Oral pathology for dental hygienists*, 5th ed, St. Louis, 2009, Saunders.)

Infectious Mononucleosis

Human herpesvirus type 4 (Epstein-Barr virus) usually causes no or mild symptoms after infecting a child but may cause infectious mononucleosis (also known as the kissing disease) in adolescents and young adults. As might be suspected, this virus is spread from person to person through contact with saliva but also occasionally through blood transfusions. Symptoms of infectious mononucleosis commonly include fever, malaise, anorexia, fatigue, sore throat, oral ulcers, and enlarged cervical lymph nodes (those under the jaw). Other oral manifestations may include palatal petechiae (small red areas, Figure 7-7), widespread erythema (reddening) of the oral mucosa, and swelling of the uvula. This virus also is associated with hairy leukoplakia (whitish

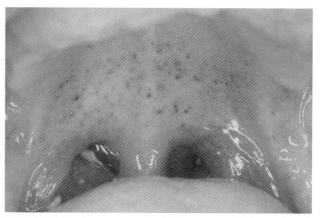

FIGURE 7-7 Infectious mononucleosis. Numerous petechiae on the soft palate. (From Newville BW, Damm DD, Allen C, Bouquot JE: *Oral and maxillofacial pathology*, 3rd ed, St. Louis, 2009, Mosby.)

lesions on the tongue) and with malignancies such as Burkitt lymphoma, B-cell lymphoma in the immunocompromised, and nasopharyngeal carcinoma.

RESPIRATORY DISEASES

Streptococcal Pharyngitis

Streptococcus pyogenes (sometimes called β-hemolytic group A *Streptococcus*) causes streptococcal pharyngitis ("strep throat") and scarlet fever. Scarlet fever is "strep throat" with a skin rash. *S. pyogenes* is spread by droplet infection from mouth to mouth, and a few persons who become infected experience poststreptococcal complications resulting in rheumatic fever or kidney damage. Each subsequent infection with *S. pyogenes* or with some other streptococci can result in progressively more damage to the heart (rheumatic heart disease) or the kidney. This is why patients with a history of poststreptococcal diseases are protected from possible reactivation by receiving antibiotics before dental or medical care.

Certain protease-producing strains of *S. pyogenes* (sometimes referred to as "flesh-eating" bacteria) can cause a condition called necrotizing fasciitis, which produces rapidly spreading damage to muscle tissue. Fortunately, only approximately 1000 cases of this disease occur each year.

Children and adults carry *S. pyogenes* in their nose and throat area without having any symptoms and can spread the organism to others in respiratory droplets (see Table 7-2). Most harmful streptococcal infections respond well to penicillin therapy.

Tuberculosis

Occurrence

Tuberculosis is a lung infection caused by the bacterium *Mycobacterium tuberculosis*. Although tuberculosis is not a particular problem among dental professionals, it is a major health problem worldwide. Approximately 10 million new cases of tuberculosis and 3 million associated deaths occur annually worldwide. In the United States, tuberculosis is increasing among racial/ethnic groups (non-Hispanic blacks, Hispanics, Asian/Pacific Islanders, Native Americans/Alaskan natives), but the overall number of cases has reached a plateau since 2009. In 1990, almost 70% of all reported cases of tuberculosis in the United States occurred among these minorities. Between 1953 and 1984, the number of reported cases of tuberculosis in the United States steadily declined. This number began to increase through 1995, when it began to level off. In 1996, the Centers for Disease Control and Prevention (CDC) indicated that approximately 22,000 active tuberculosis cases were reported in the United States. In 2006, 13,779 tuberculosis cases were reported to CDC from the 50 states and the District of Columbia, representing a 2.1% decrease from 2005.

Adverse social conditions and economic factors, the epidemic of acquired immunodeficiency syndrome (AIDS), and immigration of persons with tuberculosis are contributing factors to the occurrence of tuberculosis in the United States. Tuberculosis is a major problem among the homeless, persons infected with HIV, and drug abusers. Tuberculosis in those with HIV disease is commonly a reactivation of an earlier asymptomatic infection, as described subsequently.

Tuberculosis in the Dental Office

The risk for the dental team of acquiring tuberculosis is low because prolonged exposure to an infectious environment usually is required for infection to occur, and brief contact appears to be of little risk. Spread from one person to another relates to closeness of contact and the duration of exposure to infectious droplets. Thus the key factor in spread is the concentration of infectious particles in the inhaled air. Respiratory aerosols remain airborne for several hours, but the concentration of the infectious particles decreases with time from dilution with "clean" air and eventual settling. Nevertheless, tuberculosis is acquired by breathing in respiratory droplets from an infectious person with active pulmonary tuberculosis, and the dental team must be concerned by such transmission.

The dental office should have a protocol for identifying patients who possibly have active pulmonary tuberculosis. These patients should be referred immediately for medical evaluation and have their dental care deferred until the tuberculosis is inactive or has been treated and is no longer infectious. Dental personnel should not treat patients with active tuberculosis unless they institute special isolation precautions that are usually only available in hospital clinics. The approach to the management of possible active tuberculosis patients is that described by the CDC. The CDC has published guidelines for the prevention of tuberculosis in dental health care facilities (see Appendix C).

Box 7-1 shows the risk factors for tuberculosis and the symptoms of active tuberculosis and also describes questions on a medical history that may help identify dental patients who possibly have active tuberculosis.

BOX 7-1

Risk Factors, Symptoms, and Medical History Questions Related to Tuberculosis

Risk Factors
- Close/prolonged contact with known active tuberculosis case
- Residency in prisons, mental institutions, nursing homes, certain health care facilities
- HIV disease
- Alcoholism
- Intravenous drug abuse
- Homelessness
- Old age

Symptoms
- Malaise
- Productive cough for more than 3 weeks
- Blood in sputum
- Headache
- Fever, night sweats
- Weight loss

Medical History Questions
- Previous diagnosis of tuberculosis?
- Previous treatment for tuberculosis?
- Positive tuberculosis skin test?
- Productive cough for more than 3 weeks?
- Blood in the sputum?
- Headache, fever, chills, night sweats?
- Recent weight loss, anorexia, fatigue?
- HIV disease?
- Other systemic diseases?
- Immunosuppressive therapy?
- Alcoholism?
- Intravenous drug use?
- Relatives or close friends with active tuberculosis?
- Visited anyone in hospital with active tuberculosis?

Disease Process

If enough inhaled *M. tuberculosis* bacteria reach the lung alveoli and begin to multiply, one is said to be infected. In most persons, the inflammatory and immune responses control the infection, with the only evidence of infection being a positive tuberculin skin test (see the following discussion). Cells of *M. tuberculosis* initially resist destruction after being engulfed by macrophages during the inflammatory response. However, after immunity develops (cell-mediated immune response; see Chapter 3), the macrophages are activated to be able to kill the engulfed bacteria and the infection does not progress to active disease. However, most infected persons (even if the cell-mediated immune response initially controls the infection) cannot completely rid the body of the tuberculosis bacteria unless they take antituberculosis drugs. For this reason, those with positive tuberculosis skin tests, even if they have never had any tuberculosis symptoms, usually are placed on a course of antituberculosis drug therapy. Patients not placed on antituberculosis drug therapy retain the bacteria in their bodies and may later progress to active disease (latent tuberculosis infection or reactivation tuberculosis).

Approximately 10% of persons infected with *M. tuberculosis* progress from infection to active disease with symptoms. About half of these progress to active disease soon after the primary infection, and about half progress later in their lives. Symptomatic pulmonary tuberculosis begins with the development of an exudative condition in the lung, like pneumonia. Continued disease results in a granulomatous reaction (consolidation of tissue around the lung infection site), referred to as tubercle formation. As the disease progresses, these tubercles enlarge, may become necrotic (caseation necrosis), and break down, producing cavities (open spaces) in the lung tissue. In persons who are infected but are asymptomatic, and in those with symptomatic tuberculosis, healing may occur with or without the formation of calcified lung lesions or nodules, or development of fibrous tissue with calcium deposits.

Because *M. tuberculosis* can survive inside of macrophages early in the infection, this bacterium can be disseminated throughout the body (wherever the macrophages go). If active disease occurs, complications may develop that can involve infections in essentially any organ of the body.

Multiple Drug-Resistant Mycobacterium Tuberculosis

Another disturbing fact about tuberculosis is that strains of *M. tuberculosis* that are resistant to the drugs normally used to treat this disease recently have emerged. These strains are causing outbreaks of multiple drug-resistant tuberculosis. The CDC reported that approximately 15% of all tuberculosis cases tested involved strains resistant to at least one antituberculosis drug (e.g., isoniazid, rifampin, and ethambutol) and 4% were resistant to both of the two most effective antituberculosis drugs. Most of the patients involved in outbreaks of multiple drug-resistant tuberculosis have been AIDS patients; others include hospital patients and institutionalized inmates. Transmission of multiple drug-resistant tuberculosis to hospital workers and prison guards is documented. The key approach to managing these infections is to diagnose the infection and analyze the causative strain of *M. tuberculosis* as soon as possible so that the proper antituberculosis drugs can be administered at the earliest possible moment.

Tuberculin Skin Test

The Mantoux test, or purified protein derivative (PPD) test, is used to screen for tuberculosis infection. PPD is prepared from cultures of *M. tuberculosis* and is used in the skin testing. The testing involves injecting a small amount of the

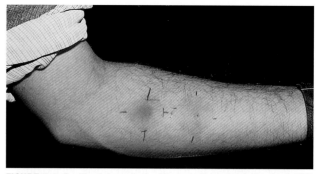

FIGURE 7-8 Positive tuberculosis skin test. (From Zitelli BJ, Davis HW: *Atlas of pediatric physical diagnosis*, 5th ed, Philadelphia, 2008, Mosby.)

PPD just under the skin (intradermally) on the underside of the forearm. The injection site is observed 48 to 72 hours later for any reaction to the PPD, although a positive reaction in some may be delayed for a week. A positive reaction is the occurrence of induration (a hardening, small nodule) at the injection site, and the degree of the positive reaction is determined by measuring the diameter of the indurated site (Figure 7-8). Box 7-2 gives the CDC guidelines for interpreting the tuberculin skin test results.

Vaccination

A vaccine for prevention of tuberculosis has not been cleared for use in the United States. However, the bacille Calmette-Guérin vaccine is used widely throughout the rest of the world. This vaccine consists of a live attenuated (weakened) bovine strain that probably causes a nonprogressing infection as a substitute for infection with virulent tuberculosis strains. Not everyone who receives the vaccine is protected, but those who are vaccinated become PPD–tuberculin skin test positive. In such persons, the skin test becomes useless as an aid for diagnosing genuine *M. tuberculosis* infection.

Streptococcus Pneumoniae

Many bacterial and viral agents can cause pneumonia, but *Streptococcus pneumoniae* is of particular importance. Until 2000, *S. pneumoniae* infections caused 60,000 cases of invasive disease each year and up to 40% of these were caused by pneumococci nonsusceptible to at least one drug. These figures have decreased substantially following the introduction of the pneumococcal conjugate vaccine for children. In the year 2002, there were 37,000 cases of invasive pneumococcal disease. Of these, 34% were caused by pneumococci nonsusceptible to at least one drug and 17% were caused by a strain nonsusceptible to three or more drugs.

S. pneumoniae normally exists in the nose and throat area of human beings and is carried asymptomatically in preschoolers and adults (see Table 7-2). The bacterium is spread by droplet inhalation of respiratory/oral droplets. This bacterium also is the leading cause of middle-ear infections in children and can cause bacterial meningitis, an inflammation

---

BOX 7-2

Centers for Disease Control and Prevention Guidelines for Interpreting PPD-Tuberculin Skin Test Reactions*

1. An induration of >5 mm is classified as positive in:
   - persons who have HIV infection or risk factors for HIV infection but unknown HIV status.
   - persons who have had recent close contact with persons who have active tuberculosis.
   - persons who have fibrotic chest radiographs (consistent with healed tuberculosis).
2. An induration of >10 mm is classified as positive in all persons who do not meet any of the criteria above but who have other risk factors for tuberculosis, including:
   - high-risk groups.
   - injecting drug users known to be HIV-seronegative.
   - persons who have other medical conditions that reportedly increase the risk for progressing from latent tuberculosis infection to active tuberculosis (e.g., silicosis, gastrectomy, or jejunoileal bypass; being >10% below ideal body weight; chronic renal failure with renal dialysis; diabetes mellitus; high-dose corticosteroid or other immunosuppressive therapy; some hematological disorders, including malignancies such as leukemias and lymphomas; and other malignancies).
   - children younger than 4 years of age.
   - high-prevalence groups.
   - persons born in countries in Asia, Africa, the Caribbean, and Latin America that have a high prevalence of tuberculosis.
   - persons from medically underserved, low-income populations.
   - residents of long-term care facilities (e.g., correctional institutions and nursing homes).
   - persons from high-risk populations in their communities, as determined by local public health authorities.
3. An induration of >15 mm is classified as positive in persons who do not meet any of the above criteria.
4. Recent converters are defined based on the size of induration and age of the person being tested:
   - Ten-millimeter increase or greater within a 2-year period is classified as a recent conversion for persons younger than 35 years of age.
   - Fifteen-millimeter increase or greater within a 2-year period is classified as a recent conversion for persons older than 35 years of age.
5. PPD skin test results in health care workers:
   - In general, the recommendations in sections 1, 2, and 3 of this box should be followed when interpreting skin test results in health care workers.
   - A recent seroconversion in a health care worker should be defined generally as a >10-mm increase in size of induration within a 2-year period. For health care workers who work in facilities where exposure to tuberculosis is unlikely, an increase of >15 mm within a 2-year period may be more appropriate for defining a recent conversion because of the lower positive-predictive value of the test in such groups.

*From Centers for Disease Control and Prevention: Guidelines for preventing the transmission of *Mycobacterium tuberculosis* in health-care facilities, 1994, *MMWR Recomm Rep* 43(RR-13):62, 1994.

---

of the membranes around the brain. A vaccine is available for the most common types of *S. pneumoniae* and is recommended for the elderly or others who may be predisposed to lung infections.

Human Herpesvirus Type 5

Human herpesvirus type 5 (cytomegalovirus) usually causes no symptoms on primary infection but occasionally causes disease in newborns and immunocompromised persons. The virus can be spread by contact with saliva, vaginal secretions, semen, breast milk, blood, and transplanted tissue. Human herpesvirus 5 can cause a congenital disease called cytomegalic inclusion disease that has a high fatality rate and causes mental retardation, neurologic problems, deafness, and possible damage to many internal organs. Infection in otherwise healthy adults is usually asymptomatic but may cause symptoms like those of infectious mononucleosis. Infection of immunosuppressed persons or those with AIDS can be devastating and may involve transplant patients receiving immunosuppressive drugs. Conditions that may develop in such persons include pneumonia, gastroenteritis, and hepatitis. Cytomegalovirus retinitis occurs in approximately 10% to 15% of AIDS patients, and cytomegalovirus colitis or cytomegalovirus esophagitis occurs in approximately 10% of AIDS patients.

Human Herpesviruses Types 6, 7, and 8

Human herpesvirus type 6 commonly is isolated from saliva and recently was identified as the cause of roseola (exanthema subitum). Roseola occurs as a high fever and a skin rash in infants. This virus also may cause infectious mononucleosis symptoms in some adults. Human herpesvirus type 7 also is isolated from saliva in as many as 70% to 80% of adults and children, but has not yet been associated clearly with any particular disease state. Human herpesvirus type 8 has been associated recently with Kaposi sarcoma, a condition seen in many AIDS patients.

Influenza

Influenza (sometimes referred to as the "flu") is a respiratory disease caused by the influenza virus of which here are two main types that infect humans, type A and type B. Symptoms can include fever, cough, sore throat, runny or stuffy nose, body aches, headache, chills, fatigue, nausea, diarrhea, and vomiting. Influenza can be transmitted through droplet exposure of mucosal surfaces by respiratory secretions from coughing or sneezing; contact, usually by hands, with an infectious patient or fomite (a surface contaminated with secretions) followed by self-inoculation of virus onto mucosal surfaces such as those of the nose, eyes, and mouth; and small particle aerosols in the vicinity of the infectious individual. Further information about influenza and related vaccinations is given in Chapter 9.

Other Respiratory Diseases

Table 7-1 lists other respiratory diseases that are spread by inhalation of infected respiratory/oral droplets. These include diseases caused by approximately 170 different types of viruses and involve the common cold, pneumonia, croup, bronchitis, erythema infectiosum, measles, mumps, and rubella. Additional bacteria are involved in causing bacterial pneumonias, meningitis, and diphtheria.

WATERBORNE DISEASE AGENTS

Many disease agents may be spread through contaminated water, including those that cause cholera, *Shigella* and amebic dysentery, salmonellosis, *Escherichia coli* colitis, cryptosporidiosis, and hepatitis A and E. Because these disease agents are not known to be spread in dental offices, they are not discussed further. However, numerous studies show that the water inside dental units and hoses for water-spray handpieces and the air/water syringes are contaminated heavily with bacteria. The level of these bacteria in dental unit water is much greater than that of tap water. When waterborne bacteria enter the dental unit, they attach to the inside walls of the water lines. These bacteria then form a biofilm on the inside of water lines that releases bacteria as the water flows out of the lines (for further discussion. see Chapter 14).

Although 30 to 40 different types of bacteria may be present in dental unit water, two are of particular interest because of their potential for causing opportunistic infections. One (*Legionella pneumophila*) causes legionnaires disease and Pontiac fever, and the other (*Pseudomonas aeruginosa*) is an opportunistic pathogen that can cause several harmful infections.

Legionnaires Disease

L. pneumophila is a gram-negative rod-shaped bacterium that causes approximately 70% of the cases of legionnaires disease. This disease is a pneumonia and was named after first being recognized among attendees of an American Legion convention in Philadelphia in 1976. *L. pneumophila* and more than 30 other species of *Legionella* commonly exist in natural and domestic waters, but most of the cases of legionnaires disease are presumed to result from inhalation of water from water-handling systems rather than from lakes or streams. Such handling systems include air conditioning cooling towers, humidifiers, ultrasonic nebulizers, vegetable misters, respiratory therapy equipment, shower heads, industrial sprayers, fountains, spas, and water distribution systems in some buildings.

One acquires lung infections with *L. pneumophila* by inhaling contaminated water or by aspirating the bacterium after it has colonized the oropharyngeal area. The infection progresses to pneumonia mostly in the elderly and those who have some weakened body defenses. Erythromycin is used for treatment, and spread of the disease from person to person has not been documented.

Pontiac fever (named after the site in Michigan of the first recognized outbreak) also is caused by *L. pneumophila*, but this disease is not a pneumonia. Instead, the disease is an acute self-limiting condition involving flulike symptoms of fever, chills, muscle aches, headache, mild cough, and sore throat.

In Rome, Italy, an 82-year-old women died in 2011 from legionnaires disease that was contracted from a dental office. During the incubation period for this disease (2 to 10 days), the woman only left her home to attend two dental appointments and apparently had no other risks of exposure to this bacterium. Testing of water in her home was negative for *Legionella*. However, three different methods of testing showed the same genetic form of *L. pneumophila* serogroup 1 in the patient's bronchial aspirate and the dental office's tap water, dental unit waterline, and high-speed handpiece turbine. No other cases of legionnaires disease or Pontiac fever were discovered among the patients of this dental practice.

Although no scientific documentation exists for spread of legionnaires disease from dental offices in the United States, approximately 10% of dental offices apparently have *Legionella* in the dental unit water used for patient care. Thus some patients possibly may be exposed to this bacterium from some dental units. Comparison of past antibody response to *Legionella* in dental personnel with the same antibody response in nondental personnel in two separate studies also revealed that dental personnel had a higher exposure incidence to *Legionella*. Thus some dental personnel at least may be exposed to *Legionella* by contact with aerosols from dental unit water coming out of high-speed handpieces, ultrasonic scalers, and air/water syringes. Approaches to maintain good quality dental treatment water are described in Chapter 14.

Pseudomonas Infection

A report from England shows that two cancer-weakened dental patients acquired oral infections with *P. aeruginosa* that originated from dental unit water. The same study also showed that an additional 78 patients treated at the same dental unit were colonized orally for 4 to 10 weeks by the *P. aeruginosa* present in the dental unit water. However, none of these patients developed harmful infections with the *Pseudomonas* bacterium, presumably because they were not cancer-weakened or otherwise compromised. *P. aeruginosa* is an important opportunistic pathogen (see Chapter 3). The bacterium occurs widely in nature and is present in low numbers in the municipal water used in a dental unit.

In addition to waterborne bacteria, dental unit water may contain low numbers of oral bacteria. Retraction of oral bacteria back into the handpiece and air/water syringes and their connecting water lines may occur when these instruments are turned off after use in the mouth. Some dental units (depending on how they are constructed) contain antiretraction valves to prevent this from occurring, but these valves fail periodically.

The CDC and the American Dental Association indicate the following:

- Dental unit water should not be used to irrigate surgical sites in which bone is exposed.
- Water lines should be flushed at the beginning of the day to reduce temporarily the number of waterborne bacteria that may have accumulated in the water overnight.
- Water lines should be flushed between patients to reduce the number of oral microorganisms that may have been retracted into the lines after each patient.

Chapter 14 gives information on how to improve the microbial quality of dental unit water.

METHICILLIN-RESISTANT *STAPHYLOCOCCUS AUREUS*

Methicillin-resistant *Staphylococcus aureus* (MRSA) is a bacterium that is resistant to certain antibiotics called β-lactams. These antibiotics include methicillin and other more common antibiotics such as oxacillin, penicillin, and amoxicillin. In the community, most MRSA infections are skin infections that may appear as pustules or boils which often are red, swollen, painful, or have pus or other drainage. They often first look like spider bites or bumps that are red, swollen, and painful. These skin infections commonly occur at sites of visible skin trauma, such as cuts and abrasions, and areas of the body covered by hair (e.g., back of neck, groin, buttock, armpit, beard area of men). More severe or potentially life-threatening MRSA infections occur most frequently among patients in health care settings and include bloodstream infections, surgical site infections, and pneumonia. The signs and symptoms will vary by the type and stage of the infection.

Fortunately, there is no evidence that the problems with hospital-associated MRSA infections, as well as those caused by *Clostridium difficile* and others, have become prominent in dentistry. However, MRSA has been shown to be present on dental operatory surfaces, student laptops, and in dental personnel. Consequently, we cannot let our guard down. MRSA infections are usually spread by having contact with someone's skin infection or personal items an infected person has used. Factors that have been associated with the spread of MRSA skin infections include close skin-to-skin contact, openings in the skin such as cuts or abrasions, contaminated items and surfaces, crowded living conditions, and poor hygiene. Procedures that help prevent the spread of MRSA and other microbes include hand hygiene, wearing appropriate personal protective equipment, cleaning and disinfecting or using surface barriers on clinical contact surfaces, and cleaning and sterilization of contaminated reusable items.

SELECTED READINGS

Centers for Disease Control and Prevention: *Drug-resistant Streptococcus pneumoniae disease* http://www.cdc.gov/ncidod/dbmd/diseaseinfo/drugresisstreppneum_t.htm. Accessed November 2007.

Centers for Disease Control and Prevention: Guidelines for prevention of the transmission of *Mycobacterium tuberculosis* in health-care facilities, *MMWR Recomm Rep* 43(RR-13):1–132, 1994.

Centers for Disease Control and Prevention: *National Center for Infectious Diseases: Infectious diseases information* http://www.cdc.gov/ncidod/diseases/index.htm. Accessed January 2012.

Centers for Disease Control and Prevention: *Tuberculosis 2006* http://www.cdc.gov/tb/surv/surv2006/pdf/FullReport.pdf. Accessed January 2012.

Depoala LG, Mangan D, Mills SE, et al: A review of the science regarding dental unit waterlines, *J Am Dent Assoc* 133:1199–1206, 2002.

Donlon RM: Biofilms microbial life on surfaces, *Emerg Infect Dis* 8:881–890, 2002.

Dunlop R, Palenik CJ, Kowolik MJ: *Presence of methicillin-resistant Staphylococcus aureus on dental student laptops*Washington, DC, 2010, American Association for Dental Research, Annual Meeting. abst # 370.

Glick M, Goldman HS: Viral infections in the dental setting, *J Am Dent Assoc* 124:79–86, 1993.

Haraszthy VI, Gerber DS, Clark C, et al: *Methicillin-resistant Staphylococcus aureus in a dental school population*Miami, 2009, International Association for Dental Research, General Session. abst #3423.

Kurita H, Kurashina K, Honda T: Nosocomial transmission of methicillin-resistant *Staphylococcus aureus* via the surfaces of the dental operatory, *Br Dent J* 201:297–300, 2006.

Miller CH: Microbes in dental unit water, *J Calif Dent Assoc* 24:47–52, 1996.

Miller CH, Cottone JC: The basic principles of infectious diseases as related to dental practice, *Dent Clin North Am* 37:1–20, 1993.

Musher DM: How contagious are common respiratory tract infections? *New Engl J Med* 348:1256–1266, 2003.

Ricci ML, Fontana S, Pinci F, et al: Pneumonia associated with a dental unit waterline, *Lancet* 379:684, 2012.

Roberts MC, Soge OO, Horst JA, et al: Methicillin-resistant *Staphylococcus aureus* from dental school clinic surfaces and students, *Am J Infect Cont* 39(8):628–632, 2011.

REVIEW QUESTIONS

Multiple Choice

1. Which of the following microbes causes thrush and denture stomatitis?
   a. Human herpesvirus type 1
   b. Coxsackievirus
   c. *Candida albicans*
   d. *Treponema pallidum*

2. Herpetic whitlow is an infection of the:
   a. hand and fingers
   b. lips
   c. genitalia
   d. mouth

3. Those who have shingles previously had:
   a. tuberculosis
   b. chickenpox
   c. syphilis
   d. diphtheria

4. Herpangina and hand-foot-and-mouth disease are caused by the same group of viruses called:
   a. varicella-zoster
   b. human herpesvirus
   c. Epstein-Barr virus
   d. coxsackievirus

5. The bacterium that causes strep throat also causes necrotizing fasciitis and:
   a. tuberculosis
   b. diphtheria
   c. scarlet fever
   d. chickenpox

6. Which of the following is not true about tuberculosis?
   a. Tuberculosis is a common occupational disease of dental workers.
   b. Tuberculosis is a major health problem worldwide.
   c. Human immunodeficiency virus disease and homelessness are risk factors for tuberculosis.
   d. A skin test is available to help diagnose tuberculosis.

7. Where does *Streptococcus pneumoniae* (causes lobar pneumonia) normally exist when it is not causing disease?
   a. In natural and domestic waters
   b. In the intestinal tract
   c. In the nose and throat
   d. On the hands

8. Where does *Legionella pneumophila* (causes legionnaires disease) normally exist when it is not causing disease?
   a. In natural and domestic waters
   b. In the intestinal tract
   c. In the nose and throat
   d. On the hands

9. What bacterium in dental unit water has been shown to cause oral disease in immunocompromised patients?
   a. *Streptococcus pyogenes*
   b. *Legionella pneumophila*
   c. *Pseudomonas aeruginosa*
   d. *Mycobacterium tuberculosis*

10. Specific oral lesions are caused by all of the following except:
    a. rhinoviruses
    b. human herpesvirus type 1
    c. *Candida albicans*
    d. *Treponema pallidum*

11. Which of the following statements about the bacille Calmette-Guérin vaccine for tuberculosis is not true?
    a. The vaccine is cleared for use in the United States.
    b. The vaccine is used widely outside the United States.
    c. Not everyone who receives the vaccine is protected.
    d. Vaccinated individuals show a positive skin test for tuberculosis.

12. Which of the following microbes are well known for causing periodic recurrences after the initial infection?
    a. Influenza viruses
    b. Rubella viruses
    c. Human herpesviruses
    d. *Neisseria gonorrhoeae*

13. An opportunistic pathogen causes disease only:
    a. when it is swallowed
    b. under special circumstances that give it an advantage to multiply to harmful levels
    c. when a person has been treated with an antibiotic
    d. in persons who have no other infectious disease

14. All of the following except one are herpesviruses. The exception is:
    a. simplex type 1
    b. varicella-zoster
    c. Epstein-Barr
    d. coxsackievirus

15. All of the following except one are sexually transmitted diseases that may produce oral lesions. The exception is:
    a. syphilis
    b. infectious mononucleosis
    c. gonorrhea
    d. herpes infection type 2

16. In the community, most MRSA infection are infections of the:
    a. lungs
    b. liver
    c. brain
    d. skin

Please visit http://evolve.elsevier.com/Miller/infectioncontrol/ for additional practice and study support tools.

Infection Control Rationale and Regulations

OUTLINE

LEARNING OBJECTIVES

After completing this chapter, the student should be able to do the following:

1. Describe the rationale for performing infection control procedures, the pathways by which microbes may be spread, and which infection control procedures can be used to interfere with the different pathways of microbial spread in the dental office.
2. Describe the goal of infection control.
3. Describe the role played by governmental and professional organizations in dental infection control.
4. Summarize the bloodborne pathogens standard from the Occupational Safety and Health Administration.
5. Summarize the recommendations for infection control in dentistry from the Centers for Disease Control and Prevention.

6. Summarize the bloodborne pathogens standard from the Occupational Safety and Health Administration.

7. Summarize the recommendations for infection control in dentistry from the Centers for Disease Control and Prevention.

KEY TERMS

American Dental Association
Association for the Advancement of
　Medical Instrumentation
Bloodborne Pathogens Standard
Centers for Disease Control and
　Prevention

Direct Contact
Droplet Infection
Environmental Protection Agency
Food and Drug Administration
Indirect Contact

Occupational Safety and Health
　Administration
Organization for Safety and Asepsis
　Procedures
Standard Precautions
Universal Precautions

RATIONALE FOR INFECTION CONTROL

The logic for routinely practicing infection control is that the procedures involved interfere with the steps in development of diseases that may be spread in the office. Chapters 6 and 7 describe the diseases that may be spread; Chapter 3 describes the steps in development of such diseases (source, escape, spread, entry, infection, and disease).

Pathways for Cross-Contamination

A total office infection control program is designed to prevent or at least reduce the spread of disease agents from the following:
- Patient to dental team
- Dental team to patient
- Patient to patient
- Dental office to community, including the dental team's families
- Community to patient
- Dental team to family

These subdivisions of infection control are based on the six pathways for cross-contamination; Table 8-1 describes their relationship to modes of disease spread and infection control procedures.

Patient to Dental Team

The opportunities for spread of patient microorganisms to members of the dental team are numerous, and this pathway is more difficult to control than the other five pathways. Direct contact (touching) with patient's saliva or blood may lead to entrance of microorganisms through nonintact skin resulting from cuts, abrasions, or dermatitis. Invisible breaks in the skin also exist, especially around the fingernails. Sprays, spatter, or aerosols from the patient's mouth may lead to droplet infection through nonintact skin; mucosal surfaces of the eyes, nose, and mouth; or inhalation. Indirect contact involves transfer of microorganisms from the source (e.g., the patient's mouth) to an item or surface and subsequent contact with the contaminated item or surface.

Examples include cuts or punctures with contaminated sharp objects (e.g., instruments, needles, burs, files, scalpel blades, and wire) and entrance through nonintact skin as a result of touching contaminated instruments, surfaces, or other items. Another opportunity for disease spread occurs by direct contact with infectious skin lesions or other nonintact skin of the patient with entrance of microorganisms through nonintact skin on the dental member's hands. This latter route of disease spread in the office is not common.

Infection control procedures to prevent patient-to-dental team spread are listed in Table 8-1 and are described in detail in subsequent chapters.

Dental Team to Patient

Spread of disease agents from the dental team to patients is a rare event but could happen if members do not follow proper procedures. If the hands of dental team members contain lesions or other nonintact skin, or if their hands are injured while in the patient's mouth, bloodborne pathogens or other microorganisms could be transferred by direct contact with the patient's mouth, and they might gain entrance through mucous membranes or open tissue. The patient may have indirect contact with bloodborne pathogens or other agents if a member of the dental team bleeds on instruments or other items that then are used in the patient's mouth. Chapter 6 describes apparent spread of bloodborne diseases from dentists to patients. Droplet infection of the patient from the dental team could occur, but this can occur in everyday life and is certainly not unique to the dental office.

Infection control procedures that interfere with this pathway of cross-contamination are listed in Table 8-1 and are described later.

Patient to Patient

Disease agents might be transferred from patient to patient by indirect contact through improperly prepared instruments, handpieces and attachments, operatory surfaces, and hands. Although, at the time of this writing, disease transmission from contaminated instruments or surfaces to dental patients has not been documented, the potential for such transfer

TABLE 8-1   **Mechanisms of Disease Spread and Prevention**

Pathway of Cross-Contamination	Source of Microorganism	Mode of Disease Spread	Mechanism or Site of Entry into Body	Infection Control Procedure
Patient to dental team	Patient's mouth	Direct contact	Through breaks in skin of dental team	Gloves/hand hygiene Immunizations
		Droplet infection	Inhalation by dental team	Mask Rubber dam Mouth rinsing
			Through breaks in skin of dental team	Gloves/hand hygiene Protective clothing Face shield Rubber dam Mouth rinsing
			Through mucosal surfaces of dental team	Mask Eyewear Face shield Rubber dam Mouth rinsing Immunization
		Indirect contact	Cuts, punctures, or needlesticks in dental team	Needle safety and waste management Heavy gloves for cleanup Ultrasonic cleaning rather than hand scrubbing Instrument cassettes to reduce direct handling during cleaning Antimicrobial holding solution Antimicrobial cleaning solution
			Through breaks in skin of dental team	Heavy gloves for cleanup Protective clothing Immunization
	Patient's skin lesions	Direct contact	Through breaks in skin of dental team	Gloves/hand hygiene Immunizations
Dental team to patient	Dental team's hands (lesions or bleeding)	Direct contact	Through mucosal surfaces of patient	Gloves/hand hygiene Care in handling sharp objects Immunizations
		Indirect contact	Bleeding on items used in patient's mouth	Gloves/hand hygiene Instrument sterilization Surface disinfection Immunizations
	Dental team's mouths (oral or respiratory fluids)	Droplet infection	Inhalation by patient	Mask Face shield
			Through oral mucosal surfaces of patient	Mask Face shield
Patient to patient	Patient's mouth	Indirect contact (instruments, surfaces, hands)	Through oral mucosal surfaces of patient	Instrument and handpiece sterilization Sterilization monitoring Surface covers Surface disinfection Hand hygiene and proper gloving Changing mask Decontaminating protective eyewear Changing protective clothing when needed Use of sterile or clean supplies Flushing dental unit water lines Monitoring water line antiretraction valves Use of disposable items

Continued

TABLE 8-1   **Mechanisms of Disease Spread and Prevention—cont'd**

Pathway of Cross-Contamination	Source of Microorganism	Mode of Disease Spread	Mechanism or Site of Entry into Body	Infection Control Procedure
Office to community	Patient's mouth	Indirect contact	Cuts, punctures, breaks in skin of dental laboratory, waste disposal, or laundry personal	Waste management Disinfection of impressions and appliances Proper management of contaminated laundry Hand hygiene
Dental team to family	Patient's mouth	Direct/indirect contact	Intimate contact	Immunization, hand hygiene, changing protective clothing before leaving the office
Community to patient	Municipal water	Direct contact	Patient's mouth	Using new and separate water source Periodically disinfecting inside of dental unit water lines Using water containing an approved antimicrobial agent Filtering the water

From US Department of Labor, Occupational Safety and Health Administration: *Controlling occupational exposure to blood-borne pathogens,* OSHA 3127 (revised), Washington, DC, 1996, OSHA.

does exist and has been documented to occur in the medical field. Conversely, transfer of the herpes simplex virus from a patient to the hands of a hygienist and then to the mouths of several patients has been documented, as described further in Chapters 10 and 11.

Patient-to-Patient Spread of Human Immunodeficiency Virus

A report indicates the apparent spread of human immuno-deficiency virus (HIV) from patient to patient in a medical/surgical practice in New South Wales, Australia. Five of nine patients seen in that medical office on the same day in November 1989 became HIV-positive, but the surgeon was HIV-negative. All five of these patients had minor surgeries that day involving the removal of moles or small cysts. Four of the five patients who became HIV-positive did not have any apparent risk factors for acquiring HIV disease (e.g., intravenous drug abuse, multiple sex partners of unknown HIV status, blood transfusions, or sexually transmitted diseases). These four patients also experienced sore throat, swollen glands under the chin, slight joint pains, and slight fever in December 1989. These are the symptoms of an HIV infection, referred to as acute retroviral syndrome, that usually occur about a month after the initial infection. The fifth patient admitted to having sex with male partners of unknown HIV status—likely his source of HIV. This patient died of *Pneumocystis jiroveci* (formerly *Pneumocystis carinii*) pneumonia (a leading cause of infectious disease death in patients with acquired immunodeficiency syndrome) in 1990. This strongly suggests that he already was infected in November 1989 when he was in the New South Wales medical office and that this patient served as the source of HIV in this incident.

The surgeon in this practice indicated that he ran the office by himself and that he did not use multiple-dose injection vials (an important mode of disease spread), did not reuse

scalpel blades but did reuse the handles, and changed gloves for every patient. He stated that he processed his contaminated instruments by soaking them in 1% glutaraldehyde, washing them in water, and placing them in boiling water for 5 to 10 minutes. These procedures have several problems (Chapter 11 describes the correct procedures for processing contaminated instruments). Because glutaraldehyde disinfectant/sterilant is commercially available only at concentrations between 2.0% and 3.4%, the surgeon apparently diluted his glutaraldehyde before using it, which saves money but also dilutes microbial effectiveness. Apparently, the instruments were not scrubbed or ultrasonically cleaned in a detergent, which suggests that blood could have remained on them after "washing in water." Although boiling likely can kill most microorganisms on instruments, if the instruments are clean, boiling is not a recognized method of sterilization. Obviously, the instruments were not wrapped before processing, so they may have become recontaminated as a result of improper handling after the boiling step but before they were reused on another patient.

The surgeon also stated that the instrument processing area was about 9 feet away from where the surgeries were performed. Without a physical separation between "clean" areas and "dirty" areas, chances increase for cross-contamination. Thus several breaches in infection control procedures are apparent in this medical practice that may have resulted in the spread of HIV from one patient to four others that day. Unfortunately, the appointment schedule for that day was not available to confirm that the HIV-positive man was an early patient of the day. The infection control procedures used to prevent patient-to-patient spread of disease agents are listed in Table 8-1 and are described in more detail later.

Patient-to-Patient Spread of Hepatitis B Virus

Although dental workers are at occupational risk of acquiring hepatitis B, there has been a decline in such cases over the last 20 years as a result of the vaccine and enhanced infection control procedures. Also, no cases of hepatitis B spread from dentist-to-patient have been reported since 1987. However, the very first report of patient-to-patient spread of the hepatitis B virus (HBV) in a dental office appeared in 2007. This incident occurred in September 2001 in an oral surgery practice in New Mexico. The investigation by the Centers for Disease Control and Prevention (CDC) and the state department of health showed that the woman who acquired hepatitis B (index patient) had 11 teeth extracted in the same operatory used earlier that day for the extraction of three teeth from a patient later found to be HBV-positive (source patient). The same doctor and assisting staff performed the surgeries on both of these patients, but none of the office workers had serologic evidence of HBV-infection. Genetic analysis and viral typing showed that the viruses from the index and source patients matched. The source patient was hepatitis B e antigen (HBeAg)-positive, which indicated a high viral load. Further investigation revealed no unusual events on that day in question. Medication vials were managed appropriately. Standard precautions for preventing the spread of bloodborne viruses were followed, including appropriate hand antisepsis. Gloves, gowns, and masks were changed for each patient. Nitrous oxide masks were cleaned and disinfected between use, and surgical instruments were hand scrubbed, rinsed, dried, packaged, and processed through a steam sterilizer between patients. High-touch areas in the operatory were covered with plastic or foil and changed for each patient. Surfaces were also disinfected between patients.

Thus, whereas the evidence indicated that patient-to-patient spread of HBV occurred, there was no evidence of a breakdown in procedures. The investigators could only speculate on the mode of transmission. One possibility was cross-contamination from an environmental surface that was inadequately cleaned and disinfected despite the good standard operating procedures detected. The use of multidose vials in general are highly suspect in transmission events, but the procedures performed in this instance were found to be totally appropriate. One interesting note is that three of the five patients were seen on that day after the source patient already had been vaccinated against hepatitis B. This may have limited the spread and prevented the investigators from identifying the mechanisms of the spread by possibly identifying common factors.

Dental Office to Community

The dental office-to-community pathway may occur if microorganisms from the patient contaminate items that are sent out or are transported away from the office. For example, contaminated impressions, appliances, or equipment needing service in turn may contaminate personnel or surfaces in dental laboratories and repair centers indirectly. Dental laboratory technicians have been infected occupationally with HBV.

This pathway may also occur if members of the dental team transport microorganisms out of the office on contaminated clothing. In addition, if a member of the dental team acquires an infectious disease at work, the disease could be spread to personal contacts outside the office.

Regulated waste that contains infectious agents and is transported from the office may contaminate waste haulers if it is not in proper containers. Immunity from hepatitis B vaccination protects the dental team from acquiring the disease and passing it along to family members. Other infection control procedures that interfere with the office-to-community pathway are listed in Table 8-1 and are described in later chapters.

Community to Patient

The community-to-patient pathway involves the entrance of microorganisms into the dental office in the water that supplies the dental unit. These waterborne microorganisms colonize the inside of the dental unit water lines and form a film of microorganisms (biofilm) on the inside of these lines. As water flows through the lines during use of the air-water syringe, high-speed handpiece, or ultrasonic scaler on some units, it "picks up" microorganisms shed by the biofilm. Although municipal water may have a dozen or so bacteria per milliliter (mL) of water as it enters the dental unit, the water exiting a dental unit through the air-water syringe or through the spray from a high-speed handpiece may contain more than 100,000 bacteria per milliliter. One milliliter is equivalent to about one-fourth of a teaspoon.

No evidence exists that this contaminated water is making individuals sick on any wide scale, but use of heavily contaminated water during dental care is not good infection-control practice. Such water certainly must not be used during surgery. Potential pathogens (e.g., *Pseudomonas aeruginosa* and *Legionella pneumophila*) may be present in the incoming water and in the dental unit water line biofilm. One report from England describes how, in 1988, two cancer-compromised patients acquired oral infections with *P. aeruginosa* that was later found to be present in water from a dental unit previously used in the care of those patients. Chapter 13 presents more details about contaminated dental unit water, and Table 8-1 suggests infection control procedures to improve the microbial quality of dental unit water.

Dental Team to Family

If disease prevention procedures are not performed, members of the dental team may transport potentially infectious agents home to family members. This may occur if hands are not decontaminated before leaving the office or if contaminated clothing is worn home.

Goal of Infection Control

After microorganisms enter the body, three basic factors determine whether an infectious disease will develop: virulence (pathogenic properties of the invading microorganism), dose (the number of microorganisms that invade the body), and resistance (body defense mechanism of the host). These factors are called determinants of an infectious disease, and their interaction determines the outcome of an infection as follows:

$$\text{Health or disease} = \frac{\text{Virulence} \times \text{Dose}}{\text{Body resistance}}$$

Health is favored by low virulence, low dose, and high resistance; disease is favored by high virulence, high dose, and low resistance. Prevention of infectious diseases involves influencing the determinants to favor health.

Unfortunately, virulence of microorganisms in their natural environments cannot be changed easily. Thus our body defenses must deal with whatever microorganism presents itself, be it one with high virulence or low virulence. We can enhance our resistance to infectious diseases through specific immunization (e.g., hepatitis B and tetanus), but immunizations are not available against all of the diseases we would like to prevent. Thus the only disease determinant we can manage effectively is the dose, and management of the dose is called infection control.

Therefore, the goal of infection control is to reduce the dose of microorganisms that may be shared between individuals or between individuals and contaminated surfaces. The more the dose is reduced, the better the chances for preventing disease spread. Procedures that minimize spraying or spattering of oral fluids (e.g., rubber dam, high-volume evacuation, and preprocedure mouth rinse) reduce the dose of microorganisms that escape from the source. Handwashing and surface precleaning and disinfection reduce the number of microorganisms that may be transferred to surfaces by touching. Barriers such as masks, gloves, and protective eyewear and clothing reduce the number of microorganisms that contaminate the body or other surfaces.

Instrument precleaning and sterilization eliminate or reduce the number of microorganisms that may be spread from one patient to another. Proper management of infectious waste by using appropriate containers for disposal eliminates or reduces the number of microorganisms that may contaminate persons or inanimate objects. Disease prevention is based on reducing the dose and increasing the resistance of the body.

RECOMMENDATIONS AND REGULATIONS

Recommendations are made by individuals or groups that have no authority for enforcement. Regulations are made by groups that do have the authority to enforce compliance, usually under the penalty of fines, imprisonment, or revocation of professional licenses.

Anyone may make recommendations, but governmental groups or licensing boards in towns, cities, counties, and states make regulations.

Infection Control Recommendations

Centers for Disease Control and Prevention

The current infection control recommendations for dentistry from the Centers for Disease Control and Prevention (CDC) are summarized in this chapter and are presented in total in Appendix B. Although the CDC began making general infection control recommendations many years ago, their first set of complete recommendations directed specifically toward dentistry was in 1986, with updates in 1993 and 2003. Most infection control procedures practiced in dentistry today are based on the 2003 recommendations. The CDC is a part of the Public Health Service, which is a division of the U.S. Department of Health and Human Services. The CDC has a Division of Oral Health that studies oral diseases, fluoride applications, and infection control in dentistry. The CDC does not have the authority to make laws, but many of the local, state, and federal agencies use CDC recommendations to formulate the laws. See Appendix B for further information on the CDC and how to access their Web site and infection control recommendations.

The CDC also has published guidelines on preventing the transmission of tuberculosis in health care settings, which include dental offices. Excerpts from these guidelines are presented in Appendices B and C.

American Dental Association

The American Dental Association (ADA) has provided detailed infection control recommendations since the 1970s and currently makes such recommendations through its Councils on Scientific Affairs and Dental Practice. The most recent detailed recommendations from the ADA were published in the August 1996 issue of the *Journal of the American Dental Association*. The ADA supports the 2003 CDC infection control recommendations as described in the ADA's *Statement on Infection Control in Dentistry* (see Appendix G). The ADA's main office is located in Chicago, and Appendix A gives its Web address.

Organization for Safety and Asepsis Procedures

The Organization for Safety and Asepsis Procedures (OSAP) (see Appendix A) is a not-for-profit professional organization composed of dentists, hygienists, assistants, university professors, researchers, manufacturers, distributors, consultants, and others interested in infection control. This broad-based group is the premier infection control education organization in dentistry. The organization provides a monthly publication to keep its members in pace with new information and also provides a newsletter, reports, position papers, announcements, and press releases. This organization also sponsors regional and national educational programs related to infection control for its members. All members of the dental team should join this organization to keep up to date in the area of infection control (see Appendices A and D).

Association for the Advancement of Medical Instrumentation

The Association for the Advancement of Medical Instrumentation (AMMI) (see Appendix A) is another voluntary organization that is composed of manufacturers, distributors, researchers, regulators, and users of medical/dental equipment. One component of this organization is devoted to developing sterilization standards, including recommended practices on how properly to use sterilizers and technical documents on the equipment. For example, two documents of particular interest to the dental team describe the proper use and monitoring of small office steam and dry heat sterilizers.

Infection Control Regulations

State and Local

Some state and local regulations exist in relation to medical waste management, instrument sterilization, and sterilizer spore testing in dentistry. Examples of states with such special dental infection control regulations include California, Connecticut, Florida, Indiana, Missouri, Ohio, Oregon, and Washington. In some instances these regulations are made by the county health departments and in others by state legislatures, state boards of dental examiners, state dental disciplinary boards, or state departments of health.

Twenty-six states also have their own division of the Occupational Safety and Health Administration (OSHA) in their state departments of labor (see Appendix A). These states must administer regional OSHA standards, including those for occupational exposure to bloodborne pathogens and for management of hazardous materials, which are at least as stringent as the federal OSHA standards.

Because infection control regulations can vary from state to state, particularly in the areas of instrument sterilization, waste management, and sterilizer spore testing, it is important for the dental team to keep in contact with the various state agencies for the latest information that may affect infection control in the dental office. Two other sources of information may be the state dental association and the infection control officer in a school of dentistry located in the state.

Food and Drug Administration

The Food and Drug Administration (FDA) (see Appendix A) is a part of the U.S. Department of Health and Human Services. In relation to infection control, the FDA regulates the manufacturing and labeling of medical devices (such as sterilizers, biologic and chemical indicators, ultrasonic cleaners and cleaning solutions, liquid sterilants [e.g., glutaraldehydes], gloves, masks, surgical gowns, protective eyewear, handpieces, dental instruments, dental chairs, and dental unit lights) and of antimicrobial handwashing agents and mouth rinses.

The purpose of the FDA is to ensure the safety and effectiveness of drugs and medical devices by requiring "good manufacturing practices" and reviewing the devices against associated labeling to ensure that claims can be supported. The FDA may require general controls, certain performance standards, or various items such as notification from a manufacturer that a device is about to be marketed to requiring certain performance standards or approval of the device before marketing. All medical devices to be sold in the United States first must be cleared by the FDA. To do this, the manufacturers submit to the FDA a 510(k) application (premarket notification) that describes the device and the manufacturing facilities and presents the results of studies conducted to support any claims of effectiveness and safety made for the device. The FDA does not control the actual use of a medical device but indicates that misuse (using an item contrary to instructions on the device) transfers any liability for problems that develop from the manufacturer to the user.

Environmental Protection Agency

The U.S. Environmental Protection Agency (EPA) (see Appendix A) is associated with infection control by attempting to ensure the safety and effectiveness of disinfectants. The EPA also is involved in regulating medical waste after it leaves the dental office. Information on the safety and effectiveness of disinfectants must be submitted by manufacturers to the EPA for review to make sure that safety and the antimicrobial claims stated for the products are supported with scientific evidence. If the claims meet the criteria, the disinfectant product receives an EPA registration number that must appear on the product label. Chapter 17 discusses EPA involvement with waste management.

Occupational Safety and Health Administration

The Occupational Safety and Health Administration (OSHA) (see Appendix A) is a division of the U.S. Department of Labor, and its charge is to protect the workers of America from physical, chemical, or infectious hazards in the workplace. Chapter 26 describes the OSHA standard for protection against hazardous chemicals. OSHA began to develop its standard for protection against occupational exposure to bloodborne pathogens in 1986 and published the final rules in 1991. The standard is known as the bloodborne pathogens standard, and it became effective nationwide in 1992. OSHA requires that a copy of the regulatory text of this standard be present in every dental office and clinic. Appendix H provides the text of the standard.

This standard indicates that the employer has the responsibility to protect employees from exposure to blood and other potentially infectious materials in the workplace and to give proper care if such exposure does occur. The standard applies to employers in any type of facility in which employees have a potential for exposure to body fluids, including dental and medical offices; dental, clinical, and research laboratories; hospitals; funeral homes; emergency medical services; nursing homes; and others.

Compliance with this standard is monitored through investigations of facilities by OSHA compliance officers after a complaint by an employee of the facility to OSHA.

Compliance officers also may investigate a facility with 11 or more employees even in the absence of an employee complaint. Noncompliance with any rule in the standard can result in a fine.

The standard is effective throughout the United States and in 26 states is administered by the state OSHA programs. In the other states, the standard is administered through regional branches of the federal OSHA (see Appendix A for details).

SUMMARY OF THE OCCUPATIONAL SAFETY AND HEALTH ADMINISTRATION BLOODBORNE PATHOGENS STANDARD

The bloodborne pathogens standard is the most important infection control law in dentistry for protection of health care workers. Box 8-1 describes general steps for employer compliance with this standard, and the seven major sections of the standard are summarized next. Appendix H gives the complete standard.

Exposure Control Plan

Each dental office, clinic, or school must prepare a written exposure control plan that contains the elements listed in Box 8-2. This plan must be reviewed and updated at least annually, and a copy must be accessible to all employees.

Exposure Determination

An occupational exposure is defined as any reasonably anticipated skin, eye, mucous membrane, or parenteral (e.g., needlestick, cut, abrasion, or instrument puncture) contact with blood or other potentially infectious material such as

saliva that may result from the performance of an employee's duties. For the exposure determinations, one must survey all tasks performed by all employees and make a list of all job classifications in the office in which all of the employees in that classification have occupational exposure (e.g., "dentist," "dental hygienist," "clinical dental assistant"); then make a second list of job classifications in which some of the employees in that classification may have occupational exposure (e.g., "receptionist," "bookkeeper," "office manager"). The employer must make these determinations as if gloves, masks, eyeglasses, and protective clothing are not being used.

Now the employer must make a list of all tasks and procedures or groups of closely related tasks and procedures in which occupational exposure occurs (without regard to personal protective equipment or clothing) and that are performed by employees in job classifications noted in the second list.

Employees in these job classifications on the first and second lists are covered under the standard.

BOX 8-1

The Occupational Safety and Health Administration Bloodborne Pathogen Standard: General Steps for Compliance

1. Review the standard.
2. Prepare a written exposure control plan.
3. Train the employees.
4. Provide employees everything needed to comply with the standard.
   a. Offer hepatitis B vaccination series.
   b. Provide, maintain, dispose of, or clean, and ensure use of personal protective equipment and/or engineering controls.
   c. Establish appropriate work practices and decontamination procedures.
   d. Establish postexposure medical evaluation and follow-up.
   e. Provide appropriate biohazard communication.
5. Maintain appropriate records.

BOX 8-2

The Occupational Safety and Health Administration Written Exposure Control Plan

Prepare a written plan that documents the components listed below:
1. Exposure determination
Determine which employees may have occupational exposure and are therefore covered under the standard.
2. Schedule of implementation
Describe how and when the provisions of the standard will be implemented, including the following:
   a. Communication of hazards to employees
   b. Hepatitis B vaccination
   c. Postexposure evaluation and follow-up
   d. Record keeping
   e. Methods of compliance such as engineering and work practice controls, personal protective equipment, and housekeeping
3. Evaluation of exposure incidents
Describe how the circumstances surrounding an exposure incident will be evaluated.
4. Prevention of sharps injuries
   a. Describe how newer medical devices that may reduce exposure will be identified and considered for adoption.
   b. Describe the methods used to evaluate the devices and the results of the evaluations.
   c. Describe the justification as to why a device was or was not selected for use.
   d. Describe how the persons directly involved in patient care are involved in the identification, evaluation, and selection processes.

Schedule of Implementation

The employer must prepare a schedule of when and how each provision of the standard will be implemented. The provisions to be included are listed in Box 8-2 and described further in this chapter. One approach in a small office is simply to make notes on a copy of the standard of when (a specific date) and how each provision will be implemented. Larger facilities may wish to prepare a more extensive document covering all health and safety provisions that includes the exposure control plan.

Evaluation of Exposure Incidents

If an employee is exposed to blood, saliva, or other potentially infectious materials, the employer must evaluate the circumstances surrounding the incident. The route of exposure needs to be documented (e.g., splash in the eyes or needlestick in the left thumb), and the source patient, types of protective barriers worn at the time of exposure, and what the employee was doing at the time of exposure should be documented. Documentation can best be accomplished by using an exposure incident report form (see an example in Appendix E). Evaluation of this information will assist in the postexposure medical evaluation (described later) of the employee and will determine whether the employee may need further training in attempts to prevent future exposures.

Evaluation and Use of Safety Devices

Each dental office must document annually the consideration and implementation of appropriate commercially available and effective safer medical devices designed to eliminate or minimize occupational exposure. An employer who is required to establish an exposure control plan shall solicit input from nonmanagerial employees responsible for direct patient care who are potentially exposed to injuries from contaminated sharps in the identification, evaluation, and selection of effective engineering and work practice controls and shall document the solicitation in the exposure control plan.

Communication of Biohazards

Informing employees of biohazards is to occur in two general ways: by giving specific information and training and by using labels and signs that identify hazards. The goal of this communication is to eliminate or minimize exposure to bloodborne and other pathogens.

Information and Training

The OSHA standard indicates that employers shall ensure that all employees with occupational exposure participate in a training program on the hazards associated with body fluids and the protective measures to be taken to minimize the risk of occupational exposure. Box 8-3 gives the minimum content of the required training program. The training is to be provided at no cost to the employee at the time of initial appointment (before the employee is placed in a position in which occupational exposure may occur) and at least annually thereafter, as well as whenever job tasks change that may reflect the employee's potential for exposure. The training must be given to full-time, part-time, and temporary employees who have a potential for exposure.

A person must conduct the training or at least be available during the training to answer questions. Training solely

---

BOX 8-3

Minimum Content of Occupational Safety and Health Administration-Required Training

- An accessible copy of the regulatory text of the bloodborne pathogen standard and an explanation of its contents
- A general explanation of the epidemiology and symptoms of bloodborne diseases
- An explanation of the modes of transmission of bloodborne pathogens
- An explanation of the employer's exposure control plan and the means by which the employee can obtain a copy of the written plan
- An explanation of the appropriate methods for recognizing tasks and other activities that may involve exposure to blood and other potentially infectious materials
- An explanation of the use and limitations of methods that will prevent or reduce exposure, including appropriate engineering controls, work practices, and personal protective equipment
- Information on the types, proper use, location, removal, handling, decontamination, and disposal of personal protective equipment
- An explanation of the basis for selection of personal protective equipment; information on the hepatitis B vaccine, including information on its efficacy, safety, method of administration, the benefits of being vaccinated, and that the vaccine and vaccination will be offered free of charge
- Information on the appropriate actions to take and persons to contact in an emergency involving blood or other potentially infectious materials
- An explanation of the procedure to follow if an exposure incident occurs, including the method of reporting the incident and the medical follow-up that will be made available
- Information on the postexposure evaluation and follow-up that the employer is required to provide for the employee after an exposure incident
- An explanation of the signs and labels or color coding required by the standard
- An opportunity for interactive questions and answers with the person conducting the training session

by means of a film or videotape or written material without the opportunity for discussion is not acceptable. Likewise, a generic computer program, even an interactive one, is not considered appropriate unless it is supplemented with the site-specific information required (e.g., the location of the exposure control plan and the procedures to be followed if an exposure incident occurs) and a person is accessible for interaction.

The OSHA standard requires that the person conducting the training be knowledgeable about bloodborne pathogens and about infection control procedures related to the dental workplace. The dentist-employer, hygienists, assistants, dental school professors, or others may conduct the training, provided they are familiar with bloodborne pathogen control and the subject matter required to be presented. The trainer must be able to answer questions related to the information presented.

The manner of the training must be at a level that is appropriate for the employee being trained (e.g., the employee's education, language, and literacy level). If an employee is proficient only in a foreign language, the trainer or an interpreter must convey the information in that language.

The required record keeping (described subsequently) on the training session includes a description of the qualifications of the person providing the training. An OSHA compliance officer will verify the competency of the trainer based on the completion of specialized courses, degree programs, or work experiences if the officer determines during an investigation that deficiencies in training exist.

Use of Signs and Labels

Warning labels containing the biohazard symbol and the word "Biohazard" are fluorescent orange or orange-red with the lettering and symbol in a contrasting color (Figure 8-1). Such labels must be affixed to containers of regulated waste, refrigerators and freezers containing blood or other potentially infectious materials, and other containers used to store, transport, or ship blood or other potentially infectious materials. Red bags or red containers may be substituted for

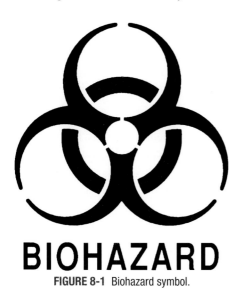

FIGURE 8-1 Biohazard symbol.

labels (if employees are trained as to the meaning of the red bags or containers). Individual containers of blood or other potentially infectious materials that are placed in a labeled container during storage, transport, shipment, or disposal are exempt from the labeling requirement. Contaminated equipment that is to be shipped for service must be labeled, however, and the label must include a description of the part of the equipment that is contaminated. Contaminated laundry also must be labeled properly, as described later in this chapter.

Hepatitis B Vaccination

Employees covered by the standard must be offered the hepatitis B vaccination series free of charge after they have received the training required by the OSHA standard and within 10 days of their employment. Booster dose or doses also must be made available free of charge if recommended by the U.S. Public Health Service. However, as yet booster doses have not been recommended. If the employee received the complete vaccine series previously, if antibody testing discloses immunity, or if the vaccine is contraindicated for medical reasons, vaccination need not be offered. The employer must not make participation in a prescreening program a prerequisite for receiving hepatitis B vaccination. The vaccine is to be administered by or under the supervision of a licensed physician or other licensed health care professional (e.g., a nurse practitioner), and this professional must be provided with a copy of the OSHA bloodborne pathogens standard (Box 8-4).

If the employee initially declines vaccination but at a later date, while still covered under the standard, decides to accept the offer, the employer must make the vaccine available at no charge at that time. Employers must ensure that employees who decline vaccination sign a specifically worded statement of declination that is printed in the OSHA standard. This statement is reproduced in Chapter 9.

To document compliance, the employer must obtain a written opinion from the physician responsible for the vaccination as to whether the hepatitis B vaccination is indicated for an employee and whether the employee received the vaccination series. The employer must retain this written opinion of employee vaccination status, giving a copy to the employee, and must make it available to a physician who later may be involved in providing a postexposure medical evaluation of the employee. This evaluation will help the evaluating physician determine the need for prophylaxis or treatment related to such an exposure. Maintenance of these records also provides documentation for the employer that a medical assessment of the employee's ability and indication to receive hepatitis B vaccination was completed.

Postexposure Medical Evaluation and Follow-up

Documentation of Exposure

After a report of an exposure incident, the employer must make immediately available to the exposed employee a confidential medical evaluation and follow-up at no cost to the employee at a reasonable time and place and performed or supervised by a licensed physician or other licensed health care professional (Box 8-5). The employer must document the exposure and surrounding circumstances, a task best accomplished by using an exposure incident report form as previously mentioned (see Appendix E). The employer gives this documentation and a job description of the employee as related to the incident, any information documenting the exposed employee's hepatitis

---

BOX 8-4

Hepatitis B Vaccination

Employer
1. Gives a copy of the OSHA standard to the health care professional
2. Provides vaccine-related training to employee
3. Offers vaccination series to employee
4a. Receives and maintains the signed statement if employee declines the offer, or
4b. Receives written opinion from health care professional on evaluation and administration of vaccine and gives copy to employee
5. Maintains written opinion or declination statement in confidential employee medical records file

Employee
1. Receives the vaccine-related training
2. Receives the offer for free vaccination from the employer
3a. Accepts the offer and sees the health care professional, or
3b. Declines the offer and signs the declination statement*
4. Is evaluated for vaccination by the health care professional and receives vaccine or explanation for not being administered vaccine

Health Care Professional†
1. Receives a copy of the Occupational Safety and Health Administration standard from employer
2. Evaluates employee for vaccination, prior immunity, or contraindication
3a. Vaccinates employee, or
3b. Explains contraindication or prior immunity to employee
4. Gives written opinion to employer on evaluation and if vaccine was administered

---

*Physician or other licensed health care professional such as a nurse practitioner. Evaluation and vaccination are provided according to recommendations from the U.S. Public Health Service.

†May later request and obtain the vaccination series free of charge.

B vaccination status (e.g., past written opinions from the health care professional), any written opinions of a health care professional from past exposure incidents, results of the source individual's blood testing, and a copy of the OSHA standard to the evaluating health care professional.

Testing of the Source Individual

The source individual is any patient whose body fluid is involved in the exposure incident. After an employee exposure, the employer must request promptly that the source individual's blood be tested (with consent) to determine HBV and HIV infectivity, unless this person already is known to be infected with HBV or HIV. If the source individual does not give consent for testing or if it is not feasible to obtain consent, the employer shall establish that this consent cannot be obtained. If consent is given, the source individual may be sent to the health care professional or an appropriate accredited laboratory or testing site for the testing. The results of the source individual's tests are confidential and are to be directed only to the health care professional evaluating the exposed employee. The employer must ensure that the exposed employee is informed confidentially of these results by the attending health care professional, but the employer does not have the right to know the source individual's test results.

Testing the Exposed Employee

The employer must make available collection and testing of blood from the exposed employee for HBV and HIV status with the employee's consent. The collection can be arranged through the health care professional. If the employee consents to blood collection but does not give consent for testing for HIV, the blood sample is to be preserved for 90 days, in case the employee later consents to testing. The health care professional is to provide medical evaluation and follow-up according to the U.S. Public Health Service recommendations and to provide the employer with a written opinion within 15 days after the evaluation. This written opinion shall include only the following information: (1) that the employee has been informed of the results of the evaluation and (2) that the employee has been told about any medical conditions resulting from exposure that require further evaluation or treatment. All other findings or diagnoses shall remain confidential and shall not be included in the written opinion.

The employer is to keep this written opinion in a confidential employee medical records file with the hepatitis B vaccination written opinion for that employee.

Record Keeping

Training Records

Records documenting that employees covered under the standard received the required training must contain (1) dates of the training sessions, (2) contents or summary of the training, (3) names and qualifications of the persons conducting the

---

BOX 8-5

Postexposure Medical Evaluation and Follow-up

Employer
1. Sends exposed employee to health care professional for testing (with consent)
2. Sends source individual to health care professional or arranges for other testing (with consent). If hepatitis B virus and HIV status is known already or consent is not given, informs the health care professional.
3. Gives the following to the health care professional:
   - Copy of OSHA standard
   - Incident report
   - Employee's job description as related to the exposure incident
   - Past written opinions on employee's hepatitis B vaccination status and any past exposure incidents
   - Results of source individual's blood testing, if available
4. Ensures that test results of source individual are given to the health care professional and that health care professional informs employee of these results, stressing confidentiality
5. Receives written opinion from health care professional
6. Maintains written opinion in confidential employee medical records file

Employee
1. Reports to the health care professional for evaluation
2. Gives or withholds consent for testing
3. Receives own and source individual's test results from health care professional
4. Is told by health care professional of any conditions resulting from exposure that require further evaluation or treatment

Health Care Professional*
1. Receives the following from the employer:
   - Copy of standard
   - Incident report
   - Employee's job description
   - Past written opinions on employee's vaccination status and any past exposure incidents
2. Arranges for testing of source individual (with consent) *or* receives test results from employer-arranged testing *or* receives other information about source individual's hepatitis B virus and human immunodeficiency virus status or that consent for testing was not given
3. Evaluates exposed employee for testing with consent and arranges for testing when indicated†
4. Informs exposed employee of:
   - Source individual's test results, stressing confidentiality
   - Results of the evaluation
   - Any condition that requires further evaluation or treatment
5. Gives written opinion to employer that employee was informed of results and of any further evaluation or treatment needed

*Physician or other licensed health care professional such as a nurse practitioner. Evaluation and vaccination are provided according to recommendations from the U.S. Public Health Service.
†If blood is drawn but consent for testing is not given, arrangements are to be made to store blood sample for 90 days should employee change his or her mind.

---

training, and (4) names and job titles of all persons attending the training sessions. The records are to be kept for 3 years from the date on which the training occurred.

Employee Medical Records

Medical records for each employee covered under the standard are to include (1) the name and Social Security number of the employee; (2) the hepatitis B vaccination status, including the dates of vaccination and the written opinion from the health care professional regarding the vaccination or the signed statement that the employee declined the offer to be vaccinated; and (3) reports documenting occupational exposure incidents, as well as the written opinion from the health care professional who made the evaluation.

These medical records are confidential and are not to be disclosed except to the employee, anyone having written consent of the employee, representatives of the secretary of labor (on request), or as required or permitted by state or federal law. The records must be maintained for 30 years past the last date of employment.

Universal Precautions

Universal precautions is the concept that all human blood and certain human body fluids that may contain blood are treated as if known to be infectious for HIV and HBV and other bloodborne pathogens. Justification for this concept is based on the inability to easily identify most of those infected with HIV, HBV, or hepatitis C virus (HCV), as described in Chapter 6. Although universal precautions still are used regarding the OSHA bloodborne pathogens standard, the CDC has expanded the concept of universal precautions into what now is called standard precautions. Standard precautions apply not just to contact with blood but also to (1) all body fluids, secretions, and excretions (except sweat) regardless of whether they contain blood; (2) nonintact skin; and (3) mucous membranes.

Engineering and Work Practice Controls

Engineering and work practice controls are to be used to minimize or eliminate employee exposure. If exposure remains after institution of these controls, personal protective equipment also is to be used.

Engineering controls generally act on the hazard itself so that the employee may not have to take self-protective action. An example is use of a sharps container. Work practice controls alter the manner in which a task is performed, reducing the likelihood of exposure, such as safe handling techniques for needles. Employers should examine and maintain or replace all engineering controls and should review work practices regularly to ensure their effectiveness.

Hand Hygiene

Readily accessible handwashing facilities are to be provided to employees. In the rare instances when this is not feasible, antiseptic towelettes or an antiseptic hand cleaner and cloth or paper towels are to be provided, with soap and water handwashing to follow as soon as feasible. Employers are to ensure that employees wash their hands as soon as possible after removal of gloves or other personal protective equipment. Hands and other skin are to be washed with soap and water, and mucous membranes are to be flushed with water as soon as feasible after contact of these body sites with blood/saliva.

Handling of Disposable Contaminated Sharps

Contaminated needles and other sharps are not to be bent, recapped, or removed unless the employer can demonstrate that no alternative is feasible or that such action is required by a specific medical procedure. Clearly, disposable needles must be removed from the nondisposable dental anesthetic syringes. Recapping is to be accomplished using a one-handed technique or a mechanical device. Shearing or breaking of contaminated needles also is prohibited.

Handling of Reusable Contaminated Sharps

Contaminated reusable sharps (e.g., special needles and sharp instruments) are to be placed in appropriate containers as soon as possible after use. The containers shall be puncture-resistant and color coded or labeled with a biohazard symbol and be leakproof on the sides and bottom. The sharps shall not be stored or processed (before decontamination) in a manner that requires employees to reach blindly into containers where these sharps have been placed.

Restricted Activities in the Work Area

Eating, drinking, smoking, applying of cosmetics or lip balm, and handling of contact lenses are prohibited in work areas where a chance exists for occupational exposure. Food and drink cannot be stored in refrigerators or freezers or kept on shelves or on countertops or in cabinets where blood or saliva is present.

Minimizing Spatter

All procedures involving blood or saliva are to be performed in such a manner that minimizes splashing, spraying, spattering, and generation of droplets of these substances. Although OSHA does not mention specific procedures that limit spatter and generation of droplets in dentistry, one might consider using a rubber dam, high-volume evacuation, and preprocedure mouth rinsing.

Specimen Containers

Specimens of blood or saliva or other potentially infectious material are to be placed in a container that prevents leakage during collection, handling, processing, storage, or shipping. The container is to be closed and color coded or labeled with a biohazard symbol for storage, transport, or shipping. A second container with the same characteristics is to be used if the outside of the primary container is contaminated. If the specimen could puncture the primary container, a second container with the same characteristics plus being puncture-resistant is to be used.

Servicing of Contaminated Equipment

Equipment that may become contaminated with blood or saliva or other potentially infectious materials is to be examined before servicing or shipping and is to be decontaminated as necessary unless the employer can demonstrate that decontamination of such equipment or portions of such equipment is not feasible. If portions remain contaminated, these portions are to be identified and labeled with a biohazard symbol. This identification and labeling information is to be conveyed to all affected employees, the servicing representative, and the manufacturer, as appropriate, before handling, servicing, or shipping so that proper precautions will be taken.

Personal Protective Equipment

When the potential exists for occupational exposure, the employer shall provide, at no cost to the employee, appropriate personal protective equipment such as gloves, protective clothing, masks, face shields or eye protection, and mouthpiece, resuscitation bags, pocket masks, or other ventilating devices. Such equipment is considered appropriate if it does not permit blood or saliva to pass through or to reach the employee's work clothes, street clothes, undergarments, skin, eyes, mouth, or other mucous membranes under normal conditions of use.

The employer is (1) to ensure that the employee uses the personal protective equipment; (2) to ensure that the regular personal protective equipment in the appropriate sizes is readily accessible in the office (including hypoallergenic gloves, glove liners, powderless gloves, or other alternatives for those who are allergic or have other reactions to the regular gloves); (3) to clean, launder, and when appropriate dispose of personal protective equipment; and (4) to repair or replace personal protective equipment as needed to maintain its effectiveness.

All personal protective equipment is to be removed before the employee leaves the work area. If blood or saliva penetrates a garment, the garment is to be removed immediately or as soon as feasible. On removal, personal protective equipment is to be placed in an appropriately designated area or container for storage, washing, decontamination, or disposal.

Gloves

Gloves are to be worn when the employee may have hand contact with blood or saliva, mucous membranes, nonintact skin, or when handling or touching contaminated items or surfaces. Handwashing is required after glove removal. Surgical or examination gloves are to be replaced as soon as practical when contaminated or as soon as feasible if they are torn, punctured, or otherwise compromised. Disposable gloves are not to be washed or decontaminated for reuse. Utility gloves may be decontaminated for reuse if the integrity of the glove is not compromised. However, they must be discarded if cracked, peeling, torn, or punctured or if they become deteriorated in any way.

Masks, Eye Protection, and Face Shields

Masks in combination with eye protection devices such as goggles or glasses with solid side shields, or chin-length face shields, are to be worn whenever splashes, spray, spatter, or droplets of blood or saliva may be generated and eye, nose, or mouth contamination may occur. If face shields are used, they need to be curved to give protection to the sides of the eyes. If regular prescription glasses are used as protective eyewear, they should have clip-on solid side shields.

Protective Clothing

Appropriate protective clothing such as gowns, aprons, lab coats, clinic jackets, or similar outer garments are to be worn in occupational exposure situations. The employer must evaluate the task to determine the appropriate nature of the protective clothing to be used. Examples of different levels of exposure given by OSHA are "soiled" (low level, requiring laboratory coats), "splashed, splattered, or sprayed" (medium level, requiring fluid-resistant garments), "soaked" (high level, requiring fluid-proof garments).

Protective clothing must not permit blood or saliva to pass through or reach the employees' work clothes, street clothes, undergarments, or skin. If an item of clothing is intended to protect the employees' person or work clothes or street clothes against contact with blood or saliva, then it would be considered as personal protective clothing. If a uniform is used to protect the employee from exposure, the uniform is considered personal protective clothing. If a lab coat or protective gown is placed over the uniform, the uniform is not protective clothing; the lab coat or gown is. Thus the outer covering is the protective clothing that the employer must provide.

The employer also is required to maintain, clean, launder, and dispose of all personal protective equipment, including protective clothing, at no cost to the employee. Furthermore, employees cannot launder the protective clothing at home. Thus employers must provide disposable protective clothing or reusable protective clothing that is laundered in the office or is cleaned by a laundry service. OSHA reasons that, with these options, the employer has control over the protective clothing to ensure proper disposal or cleaning.

Housekeeping

Employers are to ensure that the work site is maintained in a clean and sanitary condition. All equipment and environmental and working surfaces are to be cleaned and decontaminated after contact with blood or other potentially infectious materials. OSHA states that cleaning must be done "after completion of procedures, immediately or as soon as feasible when surfaces are overtly contaminated or after any spill of blood or other potentially infectious materials, and at the end of the work shift if the surface may have become contaminated since the last cleaning."

The employer must prepare and implement a written schedule for cleaning and method of decontamination of respective work sites within the facility; for example, all uncovered contaminated surfaces in the dental operatory will be sprayed with an iodophor (state the brand), wiped clean, resprayed with the iodophor, let stand for 10 minutes, and wiped dry. This will be performed immediately after care is completed for each patient.

Other statements must be written for other work sites such as the sterilizing room, x-ray room, darkroom, in-office laboratory, restroom, or any other site where surfaces may be contaminated with blood or other potentially infectious materials. OSHA does not specify which disinfectant to use, only that the disinfectant must be registered with the EPA. Although OSHA suggests that the disinfectant used should claim to kill at least HIV and HBV, the authors of this book suggest (as further discussed in Chapter 13) the use of an

EPA-registered disinfectant that is tuberculocidal, which is a stronger disinfectant.

Protective coverings (such as plastic wrap, aluminum foil, or imperviously backed absorbent paper) used to protect surfaces or equipment from contamination are to be removed and replaced as soon as possible after contamination or at the end of the work shift. Although not specified by OSHA, protective surface covers need to be replaced between patients as discussed in Chapter 13.

All reusable containers that may become contaminated with blood or other potentially infectious materials are to be inspected and decontaminated on a regular schedule and as soon as feasible if visibly contaminated.

Broken glassware that may be contaminated (e.g., an anesthetic capsule or glass beakers used in the ultrasonic cleaner) is not to be picked up directly with the hands. Mechanical means such as tongs, forceps, or a brush and dustpan should be used.

Regulated Waste

The management of regulated waste is described fully in Chapter 17. Several local, state, or federal laws may apply to various aspects of waste management in specific localities. OSHA primarily is concerned with the handling and disposal of contaminated sharps; blood or other potentially infectious materials that are in a liquid, semiliquid, or caked state; and pathologic or microbiologic wastes contaminated with blood or other potentially infectious materials.

Contaminated Sharps

Contaminated sharps (anything that could puncture the skin and contains blood or other potentially infectious materials) are to be placed in containers that are closable, puncture-resistant, and leakproof on the sides and bottom, and color-coded red or marked with a biohazard symbol. These are called sharps containers or sharps boxes. The containers are to be easily accessible and located as close as possible to where sharps are used or may be found (e.g., at chairside and in the sterilizing room). The containers are to be maintained in an upright position (so that the contents do not spill out) and are to be replaced routinely and not allowed to overflow. The containers are to be closed during handling, storage, transport, and shipment. If the outside of the container is contaminated or if the container leaks, the container is to be placed in a second leakproof, puncture-resistant, color-coded or labeled container during handling, storage, transport, or shipping.

Other Regulated Waste

Other regulated waste that is nonsharp (e.g., any item that could release liquid, semiliquid, or caked blood or other potentially infectious materials when compressed, such as a blood- or saliva-saturated gauze square) is to be placed in containers that are leakproof, closable, and color-coded or labeled with a biohazard symbol. An example is a biohazard bag. The containers are to be closed before handling, storage, transport, or shipping, and if the outside of the container is contaminated, the container is to be placed in a second closable, leakproof, color-coded or labeled container that is closed before handling, storage, transport, and shipping.

Contaminated Laundry

Contaminated laundry (e.g., reusable protective clothing, towels, and patient drapes) is to be handled as little as possible with a minimum of agitation. Laundry is not to be bagged, containerized, sorted, or rinsed in the location of use. Contaminated laundry is to be placed and transported in bags or containers that are color-coded or labeled with a biohazard symbol. When a facility uses universal precautions in handling all laundry to be cleaned, alternative labeling is sufficient if it permits all employees to recognize the containers as requiring compliance with universal precautions. If the contaminated laundry is sent off site for cleaning, it must be placed in bags or containers that are color-coded or labeled with a biohazard symbol, unless the laundry uses universal precautions in handling all soiled laundry.

Instrument Sterilization Not Covered by the Occupational Safety and Health Administration

An important area of infection control that is not covered under the OSHA bloodborne pathogens standard is instrument sterilization and associated sterilization monitoring in a clinical setting such as the dental office. These procedures are considered as patient-protection procedures rather than worker-protection procedures. Because OSHA is charged by the U.S. Congress to protect the workers of America, it cannot legally make or enforce rules that relate only to patient protection.

Appropriate procedures for processing reusable dental instruments and handpieces are described in recommendations from important organizations such as the CDC, ADA, OSAP, and AAMI. Several states, including Florida, Indiana, Ohio, Oregon, and Washington, also have passed laws requiring sterilization of all reusable instruments and handpieces between patients and monitoring of sterilization processes. Chapter 12 presents specific details for instrument sterilization and sterilization monitoring.

SUMMARY OF THE CENTERS FOR DISEASE CONTROL AND PREVENTION INFECTION CONTROL RECOMMENDATIONS FOR DENTISTRY

The CDC published its current infection control recommendations for dentistry in 2003. Many of their recommendations are the same as those in OSHA's bloodborne pathogens standard, *so only those that differ from the OSHA rules are summarized here*. Appendix B gives the complete list of the CDC recommendations.

The CDC categorizes each of their recommendations depending on the scientific evidence available to support the recommendation. These categories are included with the recommendations presented in Appendix B.

Personnel Health Elements of an Infection Control Program

A written program is to be prepared that includes policies, procedures, and guidelines for education and training; immunizations; exposure prevention and postexposure management; medical conditions, work-related illness, and associated work restrictions; contact dermatitis and latex hypersensitivity; and maintenance of records, data management, and confidentiality.

Prevention of Transmission of Bloodborne Pathogens

All dental office personnel are to be tested for antibody to hepatitis B surface antigen (HBsAg) 1 to 2 months after completion of the three-dose hepatitis B vaccination. Nonresponders are to receive a second three-dose series of the vaccine and to be retested for antibody to HBsAg. Nonresponders to this second series should be tested for HBsAg (to determine if they are HBV carriers).

Prevention of Exposures to Blood and Other Potentially Infectious Materials

Standard precautions (see the previous discussion under Universal Precautions on p.82) are to be used to protect against exposure to all body fluids, excretions (except sweat), and secretions (e.g., saliva) and against contact with nonintact skin and mucous membranes.

Hand Hygiene

If hands are visibly soiled or contaminated with blood or other potentially infectious material, they are to be washed with a non-antimicrobial or an antimicrobial soap and water. If the hands are not visibly soiled, they can be washed with a non-antimicrobial or an antimicrobial soap and water or can be decontaminated with an alcohol-based hand rub. For oral surgical procedures, before putting on sterile gloves, the hands can be washed with an antimicrobial soap and water and dried with sterile towels, or they can be washed with a non-antimicrobial soap and water, dried, and decontaminated with an alcohol-based hand rub. All liquid hand-care products are to be stored in closed containers that are disposable or can be cleaned, if refilled. When refilling, one should empty the container and wash it rather than adding the lotion or soap to top off the container. This allows for

removal of any contaminants that may have entered the container during use. Hand lotions should be used to prevent skin dryness, but they should be used at the end of the day or not contain petroleum or oil emollients that can affect the integrity of latex gloves. Fingernails are to be kept short (1/4-inch maximum), and artificial nails in general are not recommended. Hand jewelry also is not recommended, if it interferes with the donning of gloves or their fit or integrity.

Personal Protective Equipment

One should clean eyewear and reusable face shields with soap and water, or, if they are visibly soiled, one should clean and disinfect them between patients. One should wear sterile surgeon's gloves when performing surgery. (See the definition of oral surgery below.)

Contact Dermatitis and Latex Hypersensitivity

The CDC indicates that dental office personnel need to be educated about the skin reactions that can occur with frequent hand hygiene and the use of gloves. All patients also should be screened for latex allergy, and a latex-safe environment should be available for patients and office staff with a latex allergy. Latex-free dental and emergency kits are to be available at all times.

Sterilization and Disinfection of Patient Care Items

A central instrument processing area should be designated and divided into (1) receiving, cleaning, and decontamination; (2) preparation and packaging; (3) sterilization; and (4) storage. One should be careful that contaminated instruments are not intermingled with sterile instruments and should minimize the handling of loose contaminated instruments during transport. One should use automated cleaning equipment to clean visible blood and organic material from instruments and devices before sterilization or disinfection procedures. In addition to other barriers, one should wear puncture- and chemical-resistant gloves for instrument cleaning and decontamination procedures. Critical and semicritical instruments are to be packaged and heat sterilized in an FDA-cleared device (sterilizer) before use. Heat-sensitive items can be reprocessed using FDA-cleared liquid sterilants or an FDA low-temperature sterilization method. One should not use liquid sterilants for surface disinfection or as a holding solution.

One should use a container system or packaging material compatible with the type of sterilizer being used and should add an internal chemical indicator to every package. If the internal indicator cannot be seen from the outside, one should add an external indicator to each package. One should monitor each sterilizer load with mechanical monitors (e.g., time, temperature, and pressure) and should use a biologic indicator with a matched control to monitor the sterilizer at least weekly. One should allow packages to dry before removing them from the steam sterilizer.

One should check the integrity of each sterilized package before use and reclean, repackage, and resterilize the instrument, if packaging is torn or compromised in any way. Semicritical instruments that will be used immediately or within a short period of time can be sterilized unwrapped on a tray or in a container system, provided they are handled aseptically during removal from the sterilizer and transport to the point of use. Critical instruments intended for immediate use may be sterilized unwrapped provided that they are maintained sterile during removal from the sterilizer and transport.

In case of a sterilization failure (e.g., positive spore test), one should review the procedures used to determine any operator error. One should take the sterilizer out of service and retest it with mechanical, chemical, and biologic monitors. If the repeat spore test is negative and the mechanical and chemical monitoring are satisfactory, the sterilizer can be put back in service. If not, one should determine the cause of the failure and rechallenge the sterilizer with biological indicators three consecutive times before placing it back into service.

Environmental Infection Control

One should clean and disinfect clinical contact surfaces that are not barrier protected with an EPA-registered low-level (with a label claim against HIV and HBV) or an intermediate-level (has a tuberculocidal claim) hospital disinfectant after each patient. One should use an intermediate-level disinfectant if the surface is visibly contaminated with blood. Walls, floors, and sinks (housekeeping surfaces) are to be cleaned routinely with soap and water or an EPA-registered, low-level, hospital disinfectant. Reusable mop heads and cloths are to be cleaned and allowed to dry after use. Carpeting and cloth-upholstered furnishings in the dental operatory, laboratory, and instrument-processing area are to be avoided.

Dental Unit Water Lines, Biofilms, and Water Quality

One should use water that meets the EPA drinking water standard (no more than 500 colony-forming units [CFU]/mL of heterotrophic bacteria) for routine dental care. One should check with the dental unit manufacturer for appropriate procedures and equipment needed to maintain this water quality and for monitoring the water quality. One should flush the handpiece, air/water syringes, and ultrasonic scalers with water and air for 20 to 30 seconds after each patient before removing them from the water lines. One should maintain antiretraction valves in the dental units, if present.

Boil-Water Notices

One should not use dental unit water or faucet water coming from the public water system during a boil-water notice.

One should use alcohol-based hand rubs rather than an agent requiring water for hand hygiene or should use bottled water or antimicrobial towelettes. One should flush the dental unit water lines and faucets after the boil-water notice is lifted following the local recommendations or for 1 to 5 minutes in the absence of recommendation. One should consider disinfecting the dental unit water lines as recommended by the dental unit manufacturer.

Dental Handpieces and Other Devices Attached to Air and Water Lines

One should follow the manufacturers' instructions to clean and heat-sterilize handpieces and other intraoral instruments (e.g., slow-speed handpiece motors and attachments) that can be removed from the air and water lines of dental units between patients. One should not surface disinfect or use liquid sterilants or ethylene oxide gas on these items. One should not advise patients to close their lips around the tip of saliva ejectors to evacuate oral fluids.

Dental Radiology

One should use heat tolerant or disposable intraoral film-holding or positioning devices whenever possible and should clean and heat-sterilize these devices between patients. One should transport and handle exposed radiographs in an aseptic manner to prevent contamination of developing equipment. For digital radiography sensors, following the manufacturers' directions, one should heat sterilize, cover with an EPA-cleared barrier, treat with a liquid sterilant, or as last resort clean and disinfect with an EPA-registered intermediate-level (tuberculocidal) disinfectant between patients.

Aseptic Technique for Parenteral Medications

One should not administer medication from a syringe to multiple patients even if the needle is changed. One should use single-dose vials of medications when possible and should not combine the leftovers of single-dose vials for later use. If one uses multiple-dose vials, one should clean the access diaphragm with 70% alcohol before inserting a device into the vial. One should use a sterile device (needle and syringe) to enter the vial and should not touch the diaphragm. One should not reuse the syringe. One should keep the multiple-dose vial away from the treatment area to avoid accidental contamination with spray or spatter and should discard the multiple-dose vials if sterility is compromised.

Single-Use (Disposable) Devices

One should use single-use devices for one patient only and should dispose of them appropriately.

Oral Surgical Procedures

When performing oral surgery, one should perform surgical hand antisepsis before donning sterile surgical gloves, washing the hands with an antimicrobial soap and water, and drying them with sterile towels or washing them with a non-antimicrobial soap and water, drying them, and using an alcohol-based hand rub before donning sterile surgical gloves. One should use sterile surgical gloves when performing oral surgical procedures. One should use sterile saline or water as a coolant/irrigator when performing oral surgery using devices specifically designed for delivery of sterile fluids.

The CDC defines oral surgical procedures as "the incision, excision, or reflection of tissue that exposes the normally sterile areas of the oral cavity (e.g., biopsy, periodontal surgery, apical surgery, implant surgery and surgical extraction of teeth such as removal of erupted or non-erupted teeth requiring the elevation of mucoperiosteal flap, removal of bone and/or section of tooth, and suturing, if needed)."

Handling of Extracted Teeth

One should dispose of extracted teeth as regulated medical waste unless they are returned to the patient. One should not dispose of teeth containing amalgam in regulated medical waste intended for incineration. One should clean and place extracted teeth in a leak-proof container labeled with a biohazard symbol and containing an appropriate disinfectant for transport to educational institutions or to a dental laboratory. One should heat-sterilize teeth that do not contain amalgam before they are used for educational purposes.

Dental Laboratory

One should use personal protective equipment when handling items received in the laboratory until they have been decontaminated. One should clean, disinfect, and rinse all dental prostheses and prosthodontic materials (e.g., impressions, bite registrations, occlusal rims, and extracted teeth) using an EPA-registered, intermediate-level (tuberculocidal) hospital disinfectant before they are handled in the laboratory. One should consult with manufacturers regarding the stability of specific materials relative to disinfectant procedures and should include specific information as to the decontamination procedure used when laboratory cases are sent off site and on their return. One should clean and heat sterilize heat-tolerant items used in the mouth including metal impression trays and face-bow forks, following the manufacturers' recommendations for cleaning and sterilizing or disinfecting items that do not normally contact the patient (e.g., burs, polishing points, rag wheels, articulators, case pans, and lathes). If such recommendations are not available, one should clean and heat-sterilize heat-tolerant items or clean and disinfect them with an EPA-registered low- to intermediate-level hospital disinfectant, depending on the degree of contamination.

Mycobacterium Tuberculosis

Appendix C describes the CDC recommendations concerning tuberculosis.

Program Evaluation

Dental offices are to establish a routine evaluation of their infection control programs, including evaluation of performance indicators at an established frequency. (Chapter 25 gives further information on evaluation.)

SELECTED READINGS

American Dental Association: *ADA statement on infection control in dentistry,* http://www.ada.org/1857.aspx. Accessed January, 2012.

American Dental Association: Councils on Scientific Affairs and Dental Practice: Infection control recommendations for the dental office and the dental laboratory, *J Am Dent Assoc* 127:672–680, 1996.

Kohn WG, Collins AS, Cleveland JL, et al: Centers for Disease Control and Prevention: Guideline for infection-control in dental health-care settings–2003, *MMWR Recomm Rep* 52(RR-17):1–61, 2003. (http://www.cdc.gov/mmwr/preview/mmwrhtml/rr5217a1.htm. Accessed January, 2012).

Miller CH: Additions to the OSHA blood-borne pathogens standard, *Am J Dent* 14:186, 2001.

Miller CH: Averting spread of infectious disease, *Dent Prod Rpt* 40:122, 2006.

Miller CH: Complying with OSHA, *Dent Prod Rpt* 40:82, 2007.

Miller CH: Infection control strategies for the dental office. In Ciancio SG, editor: *ADA guide to dental therapeutics,* ed 3, Chicago, 2003, American Dental Association, pp 551–566.

Redd JT, Baumbach J, Kohn W, et al: Patient-to-patient transmission of hepatitis B virus associated with oral surgery, *J Infect Dis* 195:1311–1314, 2007.

US Department of Labor: Occupational Safety and Health Administration: 29 CFR Part 1910.1030: Occupational exposure to blood-borne pathogens: final rule, *Fed Regist* 56:64004–64182, 1991. (actual regulatory text, pp 64175–64182) (http://www.osha.gov/pls/oshaweb/owadisp.show_document?p_table=STANDARDS&p_id=10051. Accessed January, 2012).

US Department of Labor, Occupational Safety and Health Administration: *Controlling occupational exposure to blood-borne pathogens,* OSHA 3127 (revised), Washington, DC, 1996, OSHA.

US Department of Labor, Occupational Safety and Health Administration: *Controlling occupational exposure to blood-borne pathogens in dentistry,* OSHA 3129, Washington, DC, 1992, OSHA.

REVIEW QUESTIONS

Multiple Choice

1. Which governmental agency controls the safety and effectiveness of sterilizers?
   a. Food and Drug Administration
   b. Environmental Protection Agency
   c. Occupational Safety and Health Administration
   d. Centers for Disease Control and Prevention

2. Which governmental agency requires employers to protect their employees from exposure to blood and saliva at work?
   a. Food and Drug Administration
   b. Environmental Protection Agency
   c. Occupational Safety and Health Administration
   d. Centers for Disease Control and Prevention

3. Which governmental agency controls the safety and effectiveness of surface disinfectants?
   a. Food and Drug Administration
   b. Environmental Protection Agency
   c. Occupational Safety and Health Administration
   d. Centers for Disease Control and Prevention

4. Not doing a good job cleaning or sterilizing reusable hand instruments contributes to which pathway of cross-contamination in the office?
   a. Patient to dental team
   b. Dental team to patient
   c. Patient to patient
   d. Community to office

5. Improving the quality of dental unit water addresses which pathway of cross-contamination in the office?
   a. Community to office
   b. Dental team to patient
   c. Patient to dental team

6. The goal of dental infection control is to:
   a. eliminate all microbes in the office
   b. prevent all pathogenic microbes from entering the office
   c. sterilize all operatory surfaces between patients
   d. reduce the dose of microorganisms that may be shared between individuals

7. Which of the following is the infection control education organization in dentistry?
   a. Association for Advancement of Medical Instrumentation
   b. Organization for Safety and Asepsis Procedures
   c. Occupational Safety and Health Administration
   d. Environmental Protection Agency

8. Which of the following infection control procedures is not covered by the bloodborne pathogens standard?
   a. Wearing a surgical mask at chairside during patient care
   b. Wearing gloves during instrument processing and operatory cleanup
   c. Handwashing
   d. Cleaning and sterilizing reusable hand instruments between patients

9. According to the bloodborne pathogens standard, who pays for employee training and hepatitis B immunization?
   a. The employee
   b. The employee's insurance company
   c. The employer

10. The Centers for Disease Control and Prevention guidelines for infection control in dentistry:
    a. cover more topics than the bloodborne pathogens standard
    b. are identical to the bloodborne pathogens standard
    c. have not been updated since 1993
    d. say nothing about instrument sterilization

Please visit http://evolve.elsevier.com/Miller/infectioncontrol/ for additional practice and study support tools.

Immunization

OUTLINE

LEARNING OBJECTIVES

After completing this chapter, the student should be able to do the following:

1. State the importance of immunization in the health care field and identify vaccine-preventable diseases.
2. Describe the diagnosis, microbiology, onset and symptoms, and immunization and boosters of tetanus.
3. List the types of influenza, symptoms, process of influenza vaccinations, and the CDC recommendations for influenza vaccinations.
4. Discuss how hepatitis is transmitted, the occupational hazards of hepatitis B, and the importance and process of hepatitis B vaccinations.
5. Discuss the risks associated with missing important vaccines.

KEY TERMS

HBV Vaccination

Immunization

Influenza

Tetanus

Tetanus Toxoid

Vaccines

Health care is the second-fastest growing sector of the American economy. In the United States, an estimated 12 million persons work in the health care industry. Approximately 6.5 million persons are employed in the nation's 6000 hospitals. However, a significant portion of health care that in the past was provided only in hospitals now occurs in offices, freestanding clinics (e.g., surgery and emergency care clinics), nursing homes, and many dental specialty offices (e.g., oral surgery, periodontics, and endodontics). Health care workers in hospitals and at offsite locations are at risk for the occupational acquisition of infectious diseases. After infection, disease could be spread to patients, coworkers, household members, and possibly to the community at large.

Ensuring that dental personnel are immune to vaccine-preventable diseases is an essential part of a successful infection control plan. Optimal use of vaccines can prevent transmission of disease and can help eliminate unnecessary work restrictions. Vaccination prevents illness and is far more cost-effective than individual case management or outbreak control.

Compliance with a vaccination scheme is known to be greater when the program is mandatory rather than voluntary.

When the employer pays for the vaccinations, compliance is known to be significantly higher than if the employees must pay all or part of their immunization costs.

The types of health care provided, characteristics of the patient pool, and the age and experience of the health care workers influence the decision as to which vaccines should be included in an immunization program. In some cases, screening can help determine susceptibility to certain vaccine-preventable diseases. Hepatitis B is an example.

Dental personnel are exposed daily to a variety of communicable diseases present in their work environments. Protection is best afforded through the use of engineering and work practice controls. Also, personal protective equipment/barriers such as gloves, masks, gowns, and protective eyewear help prevent the majority of cross-infections. However, when immunization is available, it is the most effective method to reduce the chances of disease acquisition. Maintenance of immunity is an essential component of any effective infection control program. Current Occupational Safety and Health Administration (OSHA) standards require certain immunization records to be maintained for all at-risk employees.

Unfortunately, vaccines do not exist for all diseases. Important "missing vaccines" for dentistry in the United States include immunization against hepatitis C, human immunodeficiency virus (HIV) type 1, tuberculosis, and some forms of human herpesviruses.

To have the most effective and efficient office/clinic infection control program, personnel health elements must be an essential component. In addition, immunization, education and training, postexposure management, identification of medical conditions, work-related illnesses and work restriction, maintenance of records, data management, and confidentiality are important components.

Immunizations (including screenings and postexposure prophylaxis in some cases) must be combined with other elements to provide the best level of protection to health care workers. Occupational risk assessment and management, personnel health and safety education, and the proper handling of job-related illnesses and exposures are essential. Proper record keeping and data management help generate valuable information, which report the vaccination histories of the personnel and could aid in the investigation and analysis of job-related illnesses and injuries.

This chapter reviews tetanus, influenza, and hepatitis B in depth. Other vaccine-preventable diseases, however, are presented only for review in Table 9-1.

TETANUS

Tetanus ("lockjaw") is a severe disease with a high case-to-fatality ratio. Tetanus in the United States is primarily a disease of older adults, who usually are unvaccinated or are poorly vaccinated. Tetanus can be an infectious complication of any cut or puncture wound and is caused by the toxins (tetanospasmins) of *Clostridium tetani*. Proliferation of the implanted bacilli under the anaerobic conditions present in deep wounds can result in the production of the tetanospasmins.

Tetanus is usually a clinical diagnosis based on acute onset of hypertonia or painful muscular contractions (usually of the muscles of the jaw and neck first) and generalized muscle spasms. Death is often an expected outcome of infection. However, other medical problems must be ruled out first by physical and serological examination.

Worldwide, tetanus is an important disease. In many developing countries, aseptic perinatal care and vaccination schemes are suboptimal. The result is an unacceptably high infant mortality rate. In contrast, tetanus has become rare in the United States. For example, in 1947, when reporting of tetanus started, there were 560 cases. Tetanus immunization became widely available in the mid-1940s. During the period from 1991 to 1994, the Centers for Disease Control and Prevention (CDC) received notification of 201 cases. The impact of vaccination can be appreciated through a comparison of the 560 cases in 1947 to the 35 reported cases in 2001. Fifteen percent of the cases proved fatal.

Only two cases of neonatal tetanus have been reported in the United States since 1992. Worldwide, however, an estimated 600,000 annual deaths can be attributed to neonatal tetanus. Cases involving older adults who had never been vaccinated, were vaccinated improperly, or had not received booster injections are also common worldwide.

Tetanus endospores are present in the environment continually, and because they are resistant to disinfection procedures, control of their spread requires an overt effort. Meticulous handling of all wounds and the monitoring of immune status are essential. Chemoprophylaxis against tetanus is neither practical nor useful in the management of wounds.

Tetanus is a preventable disease. Tetanus toxoid (inactivated toxin) usually is given as part of a triple childhood immunization that includes diphtheria and acellular pertussis (Tdap) vaccines. The initial Tdap vaccine may be given as early as 6 weeks of age but always before the age of 7 years. A common regimen includes injections given at 2, 4, and 6 months. At least a 4-week interval must be allowed between each injection. A fourth dose is recommended at 15 to 18 months. The vaccine is designed to maintain protection during preschool years.

The scheme for boosters is straightforward and includes an injection when a child is 4 to 6 years old (which will protect through most of the school years). Another booster can be given when the child is 11 to 12 years old, if 5 years have elapsed since the last injection. If wounds are minor and uncontaminated, the CDC Advisory Committee on Immunization Practices recommends that boosters need be given only every 10 years. Efficacy is considered to be nearly 100%.

Routine tetanus booster immunization, usually combined with diphtheria toxoid, is recommended for all persons older than the age of 7 years. Traumatic injury (large, extensive wounds exposed to soil and bacterial spores) may necessitate the earlier application of a booster. Arthus-type hypersensitivity reactions to the tetanus toxoid are known, as well as adverse effects for those in their first trimester of pregnancy and for individuals who have a history of neurologic reaction or immediate hypersensitivity.

Many wounds, especially when received during the summer (when greater numbers of viable bacilli are present in the soil), can transmit organisms more readily. However, the injured often decide not to visit a physician's office or hospital for examination and possible treatment.

Protection against tetanus is based on the establishment and maintenance of adequate tetanus antitoxin levels and is achieved only through proper primary and routine booster injections. One should discuss the need for vaccination regularly with one's primary health care provider.

INFLUENZA

Influenza (the flu) is an acute respiratory disease caused by influenza type A or type B virus. Incubation ranges from 1 to 4 days. Maximum viral shedding occurs 1 day before the onset of symptoms and for the first 3 days of clinical illness.

TABLE 9-1 Strongly Recommended Immunobiologicals and Immunization Schedules for Dental Health Care Personnel

Generic Name	Primary Schedule and Booster(s)	Indications	Major Precautions and Contraindications	Special Considerations
Hepatitis B recombinant vaccine for adults	Two doses IM 4 weeks apart; third dose 5 months after the second; booster doses not necessary; doses administered IM in the deltoid	Preexposure process for those at risk of exposure to blood and body fluids	No apparent adverse effects to developing fetuses; not contraindicated in pregnancy; previous anaphylaxis to common baker's yeast is a contraindication	No therapeutic or adverse effect on HBV-infected persons; prevaccination screening is not indicated for persons being vaccinated because of occupational risk; postscreening for serologic response should be performed 1-2 months after completion of the series
Hepatitis B immune globulin	0.06 mL/kg IM as soon as possible after exposure (but no later than 7 days after exposure); a second dose should be administered 1 month later if the HBV vaccine series has not been started	Postexposure prophylaxis for persons exposed to blood or body fluids containing HBV surface antigen and who are not immune to HBV infection		
Influenza vaccine (TIV and LAIV)	Annual single-dose vaccination IM with current vaccine	All DHCP	History of anaphylactic hypersensitivity after egg ingestion; prior reaction to the vaccine	No evidence of maternal or fetal risk when vaccine was given to pregnant women with underlying conditions that render them at high risk for serious influenza complications; vaccination is recommended during second and third trimesters of pregnancy; LAIV is recommended only for healthy nonpregnant persons ages 2-49 years; health care workers caring for immunocompromised patients should receive TIV rather than LAIV
Measles live virus vaccine	One dose SC; second dose at least 1 month later	Vaccination recommended for all who lack presumptive evidence of immunity; vaccination should be considered for those born before 1957	Pregnancy; immunocompromised persons with severe immunosuppression; history of anaphylactic reactions after gelatin ingestion or receipt of neomycin or recent receipt of immune globulin	MMR[†] is the vaccine of choice if recipient is also likely to be susceptible to rubella and/or mumps; persons vaccinated between 1963 and 1967 with (1) a killed measles vaccine alone, (2) a killed measles vaccine followed by live vaccine, or (3) a vaccine of unknown type should be revaccinated with two doses of live measles vaccine
Mumps live virus vaccine	Two doses SC approximately 28 days apart	Vaccination recommended for all who lack presumptive evidence of immunity; vaccination should be considered for those born before 1957	Pregnancy; immunocompromised persons with severe immunosuppression; history of anaphylactic reactions after gelatin ingestion or receipt of neomycin	MMR[†] is the vaccine of choice if recipient is also likely to be susceptible to measles or rubella

Continued

TABLE 9-1   Strongly Recommended Immunobiologicals and Immunization Schedules for Dental Health Care Personnel—cont'd

Generic Name	Primary Schedule and Booster(s)	Indications	Major Precautions and Contraindications	Special Considerations
Rubella live virus vaccine	One dose SC; (however, because of the 2-dose requirements for measles and mumps vaccines, the use of MMR vaccine will result in most DHCP receiving 2 doses of rubella-containing vaccine)	Vaccination recommended for all who lack presumptive evidence of immunity	Pregnancy; immunocompromised state* including HIV-infected persons with severe immunosuppression; history of anaphylactic reactions after gelatin ingestion or receipt of neomycin	The risk for rubella vaccine-associated malformations in the offspring of women pregnant when vaccinated or who become pregnant within 1 month after vaccination is negligible; such women should be counseled regarding the theoretical basis of concern for the fetus
Varicella-zoster live virus vaccine	Two 0.5-mL doses SC, 4-8 weeks apart if ≥13 years of age	DHCP without reliable history of varicella or laboratory evidence of varicella immunity	Pregnancy; immunocompromised state*; history of anaphylactic reaction after receipt of neomycin or gelatin; salicylate use should be avoided for 6 weeks after vaccination	Because 71%-93% of persons without a history of varicella are immune, serological testing before vaccination may be cost-effective
Varicella-zoster immune globulin (VZIG)	The recommended dose is 125 units per 10 kg (22 lbs) body weight, up to a maximum of 625 units; the minimum dose is 125 units	Persons known or likely to be susceptible (especially those at high risk for complications, such as pregnant women) who have close and prolonged exposure to a contact case or to an infectious coworker or patient		Serological testing may help in assessing whether to administer VZIG; if use of VZIG prevents disease, person should be vaccinated subsequently
Tetanus and diphtheria (Td; toxoids) and acellular pertussis (Tdap)	1 dose IM as soon as feasible if Tdap not already received and regardless of interval from last Td; after receipt of Tdap, receive Td for routine booster every 10 years	All DHCP regardless of age	History of serious allergic reaction (i.e., anaphylaxis) to any component in Tdap; because of the importance of tetanus vaccination, persons with a history of anaphylaxis to components in Tdap or Td should be referred to an allergist to determine whether they have a specific allergy to tetanus toxoid (TT) and can safely receive TT vaccine; persons with a history of encephalopathy (e.g., coma or prolonged seizures) not attributable to an identifiable cause within 7 days of administration of a vaccine with pertussis components should receive Td instead of Tdap	Tetanus prophylaxis in wound management if not yet received Tdap

Modified from Advisory Committee on Immunization Practices; Centers for Disease Control and Prevention.: Immunization of health-care personnel, *MMWR Recomm Rep* 60(RR-7):1-45, 2011 (http://www.cdc.gov/mmwr/preview/mm wrhtml/rr6007a1.htm?s_cid=rr6007a1_e; accessed April 2012); Kohn WG, Collins AS, Cleveland JL, et al; Centers for Disease Control and Prevention: Guideline for infection control in dental health-care settings–2003, *MMWR Recomm Rep* 52(RR-17):65, 2003; and Centers for Disease Control and Prevention: *Tetanus.* http://www.cdc.gov/nip/publications/pink/tetanus.pdf, accessed May 2004.
Abbreviations: DHCP, Dental health care personnel; HBV, hepatitis B virus; HIV, human immunodeficiency virus; IM, intramuscularly; LAIV, live attenuated influenza vaccine; MMR, measles-mumps-rubella vaccine; SC, subcutaneously; TIV, trivalent inactivated split-virus vaccine.
*Persons immunocompromised because of immune deficiencies; infection with human immunodeficiency virus, leukemia, lymphoma, generalized malignancy, or immunosuppressive therapy with corticosteroids, alkylating drugs, antimetabolites, or radiation.
†The Advisory Committee on Immunization Practices recommends that the combined measles-mumps-rubella vaccine be used when any of the individual components is indicated.

Typical features of influenza include an abrupt onset of fever, coryza, a sore throat, and a nonproductive cough. Also commonly present are systemic symptoms such as headache, muscle aches, and extreme fatigue. The flu often can be confused with the common cold (Table 9-2).

Unlike other common respiratory infections, influenza can cause extreme malaise for several days. More severe disease can result if viruses invade the lungs (primary viral pneumonia) or if a secondary bacterial pneumonia occurs. Complications (including hospitalization and even death) are most common among older adults and individuals with chronic health problems such as cardiopulmonary disease. Acute symptoms usually last for 2 to 4 days. However, malaise and cough may persist for up to 2 weeks.

Influenza is transmitted via aerosolized or droplet transmission from the respiratory tract of infected persons. A less important mode of transmission is by direct contact with contaminated items. Maximum communicability occurs 1 to 2 days before the onset of symptoms to 4 to 5 days thereafter. Flu season runs from November through April in the United States with a peak of activity from late December through the end of March.

Influenza causes epidemics of severe illness and life-threatening complications almost every winter. Flu epidemics affect 10% to 20% of the population and are associated with an average of 36,000 deaths and 114,000 hospitalizations in the United States. More than 90% of deaths involve persons age 65 years and older. However, more than 50% of infections requiring a hospital stay involve persons younger than the age of 65 years. The economic impact of a severe epidemic in the United States could approach $15 billion.

Two measures available in the United States are capable of reducing the impact of influenza. These are immunoprophylaxis with vaccines and chemoprophylaxis or chemotherapy. Although antiviral drugs are available, chemoprophylaxis cannot be considered a substitute for vaccination.

Because the influenza viruses change frequently, new influenza vaccines are developed annually two times a year, one for the Northern hemisphere's flu season (November to April) and one for the Southern hemisphere's flu season (May to October). These trivalent vaccines consist of the three strains of influenza viruses (two type As and one type B) that are most likely to cause disease that season. For example, the 2011-2012 vaccine protected against an influenza H3N2 type A virus, an influenza B virus, and the H1N1 type A virus that emerged in 2009 to cause a pandemic.

There are now two types of trivalent influenza vaccines available. One is an inactivated (killed) influenza vaccine administered as a single dose intramuscularly, and the other is a live attenuated (weakened) influenza vaccine (LAIV) administered intranasally.

Individuals at high risk for influenza complications, such as persons age 50 years or older, especially those in long-term care facilities or with a serious chronic disease, should be vaccinated each year. Other individuals who are clinically or subclinically infected and who live with, attend, or treat high-risk persons can transmit the virus.

The CDC recommends that all health care workers be vaccinated annually against influenza with either the inactivated influenza vaccine or LAIV. This preventive approach will help eliminate the spread of the influenza virus from health care workers to their patients. LAIV is approved for use only among nonpregnant healthy people ages 5 years to 49 years. Health care workers who work with severely immunocompromised patients who require a protected environment should not receive LAIV. Inactivated influenza vaccine is approved for all persons older than age 6 months who lack vaccine contraindications, including those with high-risk conditions. LAIV is contraindicated for:

- Persons younger than 5 years of age or older than 50 years of age (these persons should receive the inactivated influenza vaccine)
- Persons with asthma, reactive airways disease, or other chronic disorders of the pulmonary or cardiovascular systems
- Persons with other underlying medical conditions, including metabolic diseases such as diabetes, renal dysfunction, and hemoglobinopathies
- Persons with known or suspected immunodeficiency diseases or who are receiving immunosuppressive therapies (these persons should receive the inactivated influenza vaccine)

TABLE 9-2   Differences Between a Cold and the Flu

	Cold	Flu
SYMPTOMS		
Onset	Protracted	Sudden
Fever	Rare	As high 40° C (104° F)
Headache	Rare	Prominent
General aches/pains	Slight	Common, even severe
Fatigue/weakness	Mild	Can last 2-3 weeks
Extreme exhaustion	Never	Early and prominent
Stuffy nose	Common	Sometimes
Sneezing	Usual	Sometimes
Sore throat	Common	Sometimes
Chest discomfort	Mild/moderate	Common, maybe severe
Cough	Hacking	Common
Complications	Sinus congestion and earache	Bronchitis, pneumonia; can be life-threatening
Prevention	None	Annual vaccination and antiviral medications
Treatment	Temporary relief of symptoms	Antiviral medications

- Children or adolescents receiving aspirin or other salicylates (because of the association of Reye syndrome with wild-type influenza infection) (these persons should receive the inactivated influenza vaccine)
- Persons with a history of Guillain-Barré syndrome (GBS)
- Pregnant women (these persons should receive the inactivated influenza vaccine)
- Persons who have close contact with severely immunosuppressed persons (e.g., patients with hematopoietic stem cell transplants) during those periods in which the immunosuppressed person requires care in a protective environment
- Persons with a history of hypersensitivity, including anaphylaxis, to any of the components of LAIV or to eggs

Specific recommendations from the CDC for influenza vaccination of persons who have or report a history of egg allergy are given at http://www.cdc.gov/mmwr/preview/mmwrhtml/mm6033a3.htm.

When properly administered, the influenza vaccine produces high levels of protective antibodies in most children and young adults. Some elderly recipients, especially those with chronic diseases (e.g., pulmonary or cardiovascular system diseases, diabetes mellitus, renal dysfunction, or immune suppression, even when caused by medication) develop lower postvaccination antibody titers and may remain susceptible to infection. However, current information indicates that 70% to 80% of healthy persons younger than age 65 years are protected to the point that they will not become ill.

Because the influenza viruses used in the vaccines are grown in eggs, the vaccine should not be given to persons known to have anaphylactic hypersensitivity to eggs or some component of the vaccine without first consulting a physician. In some cases, the physician may attempt desensitization.

Annual vaccination of persons at high risk (and their close contacts) for influenza-associated complications is the most effective means of reducing the impact of influenza. Because influenza viruses undergo regular antigenic shifts, vaccination must be repeated annually. The vaccine from last year may have little to no preventive ability against the prevailing influenza viruses this year. One should discuss regularly the need and regimen for vaccination with one's primary health care provider.

HEPATITIS B

The hepatitis B virus (HBV) is an infectious agent associated with acute and chronic inflammation of the liver. Worldwide, HBV is a major cause of necrotizing vasculitis, cirrhosis, and primary hepatocellular carcinoma. HBV is found primarily in blood and blood products, but also can be present in other body fluids, such as semen, tears, feces, urine, vaginal secretions, and saliva.

As discussed in Chapter 6, HBV is a bloodborne pathogen transmitted by percutaneous or mucosal exposure (e.g., intravenous drug abuse and needlestick accidents by health care workers), by sexual contact, and from mother to fetus or infant. HBV is environmentally stable, especially when surrounded by blood. This stability allows for the potential of indirect transmission such as contact with contaminated instruments.

Hepatitis B is one of the most frequently reported vaccine-preventable diseases in the United States. Each year between 15,000 and 20,000 cases of acute hepatitis B are reported. However, many persons with acute infections are asymptomatic, and many cases of symptomatic disease are not reported. Only 30% to 50% of cases have clinical symptoms indicating infection.

The CDC estimates that approximately 1000 health care workers occupationally acquired hepatitis B in 1994. This represents a 90% decline since 1985. The decrease is attributable to the use of vaccine and adherence to other preventive measures (e.g., universal and standard precautions).

Chronic HBV infection is defined as the presence of HBV viral markers in serum for at least 6 months. Risk of developing chronic infection is age dependent and is greatest for infants infected at birth (90% probability). Overall, 30% to 50% of children and 4% to 10% of adults with acute infections will develop chronic infections. Chronicity increases dramatically the chances for HBV transmission, cirrhosis, delta hepatitis virus infections, and the development of primary hepatocellular carcinoma. Approximately 1.25 million persons in the United States are estimated to be infected chronically.

Hepatitis B is a major occupational hazard for dental personnel, with attack rates among unvaccinated individuals 3 to 10 times the 4% rate present in the general population. Hepatitis B is an especially difficult problem because many dental workers have repeated intimate contact with patient body fluids and with items soiled with such fluids. HBV infection appears to be related more to the extent of exposure to blood than to the number or type of patients treated.

Personal protective barriers cannot eliminate all body fluid exposures, especially sharps injuries. Therefore the best protection against HBV infection is immunization. Two single antigen vaccines are available in the Unites States: Recombivax HB (Merck & Co., Whitehouse Station, NJ) and Engerix-B (GlaxoSmithKline Biologicals, Rixensart, Belgium). Three combination vaccines are available. One (Twinrix, GlaxoSmithKline Biologicals) is used to vaccinate adults, and two (Comvax, Merck & Co. and Pediarix, GlaxoSmithKline) are used to vaccinate infants and young children. Twinrix contains the hepatitis B surface antigen (HBsAg) and inactivated hepatitis A virus. Comvax immunizes against hepatitis B and invasive disease caused by *Haemophilus influenzae* type b (Hib). Pediarix vaccinates against hepatitis B, diphtheria, pertussis, and tetanus.

The most common adult vaccine regimen consists of three 1.0 mL doses with the second dose given 1 month after the first and the third dose 5 months after the second (see Table 9-1). Vaccination of infants (often in the delivery hospital) is common. The goals are to vaccinate at a very young age (which usually positively influences seroconversion rates) and to attempt to prevent perinatal infection from an infected mother.

Injections of the adult hepatitis B vaccine given in the deltoid muscle have produced seroconversion rates from 95% to 97% in immunocompetent, seronegative younger adults. Lower conversion rates are noted in persons older than 40 years of age, smokers, those who are overweight, and individuals who received injections in the buttocks (as low as 70% seroconversion). Recent studies indicate that genetic factors may influence seroconversion rates significantly.

All at-risk dental personnel need to be vaccinated, including clinicians, laboratory workers, and associated cleanup crews. A person such as an office receptionist may be considered as not being at risk. However, many dental offices practice multitasking because when an emergency or special patient need arises, "office workers" temporarily participate in chairside dentistry.

Unless one has some reason to suspect infection, serological screening before vaccination is not recommended. Complete protection against HBV, however, does include postscreening for antibody (anti-HBsAg) levels. This procedure should be conducted 1 to 2 months after completion of the three-dose vaccination series. If seroconversion occurs after vaccination, protective levels of antibodies have been shown to persist for at least 23 years. If a vaccine recipient fails to seroconvert, the person should, according to the CDC, receive a second series of three injections and be retested. If no response to the second three-dose series occurs, nonresponders should be tested for HBsAg, the presence of which would indicate a hepatitis B carrier state or current infection. One characteristic of a chronic HBV infection is a person's inability to produce a defensive antibody response to HBV.

The need for a booster injection still is debated. The CDC currently does not recommend boosters. This recommendation, however, is based on a proper immune response to vaccination verified through serological postscreening. The antibody levels of thousands of individuals will have to be measured for a period of years before a booster recommendation can be made. However, if an individual was vaccinated more than 5 years ago and was not evaluated serologically at that time, the best course probably would be to give a single injection and then determine the antibody titer of this person. However, one's personal physician should be consulted first over all other recommendations.

Compliance with HBV vaccination among health care workers has not been universal. Concerns expressed include vaccine safety, cost, efficacy, pregnancy-related issues, lack of information on the vaccine, and consideration of oneself to be at low risk. Hospital studies indicate that vaccination levels improve greatly when the employer pays the cost of the series. National studies show that dentists (more than 98% have been vaccinated or have been infected) are among health care worker groups with the highest rates of vaccination. Similar levels of compliance are noted for dental hygienists, with lower vaccination rates for dental assistants.

Despite the presence of a proven occupational risk and the availability of safe and effective vaccines, not all at-risk health care workers have been vaccinated. Health care workers have not been vaccinated universally for several reasons. Some still question the safety and efficacy of the vaccine. The vaccine has been shown to produce only minimal side effects. The most common complaints include transient injection site soreness and redness, headache, and fever. Individuals with severe allergies to yeast or iodine (the preservative in the vaccines) must consult their physicians before vaccination, as should individuals with pregnancy-related concerns. Another major noncompliance factor is the cost of the vaccine series ($150 to $200). The bloodborne pathogens standard of the Occupational Safety and Health Administration (29 CFR Section 1910.1030, Occupational Exposure to Bloodborne Pathogens, Final Rule, December 6, 1991) specifically recognizes the important occupational hazard that HBV presents for health care workers (see Chapter 6, Appendix H, and Box 9-1). The rule involves several employer and employee performance functions. Employers must assume all costs associated with HBV vaccination. Employees have the right to refuse vaccination. However, the employee must read and sign a declination statement. The wording must be as described in the standard. Figure 9-1 is a copy of the necessary statement.

RISK OF MISSING AN IMPORTANT OPPORTUNITY

Immunization programs have been successful in preventing diseases among children. However, most of us are not aware of the continuing need for vaccinations during adulthood. An important number of vaccine-preventable diseases occur today in the adult population. Anyone who passes through childhood without immunization or infection is at risk. Many diseases are considerably more severe when contracted as an adult. The occupations or social behaviors of adults also increase the chances of disease acquisition.

In addition to immunization against influenza, tetanus, and hepatitis B, dental personnel should discuss with their primary health care providers their immune status to other vaccine-preventable diseases. These diseases include hepatitis A, pneumococcal pneumonia, measles, rubella, mumps, and poliomyelitis. Also, whenever possible, dental personnel should make themselves available for disease screenings. Persons are screened regularly for cholesterol and blood sugar levels, blood pressure, the presence of blood in feces, and heart rate. Screenings for infectious diseases also exist. Some screenings are serologic, for example, antibody testing for hepatitides B and C, HIV, and herpesviruses. Other screenings include external monitoring for pathogen exposure; the most important of these is an annual interdermal Mantoux tuberculin skin test.

BOX 9-1

Occupational Safety and Health Administration Bloodborne Pathogens Standard (29 CFR Section 1910.1030) Hepatitis B Vaccination Performance Standards

1. The employer shall make employees aware of their occupational risk for hepatitis B through formal training.
2. The employer shall inform all at-risk employees (except those already properly vaccinated, those shown to be immune, or those for whom the vaccine is medically contraindicated) of the presence of a hepatitis B vaccine and shall make it available within 10 working days of their initial assignment. The employer shall provide information on the vaccine, including the vaccine's efficacy, safety, method of administration, the benefits of being vaccinated, and the assurance that all medical records concerning the vaccination process will be kept confidential.
3. The employer may not require the employee to be serologically prescreened prior to receiving the vaccine.
4. Any employee may decline the vaccine, but if still covered by the Standard at a later date may request to be vaccinated. Employees who decline must sign the Hepatitis B Vaccine Declination form.
5. All vaccinations must be performed under the supervision of a physician, be given in a manner according to current U.S. Public Health Service procedures, be made available at a reasonable time and place, and be of no cost to the employee. The supervising physician shall provide the employee with written assurance that the vaccination was necessary and provided in the proper manner.
6. If in the future the U.S. Public Health Service recommends booster injections, the employer shall make such boosters available.
7. Laboratory costs associated with postscreening for seroconversion will be paid by the employer.
8. The employer must maintain all medical records (e.g., dates of vaccination and laboratory serology results) concerning an employee's hepatitis B vaccination processes for the duration of employment plus 30 years.

OSHA Bloodborne Pathogens Standard (29CFR 1910.1030) Hepatitis B Vaccine Declination

I understand that due to my occupational exposure to blood and other potentially infectious material, I may be at risk of acquiring hepatitis B virus (HBV) infection. I have been given the opportunity to be vaccinated with hepatitis B vaccine, at no charge to myself. However, I decline hepatitis B vaccination at this time. I understand that by declining this vaccine, I continue to be at risk of acquiring hepatitis B, a serious disease. If in the future I continue to have occupational exposure to blood or other potentially infectious materials and I want to be vaccinated with hepatitis B vaccine, I can receive the vaccination series at no charge to me.

_____   _____
Employee signature   Date

_____   _____
Witness signature   Date

FIGURE 9-1 Employee declination statement.

SELECTED READINGS

American Dental Association: Council on Scientific Affairs and Council on Dental Practice: Infection control recommendations for the dental office and the dental laboratory, *J Am Dent Assoc* 127:672–680, 1996.

Centers for Disease Control and Prevention, Advisory Committee on Immunization Practices: *General recommended on immunization practices.* http://www.cdc.gov/mmwr/preview/mmwrhtml/rr6002a1.htm?s_cid=rr6002a1_e. Accessed April 2012.

Centers for Disease Control and Prevention: Prevention and control of influenza with vaccines: recommendations of the Advisory Committee on Immunization Practices (ACIP), 2011, *MMWR Morb Mortal Wkly Rep* 60(33):1128–1132, 2011. (http://www.cdc.gov/mmwr/preview/mmwrhtml/mm6033a3.htm. Accessed April 2012).

Centers for Disease Control and Prevention: *Seasonal influenza vaccination resources for health professionals.* http://www.cdc.gov/flu/professionals/vaccination/index.htm. Accessed April 2012.

Centers for Disease Control and Prevention: *Tetanus.* http://www.cdc.gov/vaccines/pubs/pinkbook/downloads/tetanus.pdf. Accessed April 2012.

Centers for Disease Control and Prevention: *Viral hepatitis.* http://www.cdc.gov/ncidod/diseases/hepatitis/index.htm. Accessed April 2012.

Cottone JA, Puttaiah R: Hepatitis virus infection: current status in dentistry, *Dent Clin North Am* 40(2):293–307, 1996.

Kohn WG, Collins AS, Cleveland JL, et al: Centers for Disease Control and Prevention: Guideline for infection control in dental health-care settings–2003, *MMWR Recomm Rep* 52(RR-17):1–61, 2003.

Miller CH, Palenik CJ: Sterilization, disinfection and asepsis in dentistry. In Block S, editor: *Sterilization, disinfection, preservation and sanitation*, ed 5, Philadelphia, 2001, Lippincott Williams & Wilkins, pp. 1049–1068.

Occupational Health and Safety Administration: Occupational exposure to bloodborne pathogens, final rule, 29 CFR Section 1910.1030, *Fed Regist* 56:64175–64182, 1991.

Palenik CJ: The flu season, *RDH* 23(86):88, 2003.

Palenik CJ: HIV/AIDS–thirty years on, *Dent Asep Rev* 32(8):1–2, 2011.

REVIEW QUESTIONS

Multiple Choice

1. A preventive vaccine is available in the United States against:
   a. human immunodeficiency virus
   b. hepatitis C
   c. tuberculosis
   d. tetanus

2. Usually, adults need to receive the tetanus vaccine every _____ years.
   a. 3
   b. 5
   c. 10
   d. 15
   e. 25

3. The influenza vaccine is given:
   a. three times within a given year
   b. once a year
   c. every 2 years
   d. once every 5 years

4. In what month should health care workers receive the influenza vaccine?
   a. September
   b. October
   c. November
   d. December
   e. January

5. The costs associated with hepatitis B vaccination of at-risk employees are:
   a. the responsibility of the employees themselves
   b. to be paid for by the employer
   c. usually covered by a grant from the Occupational Safety and Health Administration
   d. paid by most health insurance policies

6. Which of the following is a killed or attenuated viral vaccine?
   a. Measles
   b. Influenza
   c. Varicella-zoster
   d. Rubella
   e. Mumps

Please visit http://evolve.elsevier.com/Miller/infectioncontrol/ for additional practice and study support tools.

Hand Hygiene

OUTLINE

Hands and Disease Spread
Protective Value of Hand Hygiene
Hand Hygiene Agents

Hand Hygiene Procedures
Properties of Hand Hygiene Agents
Other Hand Hygiene Considerations

LEARNING OBJECTIVES

After completing this chapter, the student should be able to do the following:

1. Describe how the hands are a means of disease spread and differentiate between resident and transient skin flora.
2. Describe the types of products available for hand hygiene and their uses.

3. Describe the procedures for hand hygiene and when hand hygiene should be performed.
4. List properties to consider when selecting hand hygiene products and other hand hygiene considerations.

KEY TERMS

Alcohol-based Hand Rubs
Hand Hygiene

Handwashing
Resident Skin Flora

Transient Skin Flora

Normal human skin is colonized with bacteria. For example, there may be a million aerobic bacteria per square centimeter (cm: about the size of the nail on your little finger) on your scalp, approximately half a million/cm^2 in the axilla, approximately 4000/cm^2 on your abdomen, and approximately 1000/cm^2 on your forearm. Total bacteria on the hands of medical personnel have been shown to be as high as half a million, and numerous studies have shown that these hand microbes can be easily spread to others unless hand hygiene is performed.

Close your eyes for a moment, and think: How many surfaces have you touched today? Essentially every one of those surfaces contains microbes, be they environmental or on your body or on someone else's body. Microbes are ubiquitous. Did you scratch your neck, rub your eye, push back your hair, clean your teeth with your fingernail, bite your nails, rub your nose, or wipe your mouth? Did you pet the dog or cat or contact common house surfaces such as a bathroom hand towel, doorknobs, drawer pulls, flush handles, refrigerator door handle, telephone, or remote control?

These activities are a part of our normal everyday life, and usually cause no problems if we use proper hand hygiene

throughout the day, particularly before we touch food, eat, apply makeup, put on contact lenses, or do other things that transfer microbes from our hands to our mucous membranes. Microbiologically speaking, what we all do during the day is to use our hands to take samples of the various microbes on different surfaces that surround us. At the same time, we also contaminate those surfaces with the microbes already on our hands. Our hands can get "dirty" during a typical day's activity. Sometimes, we can see the dirt on our hands; and frequently, we can see the darkened water as it drips from our hands during the early stages of handwashing. Other times, the dirt is less noticeable. But even though we can't see "germs" that our hands have picked up, the germs are there.

HANDS AND DISEASE SPREAD

Our hands get contaminated and serve as a very common means of spreading microbes—but more importantly, they also can spread disease. Hands are the main route of spread of the common cold and many other respiratory diseases. During a cold, the viruses are present in our respiratory fluid and nasal secretions. When we cough into our hands or blow our nose, and then touch surfaces with these contaminated hands, others can pick up our microbes by contacting the same surfaces. When they then rub their eyes, mouth, or nose or touch food they are about to eat, the transfer of microbes is completed. That's why you should perform hand hygiene even more frequently when you have a cold or other respiratory disease. Also, stay out of the kitchen, and try not to touch common-use surfaces with unwashed hands. In addition to the cold sufferer, other members in the household or office should frequently practice hand hygiene as well. Hand hygiene is an important type of personal hygiene for everyone but is a primary disease prevention procedure for health care workers in dentistry and medicine. In fact, in the dental arena, a case report has documented that the ungloved hands of a dental hygienist suffering from dermatitis had become infected with human herpes virus from a fever blister on the lip of one patient. The hygienist then spread the virus to other patients. The soreness of her hands from the dermatitis prevented effective hand hygiene. Donning gloves interfered with the spread. Chapter 11 gives further details of this case.

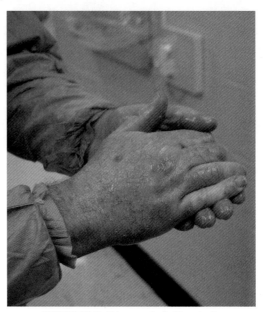

FIGURE 10-1 Using an alcohol hand rub.

PROTECTIVE VALUE OF HAND HYGIENE

Hands are one of the most important sources of microorganisms in disease spread. Hand hygiene is an important type of personal hygiene for everyone but is a primary disease prevention procedure for health care workers in dentistry and medicine.

Two types of microbial flora are on the hands: resident skin flora and transient skin flora. The resident skin flora consists of microorganisms that colonize the skin and become permanent residents. These microorganisms are always on the skin and can never be removed totally, even with a surgical scrub (likely because the resident flora can exist even several layers under the surface in the stratum corneum), but their numbers can be reduced. Although members of the resident skin flora can cause infection when directly or indirectly spread to others, they are likely less important in disease spread than the second type of skin flora, the transient skin flora. The microorganisms of this flora contaminate the hands during the touching of or other exposure to contaminated surfaces. They usually do not colonize and do not survive on the hands for long periods; thus they are called members of the transient flora (they come and go). The transient flora serves as a source of disease spread because it can contain just about any pathogenic microorganism, depending on how the hands become contaminated. Fortunately, the transient flora can be removed or greatly reduced by routine handwashing, usually because the contaminating microorganisms remain primarily on the outer layers of the skin.

Although handwashing clearly reduces the spread of disease agents, it also reduces the number of microorganisms that may contaminate and subsequently cause a harmful infection of or through the hands. Thus handwashing protects patients and the dental team.

HAND HYGIENE AGENTS

Although plain soap without antimicrobial activity performs well in removing dirt and transient microorganisms from the hands, it has little effect on the resident flora. Health care personnel handwashing products contain low to medium levels of antimicrobial agents. Their frequent use in routine handwashing procedures minimizes the number of transient microorganisms on the hands and aids in reducing the number of resident bacteria by means of their bactericidal chemical activity. Surgical scrub products contain the highest levels of antimicrobial agents and are used in a more vigorous scrubbing procedure when maximum reduction in transient and resident flora is desired, such as before surgical procedures. Nevertheless, the surgical scrub procedure will not sterilize the hands.

When the hands contain no visible soil, alcohol-based hand rubs (Figure 10-1) without water and without rinsing have been shown to be effective in hand antisepsis (Table 10-1). These hand rubs also can be used after surgical scrubbing with plain soap and water. Wall-mounted containers placed closed to where the rubs will be used are a convenient way to dispense these products (Figure 10-2).

Common antimicrobial agents in hand hygiene products include alcohols (ethanol, isopropanol, propanol), chlorhexidine digluconate, iodophor, para-chlorometaxylenol (PCMX or chloroxylenol), triclosan, and quaternary ammonium compounds (see Table 10-1). Chlorhexidine digluconate is well known for its widespread antimicrobial activity and its residual activity (prolonged antimicrobial effect). Chlorhexidine digluconate binds to the skin to give prolonged release of antimicrobial activity. Triclosan also may have a prolonged effect, whereas persistence of para-chlorometaxylenol on skin may be less. Iodophor and quaternary ammonium compounds do not exhibit prolonged activity.

TABLE 10-1   **Antimicrobial Spectrum of Some Hand Hygiene Agents**

Agent	Gram-positive Bacteria	Gram-negative Bacteria	*Mycobacteria*	Fungi	Viruses	Speed of Action	Comments
Alcohols	+++	+++	+++	+++	+++	Fast	Optimal concentration 60%-90%; no persistent activity
Chlorhexidine (2% and 4%)	+++	++	+	+	+++	Intermediate	Persistent activity, rare allergic reactions
Iodophors	+++	+++	+	++	++	Intermediate	Less irritation than iodine
Phenolics	+++	+	+	+	+	Intermediate	Neutralized by nonionic surfactants
Triclosan	+++	++	−	−	+++	Intermediate	Acceptability on hands varies
Quaternary ammonium compounds	+	++	−	−	+	Slow	Used only in combination with alcohols

Adapted from Centers for Disease Control and Prevention: Guideline for hand hygiene in health-care settings, *MMWR Recomm Rep* 51(RR-16):45, 2002.
+++, Excellent; ++, good but does not include the entire bacterial spectrum; +, fair; −, no activity.

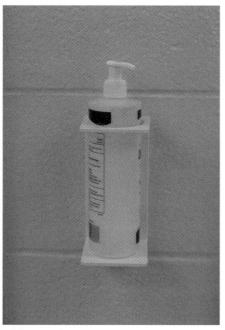

FIGURE 10-2 Wall-mounted alcohol hand rub dispenser.

Recently, more emphasis has been placed on the use of alcohol-based hand rubs. In the past these agents were recommended mainly to be most useful when no sinks were available because rinsing the hands after using the hand rubs is not necessary. A person just rubs the hands together until the gel or foam dries. However, several studies have shown that alcohol products can reduce viable bacterial counts on the hands more than plain soap or antimicrobial soap when relatively small amounts of proteinaceous material (e.g., blood or saliva) are present. Thus the hand rubs are given a more prominent role in hand hygiene procedures when no visible soil appears on the hands. Alcohol hand rubs may increase the frequency of hand hygiene because they are quick and easy to use. Alcohols dry the skin, but this effect has been reduced or eliminated by addition of emollients or other skin-conditioning agents such as glycerol in the hand rub preparations.

HAND HYGIENE PROCEDURES

The mechanical action of handwashing with a plain or antimicrobial soap is important to suspend dirt and microorganisms from the skin surface so they can be rinsed away with water. When the hands are not visibly soiled, one can use an alcohol-based hand rub for hand antisepsis. Step-by-step procedures for routine hand hygiene and surgical scrubbing are given in Procedure 10-1 and partially illustrated in Figure 10-3.

Aseptic techniques associated with hand hygiene include the use of faucets controlled by foot pedals, elbow handles, "electric eyes," or ultrasonics. If these devices are not available, then one can use plastic surface barriers to cover the faucet handles. Foot-operated or electric-eye soap dispensers also prevent contamination of the hands from multiuse soap containers. Squeeze-bottle soap dispensers facilitate cross-contamination and are not recommended. Bar soaps in soap dishes also tend to accumulate skin and environmental microorganisms and are not recommended for health care facilities. Liquid hand care products should be stored in closed containers in either disposable containers or containers that are washed and dried before refilling. Do not add soap or lotion to top off a partially empty container as this will allow any contaminants in the container to be carried over to the fresh soap. Always wash out the container before refilling it.

Box 10-1 lists times when one should perform hand hygiene. See Appendix B for the Centers for Disease Control and Prevention (CDC) recommendations on hand

PROCEDURE 10-1

Hand Hygiene

GOAL: To reduce the microbial burden on the hands so that fewer microbes will be transferred to surfaces touched and to remove chemicals from the hands that may cause irritation

Materials Needed

Non-antimicrobial liquid soap and alcohol-based hand rub

Antimicrobial handwashing agent

Hands-free soap dispenser

Soft brush to clean nails

Soft sponge for surgical scrub

Disposable towels

Sterile towels after surgical scrub

At Beginning of the Day

1. Remove jewelry; gently clean fingernails.
2. Scrub hands, nails, and forearms using a liquid antimicrobial handwashing agent and soft brush or sponge for 15 seconds.
3. Rinse with cool to lukewarm water while rubbing hands together for 10 seconds.
4. Dry hands and then forearms with clean paper towels and use towels to turn off hand-controlled sink faucets.
Rationale: This more thorough hand hygiene helps ready the hands for patient treatment for the day.

Routine Hand Hygiene During the Day
Choice 1

1. Vigorously lather hands with a liquid non-antimicrobial soap for 15 seconds.
2. Rinse with cool to lukewarm water while rubbing hands together for 10 seconds.
3. Dry hands and then forearms with clean paper towels and use towels to turn off hand-controlled sink faucets.
Rationale: To remove soil and transient microbes
Choice 2

1. Vigorously lather hands with a liquid antimicrobial soap for 15 seconds.
2. Rinse with cool to lukewarm water while rubbing hands together for 10 seconds.
3. Dry hands and then forearms with clean paper towels and use towels to turn off hand-controlled sink faucets.
Rationale: To remove soil and transient microbes and to reduce resident skin flora
Choice 3

1. Place appropriate amount of alcohol-based hand rub agent in palm of hand.
2. Vigorously rub hands together until hands are dry.
Rationale: To kill microbes when no visible soil is present on skin

Before Surgery
Choice 1

1. Remove jewelry and gently clean fingernails.
2. Scrub nails, hands, and forearms with an antimicrobial surgical scrub product and a soft sterile brush or sponge for 2 to 6 minutes using multiple scrub and rinse cycles.
3. Rinse hands and forearms with cool to lukewarm water starting with the fingers and keeping the hands above the level of the elbows. Let the water drip from the elbows, not the hands.
4. Dry with sterile towels.

PROCEDURE 10-1

Hand Hygiene—cont'd

5. Put on sterile gloves by inserting hands into the gloves held around the wrists by an assistant wearing sterile gloves.

6. Check the gloves for defects and do not touch contaminated items or surfaces before patient care.
Rationale: To remove soil and transient microbes and to kill some resident microbes
Choice 2

1. Remove jewelry and gently clean fingernails.

2. Scrub nails, hands, and forearms with a non-antimicrobial agent and a soft sterile brush or sponge for 2 to 6 minutes using multiple scrub and rinse cycles.

3. Rinse hands and forearms with cool to lukewarm water starting with the fingers and keeping the hands above the level of the elbows. Let the water drip from the elbows, not the hands.

4. Dry with sterile towels.

5. Place appropriate amount of alcohol-based hand rub agent in palm of hand.

6. Vigorously rub hands together until hands are dry.

7. Put on sterile gloves by inserting hands into the gloves held around the wrists by an assistant wearing sterile gloves.

8. Check the gloves for defects and do not touch contaminated items or surfaces before patient care.
Rationale: To remove soil and to kill transient and some resident microbes

Adapted from Miller CH: Practical barrier techniques. In Cottone JC, Terezhalmy GT, Molinari JA, editors: *Practical infection control in dentistry*, Philadelphia, 1991, Lea & Febiger; and Kohn WG, Collins AS, Cleveland JL, et al; Centers for Disease Control and Prevention: Guidelines for infection control in dental health-care setting–2003, *MMWR Recomm Rep* 52(RR-17):15, 2003.

hygiene. The importance of performing hand hygiene before gloving and after removing gloves may not be obvious. When the skin is occluded (tightly covered up) with gloves, members of the resident flora, and to a lesser extent the transient flora, dramatically increase. This increase may be as great as 4000-fold per hour. This increased growth of microorganisms in the warm, moist environment under gloves can cause skin irritation. Washing hands or using an alcohol-based hand rub before gloving reduces the number of microorganisms to begin with, and washing after removing gloves reduces the number of those that have increased, as well as the transient microorganisms that may have contacted the skin through defects in the gloves. Handwashing after removal of gloves also helps remove any powder containing latex protein, other chemicals from the gloves, and sweat. So if you use alcohol hand rubs throughout the day, periodically (e.g., after every four to five hand rubs) wash and rinse your hands to remove this build-up of debris.

PROPERTIES OF HAND HYGIENE AGENTS

Box 10-2 gives some properties to consider when selecting hand hygiene products.

Other Hand Hygiene Considerations

Dental team members can use lotions to prevent skin dryness associated with handwashing. Lotions with a base of petroleum, lanolin, mineral oil, palm oil, or coconut oil have detrimental effects on latex gloves, so these types should be used only at the end of the day. Lotions containing aloe vera, glycerin, vitamin E, or vitamin A are fine to use. Store liquid hand care products in either disposable, closed containers or closed containers that can be washed and dried before refilling. Do not add soap or lotion to (i.e., top off) a partially empty dispenser, for this will perpetuate any previous contamination inside the container. Remember when using a pump container, the return action of the pump draws microbe-laden air into the container.

One should keep nails short to allow for thorough cleaning and to prevent glove tears. One should not wear artificial nails because they can harbor microbes. One should not wear hand or arm jewelry during surgical procedures or wear hand or nail jewelry during nonsurgical procedures if they make donning gloves more difficult or compromise the appropriate fit and integrity of the gloves. Also, it's more difficult the clean the skin beneath jewelry during hand hygiene.

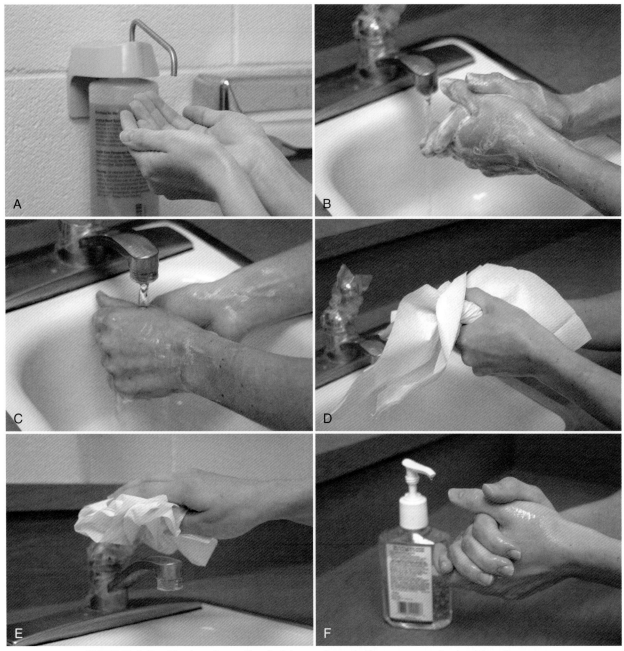

FIGURE 10-3 **Hand hygiene for routine dental procedures. A,** Dispense soap using hand-free dispenser. **B,** Vigorously lather hands. **C,** Rinse under cool tap water. **D,** Dry hands with clean paper towel. **E,** Use paper towel to turn off non–hands-free faucet, or **F,** (when no visible soil is present) use an alcohol-based hand rub and rub hands together until dry.

BOX 10-1

When to Perform Hand Hygiene at Work

- At the beginning of the day
- When hands are visibly soiled
- After bare-handed touching of contaminated objects or surfaces
- Before donning gloves
- After removing gloves
- Before eating or handling food
- Before handling contact lenses and applying makeup
- Before leaving the restroom
- At the end of the day

BOX 10-2

Properties of Hand Hygiene Agents

Consider these properties before making a selection:
- Scent
- Color
- Skin irritation
- Antimicrobial action
- Interaction with glove powder
- Time required for drying of alcohol-based hand rub
- Consistency
- Ease of lathering
- Drying of skin
- Persistence of activity
- Ease of use
- Method of dispensing
- Cost

SELECTED READINGS

American Dental Association: Councils on Scientific Affairs and Dental Practice, Instruments and Equipment, Dental Therapeutics, Dental Research and Dental Practice: Infection control recommendations for the dental office and the dental laboratory, *J Am Dent Assoc* 127:672–680, 1996.

Centers for Disease Control and Prevention: Guideline for hand hygiene in health-care settings, *MMWR Recomm Rep* 51(RR-16):1–45, 2002.

Larson E, Kumudini M, Laughton BA: Influence of two handwashing frequencies on reduction in colonizing flora with three handwashing products used by health care personnel, *Am J Infect Control* 17:83–89, 1989.

Larson EL: Effective hand degerming in the presence of blood, *J Emerg Med* 10:7–11, 1992.

Manzella JP, McConville JH, Valenti W, et al: An outbreak of herpes simplex virus type I gingivostomatitis in a dental hygiene practice, *JAMA* 252:2019–2222, 1989.

Miller CH: Hand hygiene above, under, and beyond the surface, *Dent Prods Rpt* 39:134, 2007.

Miller CH: Select and protect, *Dent Prod Rpt* 41:156–160, 2007.

Usha S, Cadnum JL, Eckstein BC, et al: Contamination of hands with methicillin-resistant *Staphylococcus aureus* after contact with environmental surfaces and after contact with skin colonized patients, *Infect Control Hosp Epidemiol* 32(2):185–187, 2011.

REVIEW QUESTIONS

Multiple Choice

1. The first handwashing of the day involves the use of:
   a. very hot water for rinsing
   b. a soft brush to clean nails
   c. surgical scrubbing for 10 minutes
   d. a simple rinsing with water only

2. When should an alcohol-based hand rub be used?
   a. Under any conditions
   b. Only following handwashing with another antimicrobial agent
   c. Only if no soil is visible on the hands
   d. Only if sterile gloves will be donned afterward

3. Which bacteria on the hands are the most important in spreading disease?
   a. Those that live on the hands permanently
   b. Those that contaminate the hands from touched surfaces

4. Which microorganisms are removed by routine handwashing?
   a. Resident flora
   b. Transient flora

5. Which of the following hand hygiene agents has a prolonged antimicrobial effect?
   a. Plain soap
   b. Chlorhexidine gluconate
   c. Iodophor
   d. Quaternary ammonium compounds

6. According to the CDC, which of the following antimicrobial hand hygiene agents acts the fastest?
   a. Iodophor
   b. Triclosan
   c. Chlorhexidine
   d. Alcohol

7. Performing hand hygiene before gloving
   a. kills all of the resident and transient skin flora
   b. makes the gloves fit better
   c. prevents the gloves from tearing
   d. reduces the number of bacteria on the skin that may multiply beneath the gloves

8. The common cold is commonly spread by
   a. used needles
   b. contaminated hands
   c. mosquitos
   d. contact with contaminated feces

9. When should an alcohol-based hand rub be used during a surgical scrub?
   a. Never
   b. After handwashing with chlorhexidine
   c. After handwashing with an iodophor
   d. After handwashing with non-antibacterial soap

10. Why should you not just top-off the soap when refilling a soap dispenser?
    a. The soap left in the dispenser will inactivate the fresh soap.
    b. Topping off will allow any contaminants in the container to be carried over to the fresh soap.

Please visit http://evolve.elsevier.com/Miller/infectioncontrol/ for additional practice and study support tools.

Personal Protective Equipment

CHAPTER

11

OUTLINE

Gloves

Protective Value

Uses and Types

Limitations

Harmful Reactions to Gloves

Masks

Protective Value

Uses and Types

Limitations

Protective Eyewear

Protective Value

Uses and Types

Limitations

Protective Clothing

Protective Value

Uses and Types

Placing and Removing Equipment Barriers

Properties of Protective Equipment

LEARNING OBJECTIVES

After completing this chapter, the student should be able to do the following:

1. Describe the protective value of gloves and list their uses, types, limitations, and harmful reactions that can occur from their use.

2. Describe the value of masks, protective eyewear, and protective clothing, and list their uses, types and limitations.

3. List the sequence of donning and removing personal protective barriers and the properties of protective equipment.

KEY TERMS

Allergic Contact Dermatitis
Irritant Contact Dermatitis

Latex Allergy
Personal Protective Equipment

Respirator
Wicking

C hapter 3 described the steps in development of an infectious disease, indicating that contamination of the body with microorganisms must occur before disease can develop. Prevention of this exposure or contamination (when possible) is always better than to rely totally on the resistance of the body to fight off disease agents after contamination. Preventing exposure means to avoid contact with the microorganisms, and one accomplishes this in two ways. One way is to prevent the microorganisms from escaping from their source (e.g., in the dental office, the main source of microorganisms is the patient's mouth). Totally preventing microorganisms from escaping the patient's mouth during care is impossible because microorganisms exit the

patient's mouth on instruments, fingers, and supplies used intraorally, and they escape in aerosols and spatter droplets generated during the use of the air-water syringe, slow- and high-speed handpieces, and ultrasonic scalers. However, use of a rubber dam and preprocedure mouth rinsing can reduce this escape of microorganisms from the patient's mouth, as described in Chapter 15.

The second way to prevent exposure is to use barriers to prevent contact with microorganisms escaping from their sources. In dentistry, this involves the use of protective barriers such as gloves, masks, protective eyewear, and protective clothing. The Occupational Safety and Health Administration (OSHA) bloodborne pathogens standard (see Chapter 8 and Appendix G) indicates that in facilities where exposure to bloodborne pathogens may occur (e.g., dental offices), the employer is responsible for providing, maintaining, cleaning/laundering, disposing of, and ensuring the use of protective barriers, sometimes referred to as personal protective equipment.

GLOVES

Protective Value

Gloves protect dental team members from direct contact with microorganisms present in patients' mouths and on contaminated surfaces; they also protect patients from microorganisms on the hands of the dental team.

Protection of the Dental Team

Although intact skin is an excellent barrier to disease agents, a small or even invisible cut appears like the Grand Canyon to microorganisms. Thus, small cuts and abrasions can serve as routes of entry of microorganisms into the body, causing a skin infection or other more widespread diseases. One study showed that fourth-year dental students had an average of four areas of trauma on their hands; 12% of the traumas became painful on contact with alcohol, suggesting open skin (cut or abrasion). Some visually intact areas also give a painful response with alcohol, particularly around the fingernails. Thus even a close visual inspection of the hands may not detect all possible portals of entry for microorganisms.

Cuts on unprotected hands are suggested by many to be an important reason for the high occurrence of hepatitis B in dental and medical personnel who do not use gloves routinely. Analyses of the disease herpetic whitlow (herpes simplex virus infection around the fingernails) before the routine gloving era of dentistry also indicate that this condition occurred more frequently in dentists than in others. Another protective value of wearing gloves in the office is protection against contact with chemicals (such as cleaners, disinfectants, sterilants, and x-ray developing solutions) and some dental materials that may irritate the skin. Heat-resistant gloves also protect against burns when heat processing instruments.

Protection of Patients

Microorganisms are present on just about every surface in the office that has not just been cleaned and disinfected. Microorganisms are there because they settle out from the air or because of contact with other contaminated surfaces. Thus ungloved hands become contaminated with microorganisms on touching just about any environmental surface and from direct contact with fluids or surfaces in a patient's mouth. If these contaminating microorganisms are not removed by handwashing (as described subsequently) or covered up with gloves, they may be transmitted to a patient.

A dental patient's blood has been shown to be retained under the fingernails of a dental team member for several days, even with handwashing. This residue could serve as a source of infection for subsequent patients. Thus routine gloving can prevent blood or saliva impaction in those areas (particularly around and under the fingernails) that are difficult to clean.

Microorganisms present in blood may exit the body through small cuts in the skin. This process probably is enhanced if these cuts are moistened, as when a dental team member does not wear gloves when working in a patient's mouth. This route of disease spread from dental team member to patient may have been important in several of the 10 reported cases of hepatitis B spread from infected dentists to patients (see Chapter 6). These infected dentists did not use gloves routinely for patient care.

One of the most clearly documented cases of disease spread in a dental office resulted from not using gloves routinely for patient care, as mentioned in Chapters 8 and 10. An ungloved hygienist with dermatitis on her hands and fingers cared for a patient with active herpes labialis (herpes simplex infection on the lips). About a week later, vesicles of herpetic whitlow developed on the hygienist's hands. Before any sign of her infection had appeared, however, she had unknowingly spread the virus to at least 20 other patients, who developed intraoral herpes lesions. When the vesicles appeared on the hygienist's hands, she began to routinely wear gloves, which prevented further spread of the virus to any more patients.

This case demonstrates three modes of disease spread in the office (as discussed in Chapters 8 and 10): first, from patient to dental team member; second, from dental team member to patient; and third, from patient to patient. In this instance, all three modes of disease spread could have been prevented by routine gloving with every patient. Another important point demonstrated by this case is that dermatitis greatly reduces the effectiveness of handwashing in removing contaminating disease agents. Less-vigorous handwashing is performed because of the painful dermatitis, and the dermatitis itself provides additional places on the hands where microorganisms can "hide" from the mechanical action of handwashing.

Uses and Types

Box 11-1 lists the several types of gloves available for various uses in the dental setting. Some have specific uses, and others have multiple uses (Figure 11-1).

Patient Care Activities

Dental professionals should wear disposable gloves during all patient care activities where a potential exists for direct hand contact with saliva, blood, or other oral fluids, mucous membranes, and nonintact skin and when handling items or surfaces contaminated with body fluids or potentially infectious materials.

Gloves used for patient care are not to be reused on a subsequent patient. Dental professionals also should not wash patient care gloves with any detergent or chemical; washing

BOX 11-1

Types of Gloves in Dentistry

Patient Care Gloves
- Sterile latex surgical gloves
- Sterile neoprene surgical gloves*
- Sterile styrene surgical gloves*
- Sterile synthetic copolymer gloves*
- Sterile reduced-protein latex surgeon's gloves
- Latex examination gloves
- Synthetic copolymer examination gloves*
- Nitrile examination gloves*
- Styrene-butadiene examination gloves*
- Polyurethane gloves*
- Powderless gloves
- Flavored gloves
- Low-protein gloves

Utility Gloves
- Heavy latex gloves
- Heavy nitrile gloves
- Thin copolymer gloves
- Thin plastic ("food handlers") gloves

Other Gloves
- Heat-resistant gloves
- Dermal (cotton) gloves

*Nonlatex gloves; one should review the labeling or check with the manufacturer to confirm.

may weaken stabilizers in the glove material or enhance penetration (causing **wicking**) of material through inherent defects. One may rinse off powder (cornstarch) on fresh gloves with plain water before patient care, if desired.

If the dental professional leaves the chairside during patient care, the best procedure is first to remove the gloves and don a fresh pair on returning to chairside. This change prevents contamination of any surfaces one may touch when away from chairside and prevents contaminating the patient with microorganisms already present on those same surfaces. One also should remember that any surface at chairside that is touched with contaminated gloves and also may be touched during the care of the next patient must have been covered previously to prevent cross-contamination or must be precleaned and disinfected before care of the next patient (see Chapter 13 on surface asepsis). An alternative to changing gloves in these situations is to use inexpensive copolymer or plastic gloves or a sheet of plastic wrap over the patient care gloves (overgloving) to prevent spread of the patient's microorganisms to surfaces that are touched. One then removes the overgloves before resuming care on the patient.

Another important aspect of glove use during patient care is that one must remove torn or punctured gloves as soon as possible, followed immediately by hand hygiene and donning of fresh gloves.

Sterile latex or vinyl gloves are used during surgical procedures, but nonsterile gloves are appropriate for most other dental procedures. Surgeon's gloves are provided in half-sizes ranging from 5 to 9 and usually provide the best fit because the gloves are made for the right hand and left hand. Most examination gloves are ambidextrous in that any glove can be used on the right or left hand. These gloves usually are provided in extra-small, small, medium, and large sizes, but some brands may be sized from 5 to 9. Latex gloves are thought by most to give a better fit than vinyl gloves, but this may not always be true. Use of gloves that fit properly is important to ensure efficient handling of items and to prevent fatigue of the hands.

Use of powderless gloves, reduced-protein latex gloves, nonlatex gloves, and dermal gloves relates to the irritations and allergic reactions some persons have to gloves. See the discussion under Harmful Reactions to Gloves below.

Operatory Cleanup and Instrument Processing

To provide more protection for the hands during operatory cleanup and handling of instruments than that provided by the thin latex or vinyl patient care gloves or thin copolymer or plastic gloves, one should use utility gloves of nitrile or heavy latex when preparing and using chemicals, precleaning and disinfecting contaminated surfaces, and handling contaminated items during instrument processing. Each person in the office needing these gloves should have his or her own pair or pairs of gloves. The heavy utility gloves are reusable and can be washed with an antimicrobial handwashing agent, rinsed, and dried.

One should use heat-resistant gloves for handling hot items when unloading sterilizers or whenever a risk of burning the hands or forearms exists.

Other Activities

The dental professional should wear gloves whenever a chance exists for contact with items potentially contaminated with pathogenic microorganisms, such as when handling appliances or equipment in the dental laboratory that have not been decontaminated; contaminated laundry; contaminated waste, tissue, or teeth; and containers of blood, saliva, or other infectious material if a risk of spilling or splashing exists.

Limitations

The manufacturing process for patient care gloves may result in a low level of pinholes; however, the U.S. Food and Drug Administration (FDA) has placed strict requirements on glove manufacturers to help ensure a high quality of these medical devices. Some manufacturers even test each glove for defects before selling them.

Although gloves provide a high level of protection against direct contact with infectious agents through touching, they offer little protection against injuries with sharp objects such as instruments, needles, and scalpel blades. Thus one still

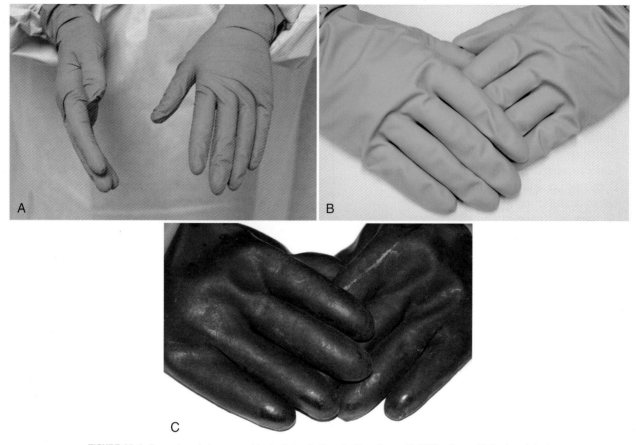

FIGURE 11-1 Examples of gloves used in dentistry. **A,** Examination gloves. **B,** Utility gloves. **C,** Heat-resistant gloves.

must handle contaminated sharps safely, even while wearing gloves. Sharps injuries also can and do occur through the heavy utility gloves during instrument processing.

One should not use gloves that are torn or have other noticeable defects. One should not reuse heavy utility gloves if they are peeling, cracking, discolored, torn, punctured, or show any other signs of deterioration.

One should not store gloves in direct sunlight or in high dust areas.

Harmful Reactions to Gloves

Some health care workers and patients have harmful reactions when they come into contact with latex gloves or with airborne glove materials. Because these reactions result from contact with latex proteins or other chemicals in the gloves, a brief description of glove manufacturing may help explain the origin of these chemicals.

Latex gloves are manufactured from latex extracted from the rubber tree *Hevea brasiliensis*, which grows in tropical areas throughout the world. The latex is in the form of a milky fluid to which anticoagulants and preservatives are first added. The latex fluid itself contains the rubber material (*cis*-1,4 polyisoprene), along with proteins, lipids, and carbohydrates. This latex material then is compounded by

adding up to 200 different chemicals, depending on the desired characteristics of the final product. These chemicals are antidegradants, vulcanizing agents that make the latex elastic, accelerators, retarders, promoters, pigments, activators, and mold-releasing agents and also may include fragrances, emulsifiers, stabilizers, biocides, and ultraviolet light absorbers. Hand-shaped porcelain formers coated with more chemicals and with cornstarch powder as a releasing agent are dipped into the compounded latex. The formers then are passed through ovens and a warm-water leaching bath to remove some of the latex proteins and other chemicals. Further treatments include adding more cornstarch or a special chlorination treatment if powder-free gloves are desired. Items manufactured from natural latex are referred to as natural rubber latex (NRL) products.

Although allergies to the NRL in gloves are the major area of concern, contact with other latex-containing products (Box 11-2) besides gloves also may induce a reaction. Currently, about 1% to 6% of the general population and 8% to 12% of regularly exposed health care workers are estimated to be sensitive to latex.

Three types of reactions may occur with gloving. One is a skin reaction to irritants in the gloves called **irritant contact dermatitis**, and the other two are the immunological reactions of **allergic contact dermatitis** and **latex allergy**.

BOX 11-2

Examples of Items That May Contain Latex*

Dental Products
- Gloves
- Rubber dams
- Prophylaxis cups
- Anesthetic carpules
- Nitrous oxide masks
- Orthodontic rings
- Bite blocks
- Mixing bowls
- Liquid droppers
- Blood pressure cuffs
- Elastic bands
- Suction adapters
- Some masks

Other Products
- Stethoscopes
- Tourniquets
- Electrode pads
- Rubber aprons and sheets
- Intravenous ports
- Catheters and ventilator tubing
- Syringe plunger tips
- Automobile tires
- Handlebar grips
- Carpeting and adhesives
- Racquet handles
- Dishwashing gloves
- Elastic bands
- Condoms and diaphragms
- Balloons and rubber toys
- Baby bottle nipples and pacifiers
- Hot-water bottles and raincoats
- Erasers and rubber bands

*Some of these items are available in latex-free forms.

Irritant Contact Dermatitis

Most reactions from wearing gloves result from a nonimmunological irritation of the skin from nonlatex chemicals in the gloves or applied to the hands. In these instances, the skin on the hands becomes dry, reddened, itchy, and sometimes cracked in severe cases.

Conditions that may initiate or aggravate this dermatitis include handwashing with irritating cleaners or antiseptics, failure to rinse completely, failure to dry hands thoroughly after rinsing, excessive perspiration on the hands, and irritation from cornstarch powder.

To reverse and prevent recurrence of irritant contact dermatitis, one should attempt to identify the irritant by first making sure one is performing proper hand hygiene. One also should consider changing gloves or handwashing agent

brands. When changing glove brands, one should be sure to determine whether a different brand is really a different type of glove. Because the same glove may be sold under many different brands, one should compare samples before purchasing "new" gloves in large volumes.

Allergic Contact Dermatitis

Four types of immunological hypersensitivities or allergies (I to IV) occur. Two of these types (I and IV) involve reactions to gloves, and both types require a person first to become sensitized to an agent (called an allergen) that on subsequent contact causes a harmful reaction. Allergic contact dermatitis is type IV hypersensitivity, also called delayed hypersensitivity, and is the most frequently occurring immunological reaction to gloves, accounting for about 80% of the cases. Type I hypersensitivity to glove latex is described subsequently.

Allergic contact dermatitis is almost always limited to the areas of contact and is characterized by initial itching, redness, and vesicles within 24 to 48 hours, followed by dry skin, fissures, and sores. The reaction to poison ivy also is a type IV hypersensitivity. Allergic contact dermatitis caused by contact with gloves results from exposure to one of the many chemicals added during latex harvesting, processing, or glove manufacturing. The most common chemical sensitizers are the accelerators used in vulcanization: thiurams, carbamates, and mercaptobenzothiazoles. Vulcanization is the polymerizing process that makes the latex elastic. In two studies of patients with allergic reactions to gloves, 72% and 83% of patients were patch-test-positive for thiurams and 25% and 22% were positive for carbamates. The patch test contains small amounts of different chemicals that when applied to the skin of an allergic person will produce a small reaction indicating the specific causative agent.

Eliminating contact with the sensitizing agent is the only way to prevent allergic contact dermatitis. Glove manufacturers attempt to control the addition of chemicals to latex products, but a confusing point is the labeling of gloves as "hypoallergenic" just because they may contain reduced levels of certain chemicals. Such gloves are not free of all potentially sensitizing chemicals and may still be able to induce harmful reactions. The FDA now prohibits such labeling.

In 2011, the FDA issued a document titled "Draft Guidance for Industry and FDA Staff—Recommended Warning for Surgeon's Gloves and Patient Examination Gloves that Use Powder." The FDA recommended that manufacturers of powdered gloves include the following change to their product labeling no later than 6 months after issuance of final guidance based on this draft, and sooner if possible:

"Warning: Powdered gloves may lead to foreign body reactions and the formation of granulomas in patients. In addition, the powder used on gloves may contribute to the development of irritant dermatitis and Type IV allergy, and on latex gloves may serve as a carrier for airborne natural latex leading to sensitization of glove users."

Latex Allergy

Mechanisms

Latex allergy is the third type of reaction to gloves and the second type involving an immune response. Latex allergy is a type I hypersensitivity, also called an immediate hypersensitivity. In this instance, a person is allergic to the naturally occurring proteins present in latex. A person who develops a latex allergy first becomes sensitized by one or more exposures to latex protein allergens before reaction to a subsequent exposure can occur. In sensitization, immunoglobulin E antibodies develop after exposure to the latex protein allergens. These antibodies bind to special cells in the body called mast cells, but a harmful reaction does not occur yet. When more latex protein allergens enter the body (with subsequent exposure), the mast cells are stimulated to produce substances that can cause skin reactions and occasionally more serious systemic reactions that affect blood flow and breathing or cause anaphylaxis.

Symptoms

The symptoms of a latex allergy reaction usually begin within 20 minutes or so after contact with NRL products and may include skin reactions of urticaria (hives), redness, burning, and itching. More severe reactions may involve respiratory symptoms such as runny nose; sneezing; watery, itchy eyes; scratchy throat; and asthma (difficult breathing, coughing spells, and wheezing). Anaphylactic shock rarely occurs as the first sign of latex allergy but could occur with subsequent exposures. Of the 80 cases of anaphylactic shock to NRL products reported in the medical literature up to 1995, 15 persons died.

Airborne latex proteins

Of particular concern in latex allergy is the potential for exposure to the NRL protein allergens present in the glove cornstarch powder. These proteins can migrate from the glove into the cornstarch, which causes more protein to be associated with the skin. This cornstarch becomes aerosolized when gloves are removed from boxes and when they are "snapped" during donning or removal. If a latex-sensitive person inhales airborne latex proteins, that person may have a serious respiratory or systemic reaction. Another important aspect of protein-laden cornstarch is that after it is airborne, it can travel extensively throughout the office, clinic, or building and expose many persons to these allergens. Studies of other allergy-causing substances have shown that the higher the overall exposure in a population, the greater the likelihood that more individuals will become sensitized. Unfortunately, the amount of latex exposure needed to produce sensitization or to produce a reaction is not known. However, reductions in exposure are known to decrease sensitization.

Prevention or Management of Latex Allergies

Allergies in the dental worker

As with all other NRL allergies, avoiding contact/exposure with latex protein is necessary to prevent reactions in a sensitive person. In the dental setting, this is accomplished by use of non-latex gloves and other items and establishment of a "latex safe" environment (or at least a reduced presence of latex). If the dental team uses latex gloves, the gloves should be the powder-free, reduced-protein type to eliminate airborne latex protein allergens. The National Institute for Occupational Safety and Health (NIOSH), a division of the Centers for Disease Control and Prevention, has issued recommendations for preventing latex allergies (Box 11-3).

Allergies in patients

The first approach to addressing latex allergies in dental patients is to include appropriate questions in the medical history (Box 11-4). Sensitivities to NRL proteins are greater in certain individuals, and this includes persons who have occupational exposure to latex. Persons with spina bifida, urogenital anomalies, and spinal cord injuries are considered at high risk. A history of allergies in the patient or patient's family is also important to consider. The same is true if a person is allergic to foods, particularly bananas, chestnuts, avocados, or kiwis. Provision of dental care for a latex-allergic patient should be done in an environment with latex as low as reasonably possible (known as ALARP). The following will help the dental team achieve this:

1. Provide treatment in a specially prepared room as first patient of the day.
   a. Staff members are not to wear latex while preparing treatment room.
   b. They are to handle all items that will contact patient with nonlatex gloves.
   c. No one who has worn latex gloves that day should enter the treatment room.
2. Minimize previous contact of patient care items with latex-containing materials.
3. Prevent latex from directly contacting the patient during treatment (use latex alternatives).
4. Eliminate patient exposure to airborne latex protein in glove powder.
5. Have dental team members wear non–latex-containing items that may contact the patient.

MASKS

Protective Value

Masks were developed originally to reduce the chances of postoperative infections in patients that were caused by microorganisms in the respiratory tracts of the surgeons. Although some controversy exists as to the ability of masks to accomplish their original purpose, wearing a mask is still standard practice during surgery or at any other time when reducing the spread of potential respiratory disease agents may be important. In recent years, a face mask also has been viewed as a means to protect the one who wears the mask from disease agents that might be present in sprays, spatter, or even some aerosol particles of body fluids or other

---

BOX 11-3

Recommendations from NIOSH for Preventing Latex Allergies in the Workplace

What Workers Should Do

- Use nonlatex gloves when appropriate.
- If one uses latex gloves, use powder-free gloves with reduced protein content.
- If one uses latex gloves, do not use oil- or petroleum-based hand lotions unless they have been shown to reduce latex-related problems.
- After removing latex gloves, wash hands with a mild detergent and dry thoroughly.
- Frequently clean areas that may be contaminated with latex powder (upholstery, carpets, ventilation ducts, and plenums).
- Frequently change ventilation filters and vacuum bags used in latex-contaminated areas.
- Take advantage of latex allergy training provided by your employer and learn about procedures for preventing latex allergies and about latex allergy symptoms (skin rash; hives; flushing; itching; nasal, eye, or sinus symptoms; asthma; and shock).
- If symptoms of latex allergy develop, avoid direct contact with latex-containing gloves and other items until after seeing a physician.
- If a latex allergy develops, consult a physician regarding the following precautions: avoid contact with latex-containing products; avoid areas where powder may be inhaled from latex gloves; tell employer about the latex allergy; and wear a medical alert bracelet.
- Carefully follow physician's instructions for dealing with allergic reactions to latex.

What Employers Should Do

- Provide workers with nonlatex gloves.
- If workers choose latex gloves, provide reduced-protein, powder-free gloves.
- Ensure that workers use good housekeeping practices to remove latex-containing dust from the workplace: identify areas contaminated with latex dust for frequent cleaning (upholstery, carpets, ventilation ducts, and plenums), and make sure that workers change ventilation filters and vacuum bags frequently in latex-containing areas.
- Provide workers with education programs and training materials about latex allergy.
- Periodically screen high-risk workers for latex allergy symptoms. Detecting symptoms early and removing symptomatic workers from latex exposure are essential to preventing long-term health effects.
- Evaluate current prevention strategies whenever a worker is diagnosed with latex allergy.

From Centers for Disease Control and Prevention, National Institute for Occupational Safety and Health. *NIOSH alert: preventing allergic reactions to natural rubber latex in the workplace*, Cincinnati, OH , 1997, US Department of Health and Human Services, Public Health Service, CDC, National Institute for Occupational Safety and Health, Pub No 97-135.

---

potentially infectious materials. In dentistry, masks mainly protect mucous membranes of the nose and mouth of the dental team from contact with sprays or spatter of oral fluids from the patient or from items contaminated with patient fluids. A much lesser degree of protection to the dental team occurs against inhalation of aerosolized particles of oral fluids that may contain infectious disease agents. Masks worn by the dental team may give some protection to the patients.

Uses and Types

The dental team should wear surgical masks any time a risk exists of spraying or spattering of fluids that may contain potentially infectious disease agents. This may occur during patient care activities involving high-speed or low-speed handpieces, ultrasonic scalers, air/water syringes, or oral irrigators and during grinding or polishing of items that may be contaminated with patient fluids. The mask should be changed with every patient because its outer surface becomes contaminated with droplets from sprays of oral fluids from the previous patient or from touching the mask with saliva-coated fingers. A mask also protects from splashes during instrument processing. Contamination of ultrasonic or other cleaning solutions may occur if the cleaning basket or instruments are accidentally dropped into the solution. Rinsing of instruments under tap water also may cause splashing.

Face masks are composed of synthetic material that serves to filter out at least 95% of small particles that directly contact the mask. In 1995, the NIOSH (a part of the Public Health Service) indicated that it would certify three classes of filters—N-, R-, and P-series—with three levels of filter efficiency—95%, 99%, and 99.97%—in each class. All filter tests are to use particles of aerosol size: 0.3-mm aerodynamic mass median diameter. The filterability of masks is referred to as Bacterial Filtration Efficiency (BFE) or Particle Filtration Efficiency (PFE). The surgical masks commonly used in dentistry are dome shaped or pliable. They may be secured with an elastic band, ear loops, or ties (Figure 11-2). Although these masks protect the mucous membranes of the mouth and nose from direct contact with droplets of oral fluids, they give limited protection against small aerosol particles important in airborne infections such as severe acute respiratory syndrome (SARS). Even though the masks are form fitting over the bridge of the nose to reduce fogging

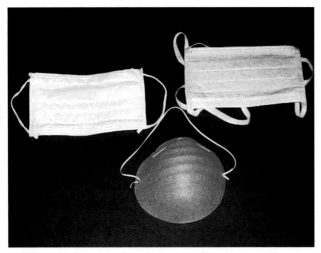

FIGURE 11-2 Examples of surgical masks. Other types not shown are available.

of eyewear, they still "leak" around the edges. Protection against airborne infection requires the use of a respirator (e.g., N-95 respirator, Figure 11-3) that fits in such a way that forces inhaled air to pass through the filter rather than around the edge of the mask. Respirators are more difficult to breathe through, and their use must be preceded by

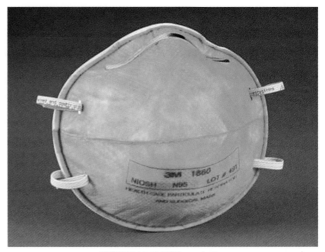

FIGURE 11-3 N95 respirator.

training and by fit testing to ensure safe use and proper functioning. Because patients with serious airborne disease (e.g., SARS) should be treated in special facilities, respirators are not part of the normal personal protective equipment needed in dental offices.

Limitations

Because surgical masks do not provide a perfect seal around the edges, unfiltered exhaled and inhaled air can pass through these sites. Thus selection of a mask that fits the face well is important to minimize passage of unfiltered air. In addition, when a mask becomes wet from moist, exhaled air, the resistance to airflow through the mask increases, causing more unfiltered air to pass by the edges of the mask. Thus one should replace wet masks approximately every 20 minutes to maintain high filterability.

PROTECTIVE EYEWEAR

Protective Value

A variety of disease agents may cause harmful infection of the eyes or enter the associated mucous membranes and cause systemic infections. An example is the herpes simplex virus, which may be present in sprays, spatter, or aerosols of oral fluids from a patient. Another example is the hepatitis B virus, which may use the eye as a portal of entry into the body and cause hepatitis B.

Besides protecting against infectious disease agents, eyewear also protects against physical damage to the eyes by propelled objects such as tooth fragments or small pieces of a restorative material exiting a patient's mouth during cavity preparation. Impact damage to the eyes can occur from any polishing, grinding, or buffing procedure, whether performed in a patient's mouth, at chairside, or in the dental laboratory. Eyewear also can protect against eye damage from ultraviolet irradiation and from splashes of chemicals

TABLE 11-1   **Comparison of Eye Protection Devices**

Type	Front Splash Protection	Side Splash Protection	Front Impact Protection	Side Impact Protection	Neck and Face Protection
Goggles	Excellent	Excellent	Excellent	Excellent	Poor
Glasses (no shields)	Good	Poor	Excellent	Poor	Poor
Glasses (with shields)	Good	Good	Excellent	Fair	Poor
Face shield*	Excellent	Good to Excellent	Variable (depends on thickness)	Variable (depends on thickness)	Variable (depends on type/length)

Adapted from American National Standards Institute: *Occupational and educational eye and face protection: Z87.1-1989*, New York, 1989, American National Standards Institute; and Palenik CJ, Miller CH: Protecting your eyes: it's the law, *Trends Tech Contemp Dent Lab* 8:69-74, 1991.
*Should include solid side and top protection.

used at chairside or for cleaning instruments and surfaces, disinfecting surfaces, developing radiographs, or working in the dental laboratory.

The dental team should offer patients eye protection during treatment. Reports of eye damage to patients include impalement of a patient's eye by an excavator, corneal abrasion from an exploding anesthetic carpule and from a piece of acrylic denture tooth, and subconjunctival hemorrhage after a dentist hit a patient's eye with his thumb. Instruments and chemicals should not be passed over the head of the patient. If a patient wears prescription eyeglasses, the patient should be allowed to continue to wear them during care; other patients should be provided with eye protection. Disposable eyewear should be provided, or patient eyewear can be decontaminated between uses.

Uses and Types

One should wear protective eyewear whenever contamination of the eyes with aerosols, sprays, or splashes of body fluids or chemicals is possible and whenever projectiles may be generated during any grinding, polishing, or buffing procedure with rotary instruments or equipment. Protective eyewear worn by the dental team should be decontaminated thoroughly before reuse with subsequent patients. Appropriate eye protection also should be used with ultraviolet irradiation. Table 11-1 compares different types of eye protection in relation to the American National Standard for Occupational and Educational Eye and Face Protection, Z87.1-1989. The design, construction, testing, and use of eye and face protection devices should be in accordance with this standard developed by the American National Standards Institute.

Limitations

Goggles that may be used by themselves or over prescription glasses may not be attractive, but they give the greatest eye protection against front and side splashes and impacts. Although glasses give protection against front splashes and impacts, side protection is poor unless they have solid side

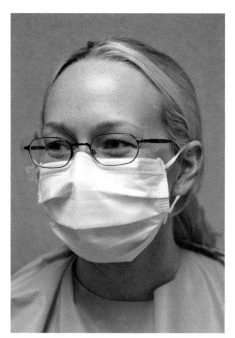

FIGURE 11-4 Prescription eyeglasses with side shields.

shields (Figure 11-4). The degree of impact protection from projectiles depends on the strength of the lenses as determined by the American National Standards Institute standard. Some protective eyeglasses have replaceable lenses (if scratching occurs), have antifogging properties, and are autoclavable. The OSHA bloodborne pathogens standard (see Chapter 8 and Appendix G) indicates that appropriate protective eyewear, in relation to splashes or sprays of body fluids, provides protection to the front and the sides of the eyes. So, eyewear should have side shields (Figure 11-5). Masks with attached eye protection are also available (Figure 11-6).

If one uses face shields, the shields should be chin length, provide top protection, and be curved to provide side protection. Some face shields are made of thin plastic and may not offer adequate protection against particles with a high-impact velocity. One also should wear masks with face shields to reduce inhalation of fluid aerosols and dust particles.

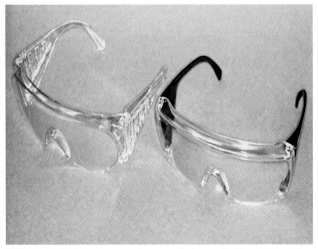

FIGURE 11-5 Protective eyeglasses with top and side shields. Other types not shown are available.

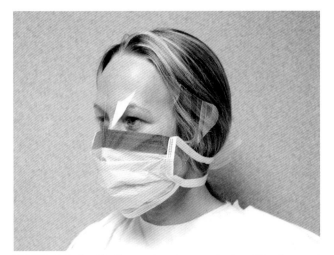

FIGURE 11-6 Combination mask and eye protection. Other types not shown are available.

PROTECTIVE CLOTHING

Protective Value

Potentially infectious microorganisms may be present in the aerosols, sprays, spatter, and droplets from the oral fluids of patients. These microorganisms not only contaminate unprotected eyes and mucous membranes of the mouth and nose but also contaminate other body sites of the dental team, including the forearms and chest area. Larger droplets also may settle on the lap while one is seated at chairside. Outer protective clothing can protect against this contamination, which otherwise may lead to infection through nonintact skin or at least to spread of the contamination from office to home or elsewhere on unprotected clothing. Changing of obviously contaminated protective clothing before providing care for the next patient is perceived as providing patient protection. Covering up microorganisms present on street clothes with protective clothing also is perceived to provide some degree of patient protection.

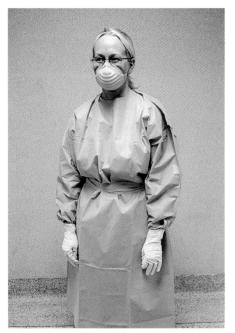

FIGURE 11-7 Disposable protective clothing.

This action prevents shedding of microorganisms from street clothes into the air near a patient who may have open tissue. Although it seems reasonable to use protective clothing for dental team and patient protection, little evidence is available on the extent to which this prevents disease spread.

Uses and Types

Dental team members should wear protective clothing whenever a chance exists for contamination of skin or other clothing with spray or splashes of saliva, blood, or other potentially infectious materials. Thus the same conditions at chairside that require use of masks and protective eyewear also require use of protective clothing. If this clothing becomes visibly soiled, the person should change clothing before caring for the next patient and should put on fresh protective clothing before surgery. One should remove protective clothing when leaving clinical areas and should not wear such clothing in lunch rooms, restrooms, or outside the office. The OSHA bloodborne pathogens standard also indicates that employees cannot take home contaminated clothing and linens for laundering. Laundering is the responsibility of the employer through laundering in the office or by contracting with a commercial laundering service. Although not required by any law, dental team members also should consider having work shoes to wear only in the office.

Protective clothing is the outer layer of clothing that protects/covers underlying work clothes, street clothes, undergarments, or skin. Examples include uniforms, clinic jackets, lab coats, aprons, and gowns. This clothing should protect against contamination of underlying clothes or skin, and materials with the greatest resistance to fluids provide the greatest protection. Few, if any, chairside dental procedures require

BOX 11-5

Putting on and Removing Equipment

Putting on
1. Protective clothing
2. Mask
3. Protective eyewear
4. Gloves

Removing*
1. Disposable gown
2. Gloves
3. Protective eyewear
4. Mask

*See Figure 11-8.

fluid-proof clothing. Head covers and shoe covers also are not mandated for use in dentistry, but head covers may be appropriate to give maximum patient protection during surgery.

A convenient approach to office management of protective clothing involves use of disposable gowns with long sleeves and a high neck to cover regular work clothes (Figure 11-7). For routine dental procedures, one may change these clothes at least once a day (e.g., over the lunch hour) or more frequently if they become visibly soiled. Another approach is use of reusable protective clothing such as uniforms, lab coats, or other attire that may be put on at the beginning of the day, but it must be changed for lunch, changed when it becomes visibly soiled, and removed before one leaves the office. Use of protective clothing that is pulled on and removed over the head is not wise because removal may contaminate the face and head with the outside of the clothing.

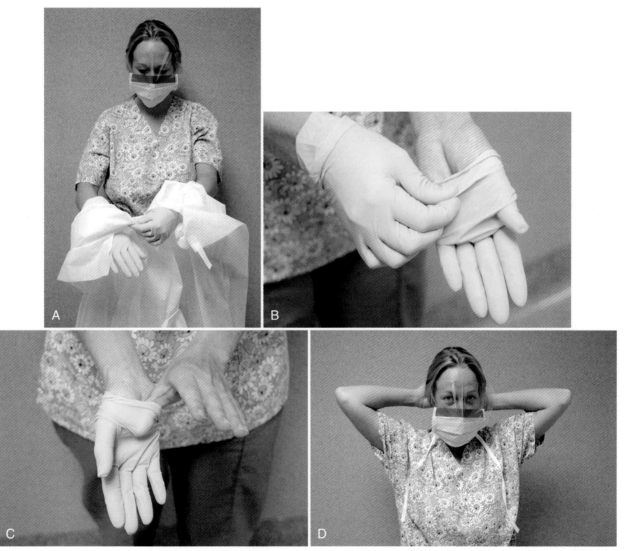

FIGURE 11-8 Removing personal protective equipment (also see Box 11-5). **A,** Remove gown by reaching back and pulling it off over the gloves, turning it inside out. **B,** Remove the first glove by pinching it at the wrist and pulling it off toward the fingers. **C,** Remove the other glove by slipping the thumb under it and pulling it off toward the fingers. **D,** Remove eyewear by grasping the ear rests, and remove the mask by touching only the elastic bands or ties.

PLACING AND REMOVING EQUIPMENT BARRIERS

Chapter 19 presents all of the steps involved in chairside asepsis. However, procedures for putting on and taking off barriers are discussed further in this section. Putting on and taking off barriers should be done in a sequence that limits further spread of microorganisms. This is true when preparing for routine and surgical procedures. For this discussion, it is assumed that the operatory has been cleaned and disinfected and that surface covers have been placed, sterilized instrument packages or cassettes have been placed on the bracket table or cart, the patient has been seated, and the history and any discussions have been completed. The important point to remember about the sequence of putting on protective barriers is to put on gloves last to avoid contaminating the gloves before they are used in the patient's mouth.

The first step is to put on protective clothing (Box 11-5) and place the patient's bib. One then unpackages the instruments and supply items without directly touching them and next puts on mask and eyewear. Just before performing treatment, one washes, rinses, and dries the hands and puts on gloves. One should not touch any contaminated items or surfaces with the gloves before they go into the patient's mouth.

After patient treatment, one considers two key issues when removing the now-contaminated protective barriers.

- The gloves can contaminate anything they touch.
- The hands may become contaminated if one touches certain parts of the protective barriers with ungloved hands.

Recent studies show that viruses may survive on objects of personal protective equipment (PPE) for hours, so care is necessary to prevent spread of that contamination during removal of used PPE. One approach to removing contaminated equipment is given in Box 11-5 and illustrated in Figure 11-8. If one is going to remove contaminated protective clothing, this step is first. To remove a disposable gown, one pulls it off over gloved hands, turning it inside out and immediately placing it into a waste receptacle. When removing disposable or reusable protective clothing, one should not touch underlying clothes or skin with the contaminated gloves (see Figure 11-8, *A*). Next, one removes gloves and washes the hands. When removing the gloves, one should not touch the skin but rather pinch the gloves in the wrist area on one hand, stretch the glove out away from the wrist, and pull the glove off (see Figure 11-8, *B*). One then places the ungloved thumb under the edge of the other glove, stretches the glove out away from the hand, slides it completely off, and places it into the waste receptacle (see Figure 11-8, *C*). One removes eyeglasses by touching them only on the ear rests (which usually are not contaminated) and placing them in an appropriate area for subsequent decontamination. One removes the mask by touching only the elastic bands around the head or ears or only the ties in back of the head (see Figure 11-8, *D*). One immediately should discard the mask into the waste receptacle. One then washes, rinses, and dries

the hands. These barriers need not be managed as regulated waste unless they are for some unusual reason dripping wet with blood or saliva. One can just place them in the regular waste receptacle.

PROPERTIES OF PROTECTIVE EQUIPMENT

Box 11-6 gives properties to consider when selecting gloves, masks, eyeglasses, and gowns.

BOX 11-6

Properties of Protective Equipment

Consider these properties before making a selection.

Gloves
- Fit
- Scent
- Powder presence
- Texture
- Flexibility
- What gloves are made of
- Color
- Protein content
- Length of cuff
- Skin irritation

Masks
- Fit around edge
- Fit over bridge of nose
- Bacterial Filtration Efficiency
- Ear loops, ties, or head band
- Scent
- Color

Eyeglasses
- Solid side shields
- Fit
- Nondistortion
- Fog resistance
- Weight
- Top shield
- Clarity
- Scratch resistance
- Color
- Size

Protective Clothing
- Coverability
- Velcro versus tie closure
- Weight
- Strike-through properties
- Color
- Thickness

SELECTED READINGS

American Dental Association: Councils on Scientific Affairs and Dental Practice, Instruments and Equipment, Dental Therapeutics, Dental Research and Dental Practice: Infection control recommendations for the dental office and the dental laboratory, *J Am Dent Assoc* 127:672–680, 1996.

Balazy A, Toivola M, Adhikari A, et al: Do N95 respirators provide 95% protection level against airborne viruses, and how adequate are surgical masks? *Am J Infect Cont* 34:51–57, 2006.

Belkin NL: Gowns and drapes for the level of exposure anticipated, *Bull Am Coll Surg* 87:20–22, 2002.

Centers for Disease Control and Prevention: Guideline for hand hygiene in health-care settings, *MMWR Recomm Rep* 51(RR-16):1–45, 2002.

Food and Drug Administration: *Draft Guidance for Industry and FDA Staff—Recommended warning for surgeon's gloves and patient examination gloves that use powder*, http://www.fda.gov/MedicalDevices/DeviceRegulationandGuidance/GuidanceDocuments/ucm228557.htm. Accessed December 2011.

Hamann CP, DePaola LG, Rodgers PA: Occupation-related allergies in dentistry, *J Am Dent Assoc* 136:500–510, 2005.

Larson EL: Effective hand degerming in the presence of blood, *J Emerg Med* 10:7–11, 1992.

Manzella JP, McConville JH, Valenti W, et al: An outbreak of herpes simplex virus type I gingivostomatitis in a dental hygiene practice, *JAMA* 252:2019–2222, 1989.

Miller CH: Select and protect, *Dent Prod Rpt* 41:156–160, 2007.

Rutala WR, Weber DJ, Sobsey MD: Coronavirus survival on healthcare personnel protective equipment, *Infect Hosp Epidemiol* 31:560–561, 2010.

REVIEW QUESTIONS

Multiple Choice

1. Wearing gloves at chairside helps prevent which of the following routes of entry of patient's microbes into the body?
   a. Inhalation
   b. Ingestion
   c. Mucous membranes
   d. Percutaneous

2. Heavy utility gloves should be used:
   a. for all intraoral procedures
   b. to rebag a dental unit with fresh surface covers
   c. to work with contaminated instruments
   d. to chart

3. Masks should be used when:
   a. spattering of contaminated fluids is possible
   b. seating a patient
   c. handling sterile packaged instruments

4. A mask should be replaced:
   a. just before going to lunch
   b. with every patient
   c. only if it becomes wet

5. The last of the personal protective barriers to be put on before patient treatment begins are:
   a. gowns
   b. masks
   c. gloves
   d. eyeglasses

6. The most common type of skin reaction to gloves is:
   a. latex allergy
   b. irritant contact dermatitis
   c. allergic contact dermatitis

7. When leaving chairside to get a new package of sterile instruments from the sterilizing room, what barrier should be removed and then replaced on returning to chairside?
   a. Gloves
   b. Mask
   c. Gown
   d. Eyeglasses

8. Wet masks should be changed because they:
   a. collect dust on the outer surface
   b. become too heavy to wear
   c. cause more air to enter around the edges
   d. begin to dissolve and fall apart

9. Gloves worn by dental personnel protect the:
   a. dental personnel
   b. patients
   c. operatory environment.
   d. dental personnel and patients

10. The mechanism of allergic contact dermatitis is the same as:
    a. hay fever
    b. the reaction to poison ivy
    c. asthma

11. Powder-free gloves are used to:
    a. prevent irritant contact dermatitis
    b. eliminate the need for hand hygiene after removing gloves
    c. limit the spread of latex protein allergens
    d. make the gloves easier to put on

12. Protective eyewear should have:
    a. extra thick lenses
    b. tinted lenses
    c. spring-loaded ear rests
    d. solid side shields

OUTLINE

Sterilization Versus Disinfection
  Sterilization
  Disinfection
  Categories of Patient Care Items
  Sterility Assurance for Patient Protection
Instrument Processing Procedures
  Holding (Presoaking)
  Precleaning
  Corrosion Control, Drying, and Lubrication
  Packaging
  Sterilization

Sterilization Monitoring
Handling of Processed Instruments
Design of the Instrument Processing Area
  General Location and Utilities
  Workflow Design
Instrument Sharpening
Instrument Protection
Handpiece Asepsis
Sterilization of Heat-Labile Items
Other Methods of Sterilization
Properties of Decontamination and
Sterilization Equipment and Products

LEARNING OBJECTIVES

After completing this chapter, the student should be able to do the following:

1. Differentiate between sterilization and disinfection; differentiate between critical, semicritical, and noncritical patient care items and describe differences in how such items are processed; and, define sterility assurance.
2. Do the following regarding instrument processing procedures:
   - List the steps involved in instrument processing and describe the rationale for each step.
   - Describe the three methods for instrument cleaning and the techniques for performing this task safely.
   - Determine which packaging materials are used for which methods of sterilization.
3. Describe the physical conditions, advantages, and precautions related to steam, dry heat, and unsaturated chemical vapor sterilization.

4. Compare the three methods of sterilization monitoring and describe how to perform each method, and describe what causes sterilization failure and what to do when failure is detected.
5. Describe how to handle, store, and distribute sterilized instruments to maintain sterility.
6. Describe the factors to consider when designing a sterilization facility within a dental office..
7. List considerations of infection control when sharpening instruments and tips for protecting dental instruments.
8. Describe how to sterilize handpieces and heat-sensitive instruments.
9. List other methods of sterilization and properties of decontamination and sterilization equipment and products.

KEY TERMS

Bioburden
Biological Indicators (Bls)
Biological Monitoring
Chemical Indicators

Chemical Monitoring
Disinfectant
Disinfection
Event-related Storage

Flash Sterilization
Gravity Displacement Steam
  Sterilizer
High-level Disinfectant

Instrument processing is a collection of procedures that prepares contaminated instruments for reuse. Box 12-1 presents the major steps for instrument processing and the explanations for each step. One must perform the processing carefully so that disease agents from a previous patient, from a member of the dental team who handled the instruments, or from the environment are not transferred by the instruments to the next patient. One also must perform processing correctly to keep instrument damage to a minimum. The overall process consists of seven steps, which are described in this chapter. Although the steps are not particularly difficult to perform, each must be performed properly in a routine, disciplined manner to ensure the desired outcome of patient protection with minimal instrument damage.

STERILIZATION VERSUS DISINFECTION

Because killing of microorganisms is an important step of instrument processing, an important first step is to have a general understanding of microbial killing methods before other steps in the process are described.

BOX 12-1

Instrument Processing

1. **Holding (presoaking):** facilitates the cleaning process by preventing debris from drying
2. **Precleaning**: removes as much of the bioburden as possible to give the subsequent sterilization step the best chance to work
3. **Corrosion control, drying, lubrication**: reduces damage to instruments and helps ensure proper functioning of the instruments
4. **Packaging**: helps maintain sterility of instruments after sterilization and before they are presented to a subsequent patient
5. **Sterilization or high-level disinfection**: kills all microbes remaining on the instruments to help ensure patient safety
6. **Sterilization monitoring**: measures the use and functioning of the sterilizer
7. **Handling processed instruments**: helps maintain the sterility of the instruments during storage and until they are used on a subsequent patient

---

Sterilization

Sterilization is a process intended to kill all microorganisms and is the highest level of microbial kill that can be achieved. Because routinely determining whether a microbial killing process actually kills all microorganisms is not possible, a highly resistant microorganism is selected as the standard challenge. If the process kills this microorganism, the process is considered to be a sterilization process. The bacterial endospore is selected as the standard challenge for sterilization because of its high resistance to killing by heat and chemicals (Figure 12-1). Spores are described more fully in Chapter 2 and in Sterilization Monitoring in this chapter. These spores are more difficult to kill than all of the common pathogenic microorganisms, including *Mycobacterium tuberculosis*, hepatitis viruses, human immunodeficiency virus type 1, fungal spores, herpesviruses, *Staphylococcus aureus*, and the thousands of other microorganisms. Thus a process cannot be called a sterilization process unless it is capable of killing high levels of bacterial endospores (i.e., is sporicidal). Three types of sterilization processes are used in dentistry: (1) heat sterilization, (2) gas sterilization, and (3) liquid chemical sterilization. Other types of sterilization procedures exist, but they have not been applied to the field of dentistry or have not yet been made practical for use in the dental office. Heat sterilization involving steam, dry heat, and unsaturated chemical vapor is the most common type of sterilization used in offices today.

The heat sterilizers operate at 121° C (250° F) to 190.6° C (375° F), and their sterilization processes can be monitored routinely for effectiveness using bacterial spores (called biological monitoring).

One also can monitor ethylene oxide gas sterilizers that operate at 22° C (72° F) to 60° C (140° F) (much lower than heat sterilizers) with bacterial endospores, but this type of sterilization is not commonly used in dental offices because of the long exposure time required for sterilization, the high cost of gas sterilizers, and the required special handling of the ethylene oxide gas sterilant.

Liquid chemical sterilization at room temperature is used on items that are damaged by heat sterilization. Examples of liquid chemical sterilants/high-level disinfectants used are glutaraldehyde, glutaraldehyde-phenate, special hydrogen peroxide, and hydrogen peroxide–peracetic acid. Although these liquid sterilants can be shown to be sporicidal in controlled laboratory testing, the microbial killing that occurs during actual use in the office cannot be monitored routinely as it can for heat sterilization. Spore tests for biological monitoring have not been developed yet for office testing of liquid sterilants. The best that can be done is to estimate chemically the concentration of active sterilant remaining in the used solution. The sterilant slowly becomes inactive. More information about sterilization is given later in this chapter.

Disinfection

Disinfection is a less-lethal process than sterilization and is intended to kill disease-producing microorganisms but not bacterial endospores. Disinfection usually refers to the use of liquid chemicals to kill microorganisms at room temperature on surfaces. If the chemical is not sporicidal but can kill other microorganisms, it is called a disinfectant. Several types of disinfectants are available—for example, synthetic phenolics, phenol, iodophors, alcohol-phenolics, sodium hypochlorite, quaternary ammonium compounds, alcohol, and alcohol–quaternary ammonium compounds. Chemicals classified as disinfectants cannot be expected to achieve sterilization. Chapter 13 gives details on these disinfectants and their uses, but an important point to understand is that one cannot determine routinely the level of microbial killing actually achieved by these disinfectants during use in the office. Thus one never knows how well disinfectants are working.

Some liquid chemicals can serve as a sterilant or a high-level disinfectant, depending on how they are used. Chapter 13 explains this use further, but in general, these chemicals are sterilants (kill high levels of bacterial spores) when used for long exposure times and are high-level disinfectants (kill low levels of bacterial spores) when used for shorter exposure times. For example, 2.0% to 3.4% glutaraldehyde is a sterilant when precleaned items are submerged for 10 hours of contact time, but is a high-level disinfectant when contact time is less than 10 hours. When used at lower concentrations or for shorter times, glutaraldehyde can achieve only disinfection. Also, as already mentioned, one cannot determine microbial killing by liquid chemicals in the office.

Categories of Patient Care Items

The Centers for Disease Control and Prevention (CDC) categorizes patient care items as critical, semicritical, or noncritical based on the potential risk of infection during use of the items (Table 12-1). These categories are referred to as the Spaulding classification, having been first proposed by Spaulding in 1968. The CDC indicates the following:
- Critical and semicritical items are to be cleaned and sterilized by heat.
- Semicritical items that are heat sensitive must, at a minimum, be cleaned and treated with a high-level disinfectant.
- Noncritical items are cleaned and treated with a low-level disinfectant (if no blood is visible on the item) or an intermediate-level disinfectant (if blood is visible).

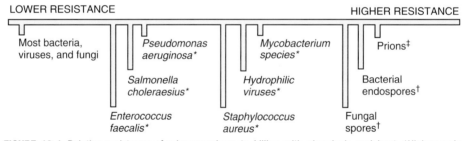

FIGURE 12-1 Relative resistance of microorganisms to killing with chemicals and heat. *Higher resistance to killing with chemicals; †higher resistance to killing with chemicals and heat; ‡are proteins, not microorganisms.

TABLE 12-1   **Categories of Patient Care Items as Identified by the Centers for Disease Control and Prevention**

Category	Definition	Examples
Critical	Penetrates soft tissue, contacts bone, enters into or contacts the bloodstream or other normally sterile tissue of the mouth	Surgical instruments, scalers, blades, surgical dental burs
Semicritical	Contacts mucous membranes but will not penetrate soft tissue, contacts bone, enters into or contacts the bloodstream or other normally sterile tissue of the mouth	Dental mouth mirror, amalgam condenser, reusable dental impression trays, dental handpieces*
Noncritical	Contacts intact skin	Blood pressure cuff, stethoscope, pulse oximeter

Adapted from Kohn WG, Collins AS, Cleveland JL, et al; Centers for Disease Control and Prevention: Guidelines for infection control in dental health-care settings–2003, *MMWR Morb Mortal Wkly Rep* 52 (RR-17):20, 2003.
*Although dental handpieces are considered a semicritical item, heat sterilization is recommended.

Sterility Assurance for Patient Protection

Universal sterilization means that all reusable instruments and handpieces are sterilized (rather than just disinfected) between use on patients. This provides the highest level of patient protection. If an item used in the patient's mouth cannot be sterilized or cannot withstand the conditions of sterilization or cannot be prevented from becoming contaminated during use, the item should not be used or should be discarded after use on one patient.

Maximum patient protection with universal sterilization can be achieved only by practicing sterility assurance. Because the sterility of each processed instrument cannot be measured routinely, one must depend on the reliability of the instrument processing procedures being performed. Thus sterility assurance is the correct performance of the proper instrument processing steps and monitoring of the sterilization step with biological, mechanical, and chemical indicators. This assurance program requires taking four steps.

1. Select the proper procedure and confirm the correct way to perform that procedure.
2. Prepare a written step-by-step description of the correct procedure to be used as a reference in training and to document patient safety techniques used in the office.
3. Incorporate the procedure into the office training program to ensure that new employees learn the correct procedure.
4. Monitor the performance of the procedure to ensure its routine use and, when possible, measure the results of the procedure.

The statement that "instruments have been sterilized" is true only if sterility assurance is practiced, that is, showing by frequent biological, mechanical, and chemical monitoring that the process used kills bacterial endospores.

INSTRUMENT PROCESSING PROCEDURES

Procedure 12-1 presents suggested step-by-step procedures and rationales for instrument processing. One must handle contaminated instruments carefully to avoid cuts and punctures from sharp items, any of which constitutes an exposure. One should always use personal protective equipment, including utility gloves, mask, and protective eyewear and clothing during these procedures, as described in Chapter 11.

Holding (Presoaking)

If instruments cannot be cleaned soon after use, they should be placed in a holding solution to prevent drying of the saliva and blood and to facilitate the actual cleaning. Some plastic/resin cassette manufacturers do not recommend presoaking, so one should follow their instructions for cleaning. Extended presoaking for more than a few hours is not recommended because this may enhance corrosion of some instruments. The holding solution may be the same detergent as that to be used for subsequent cleaning or may be water or an enzyme solution. One should place loose instruments in a perforated cleaning basket and then place the basket in the holding solution. Use of the basket reduces direct handling of instruments through the subsequent rinsing, cleaning, and rinsing steps. The presoaked instruments and the holding solution must be considered contaminated. One should discard the solution at least once a day (or more often if visibly soiled) while wearing protective equipment.

Precleaning

Precleaning is an essential step before any sterilization or disinfection procedure. Instruments become contaminated with blood, saliva, tissue fluids, and dental materials. Mixed in with these are microbes from the patient's saliva and blood. This microbe-laden debris is referred to as bioburden. The organic components in the blood and saliva (e.g., proteins, fats) coat the microbes and provide insulation from sterilizing agents in steam, dry heat, and unsaturated chemical vapor sterilizers, and from chemicals in sterilants and disinfectants. Precleaning reduces the bioburden and gives the subsequent sterilization or disinfection step the best chance to work. A "dirty" instrument may in some instances become sterile during subsequent processing, but one cannot confirm this. (Besides, a patient will never be convinced that a visibly dirty instrument is safe for use, even if it really is sterile.) Two basic types of dental instrument cleaning systems that have been cleared by the Food and Drug Administration (FDA) for safety and effectiveness are ultrasonic cleaners and instrument washers or washer-disinfectors.

Ultrasonic Cleaning

Ultrasonic cleaning, compared with scrubbing instruments by hand, reduces direct handling of the contaminated instruments and the chances for cuts and punctures. Ultrasonic cleaning is also an excellent cleaning mechanism, and staff can do other tasks while the instruments are being cleaned. The ultrasonic energy produces billions of tiny bubbles in the cleaning solution that collapse and create high turbulence at the surface of the instruments. This turbulence dislodges the debris and suspends it in the solution or dissolves it. Few instruments cannot be cleaned ultrasonically. One exception is some high-speed handpieces, although others can withstand ultrasonic cleaning. One should check the handpiece manufacturer's instructions for cleaning.

Ultrasonic cleaning units come in several sizes that are freestanding (Figure 12-2) or can be built into countertops. Many ultrasonic cleaners have automatic drains that eliminate having to lift the cleaner and pour the used cleaning solution into the sink. Some cleaners can be connected directly to water lines and have automatic rinsing cycles. These cleaners can accommodate any office or clinic and can process instruments that are loose or are in cassettes. One always should use a cleaning basket or cassette rack

PROCEDURE 12-1

Instrument Processing

GOAL: To provide sterile instruments at chairside for use on subsequent patients

Materials Needed
See Table 12-6.

1. Put on heavy utility gloves, protective eyewear, mask, and protective clothing.
   Rationale: These barriers provide personal protection from contaminants on the instruments and from chemicals used.

2. One may remove gross debris from instruments by wiping at chairside but only if one takes great care to avoid sharps injuries.
   Rationale: Wiping aids cleaning but must be performed carefully.

3. Place loose, contaminated instruments in ultrasonic cleaning basket or washer basket and place basket in holding solution until ready to clean thoroughly. If using cassettes, remove and dispose of waste and rinse cassette/instruments with water.
   Rationale: This step aids the subsequent cleaning process by removing gross debris.

4. Remove basket of instruments from holding solution, rinse with minimum splashing, and place in ultrasonic cleaner or washer, or place cassettes in cleaning rack and place in ultrasonic cleaner or washer.
   Rationale: Using baskets or cassette racks facilitates cleaning and reduces the direct handling of the instruments and cassettes.

5. Make sure ultrasonic cleaning unit or washer has been filled to proper level with cleaning solution.
   Rationale: Using the appropriate amount and type of cleaning solution ensures the best cleaning.

6. Place cover on ultrasonic cleaner or close washer door and operate for the time recommended by the cleaning unit manufacturer or cassette manufacturer. In general, these times are 4 to 16 minutes in ultrasonic cleaners. The time is set automatically in washers.
   Rationale: Thorough cleaning requires the appropriate amount of time.

7. Remove cleaning basket or cassette rack from ultrasonic units and rinse under tap water with a minimum of splashing. Rinse cassettes individually and thoroughly. Rinsing is usually automatic in washers.
   Rationale: Rinsing removes the residual cleaning solution that contains microbes.

8. Check instruments for broken tips and cleanliness, and dry loose instruments with a towel or let cassette drain. Replace or reclean items as needed. Apply rust inhibitor as needed for nonstainless items to be processed in steam.
   Rationale: Checking instruments helps monitor the effectiveness of the cleaning process and determines when cleaning equipment repair may be needed.

9. Place instruments into functional sets or add desired items to cassettes, including the appropriate biological and internal and external chemical indicators. Use packaging material that is compatible with the method of sterilization. Seal the package or wrap the cassette and label for content identification and sterilization date. Make sure chemical indicators are present or visible on the outside of the packages.
   Rationale: Indicators monitor the effectiveness of the sterilization process, and packaging maintains the sterility of the instruments after they are removed from the sterilizer.

10. Sterilize following manufacturer's recommendations for loading, sterilizing time, temperature, and drying.
    Rationale: Sterilizers must be operated at the proper time and temperature for sterility assurance.

11. Carefully remove items from the sterilizer but wait until after the dry cycle with steam sterilizers.
    Rationale: Exposing wet packs after steam processing to the external environment facilitates wicking and contamination of the internal contents. Handling of wet packs after steam processing also can tear the packaging material.

12. Observe external chemical indicators for proper reaction, retrieve biological indicators for analysis, observe internal chemical indicators, and store or distribute packages to chairside with minimal handling.
    Rationale: Chemical monitors give an immediate indication of instrument safety. Biological indicators show the main guarantee of instrument safety. Careful handling of sterile packs prevents tearing and helps maintain sterility.

PROCEDURE 12-1

Instrument Processing—cont'd

13. Maintain sterility assurance records on date and conditions of sterilization and results of mechanical, biologic, and chemical indicators.
Rationale: Maintaining sterilization monitoring records documents compliance with rules and recommendations relating to patient safety.

14. Sterilize reusable heat-labile items (e.g., some plastic items) in a liquid sterilant, rinse, and package in clean packaging material.
Rationale: Sterilization monitoring records document the performance of proper instrument sterilization and establish accountability in assurance of patient safety.

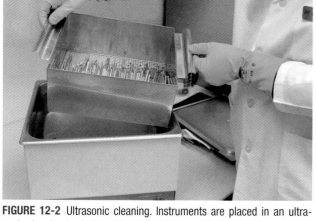

FIGURE 12-2 Ultrasonic cleaning. Instruments are placed in an ultrasonic cleaning basket, and the basket is placed in the cleaning solution.

to suspend the items in the cleaning solution because better cleaning is achieved when items are off the bottom of the chamber. In addition, use of the basket or rack eliminates the need to scoop up the instruments by hand at the end of the cycle. Operate the unit with the cover in place to reduce the noise level and keep dust from further contaminating the cleaning solution. Follow the manufacturer's directions for proper use.

One should use a cleaning solution designed for use on dental or medical instruments and recommended for use in ultrasonic cleaners. Maintain the solution at the proper level in the cleaning chamber, ensuring that all items being cleaned are submerged completely. Cleaning solutions that also have antimicrobial activity will reduce the buildup of microorganisms in the solution as it is used repeatedly. However, one should not use common disinfectants in place of a detergent solution unless they are designed for this use. One should process instruments in the cleaner until they are visibly clean. This time may vary, depending on the instruments, the amount or type of material on the instruments, and the efficiency of the ultrasonic unit. This time ranges from approximately 4 to 16 minutes. One determines the time by the visible cleanliness of the instruments. Instruments in plastic/resin cassettes require longer cleaning times

because the plastic/resin absorbs some of the ultrasonic energy.

After cleaning, one removes the basket or cassette rack and thoroughly rinses the instruments under tap water with a minimum of splashing (unless the cleaner has automatic rinsing). Used ultrasonic cleaning solutions can contain large numbers of microbes; the rinsing removes the residual cleaning solution and further reduces the bioburden. The cleaned and rinsed instruments and cassettes still are contaminated and must be handled with gloves. One should drain or otherwise discard the cleaning solution at least daily, earlier if it becomes visibly soiled. One should rinse, disinfect, rinse, and dry the cleaning chamber at the end of the day while wearing protective equipment.

One can test the functioning of an ultrasonic unit using the aluminum foil test as follows: Cut a piece of lightweight aluminum foil about 1 inch shorter than the length of the chamber and 1 inch longer than the depth of the solution in the chamber. Insert the foil vertically into the filled chamber with the length of the foil running the length of the chamber and the bottom of the foil about 1 inch above the bottom. Do not let the foil touch the bottom of the tank. Operate the unit for 20 seconds. Remove the foil and observe for small indentations (pebbling) on the foil (Figure 12-3). This pebbling should be distributed fairly evenly over the entire submerged part of the foil. If areas greater than ½ square inch have no pebbling, the unit may need servicing. Some ultrasonic unit manufacturers may use variations of this aluminum foil procedure described here; one should follow their specific directions.

Instrument Washers

Instrument washers designed to clean medical and dental instruments are used in hospitals, dental schools, and in some smaller dental offices. Like ultrasonic cleaners, these washers remove bioburden, reduce the direct handling of instruments, and can clean loose instruments in baskets or instruments in cassettes. Three different sizes of instrument washers are available: a bench top model, a floor unit, and a large production model (Figure 12-4). These washers automatically provide cleaning and rinsing, and some (called washer-disinfectors) use hot water and achieve disinfection of the instruments with cleaning. One should be sure to use the detergent recommended by the washer manufacturer.

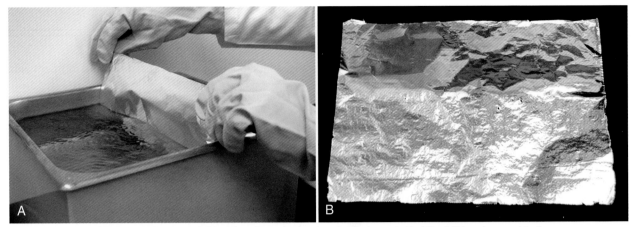

FIGURE 12-3 Aluminum foil test for ultrasonic cleaners. **A,** The lower half of the foil is submerged in the cleaning solution for 20 seconds of operation. **B,** Note the indentations and some holes evenly distributed over the submerged portion of the foil.

Instrument washers are FDA-regulated medical devices. Household dishwashers are not recommended for use on contaminated instruments because their manufacturers did not design them for this purpose and have not sought FDA assurances of safety and effectiveness.

Manual Scrubbing of Instruments

Scrubbing contaminated instruments by hand is dangerous even though the procedure is an effective method of removing debris, if performed properly. One should thoroughly brush all surfaces of all instruments while the instruments are either submerged in a cleaning solution to avoid spattering or at least scrubbed near the bottom of a deep sink. Use of a long-handled brush is best to keep the scrubbing hand as far away from the sharp instrument tips as possible. One follows the scrubbing with thorough rinsing with a minimum of splashing.

Routine manual scrubbing of instruments is not recommended because it requires maximum direct contact with the contaminated instruments, increasing the chances for cuts or punctures through the gloves. One also should not hand scrub instruments before processing them through ultrasonic cleaners or instrument washers. If the mechanical cleaners are working properly, hand scrubbing is unnecessary.

Corrosion Control, Drying, and Lubrication

Instruments or portions of instruments and burs made of carbon steel will rust during steam sterilization. Examples include non–stainless steel cutting or scraping instruments such as burs, scalers, hoes, hatchets, the cutting surfaces of orthodontic pliers, and the grasping surfaces of forceps. Although one can spray rust inhibitors (e.g., sodium nitrite) on the instruments or use a dip to reduce rusting of some of these items, the best approach is not to process such items through steam. Instead one should dry the instruments thoroughly and use dry heat or unsaturated chemical vapor sterilization on the items most susceptible to rusting in steam.

Another alternative is to switch to stainless steel-type instruments, if available.

Instruments to be processed through a steam sterilizer should at least be shaken to remove excess water or dried more thoroughly if they will be packaged in paper or paper-plastic sterilization wrap. This avoids accidental tearing of wet paper during packaging. Some hinged instruments may need to be lubricated to maintain proper functioning, but one should remove as much excess lubricant as possible before heat processing. Hinged instruments should be opened before packaging to facilitate access of the sterilizing agents to all parts of the instruments. Drying equipment for cleaned unwrapped instruments is available.

Packaging

Proper instrument processing is more than just sterilizing instruments between patients; it is delivering sterile instruments to chairside for use on the next patient. To do this, one must maintain the sterility of the instruments after they are processed through the sterilizer. Packaging instruments before processing through the sterilizer prevents them from becoming contaminated after sterilization during storage or when being distributed to chairside. Unpackaged instruments are exposed completely to the environment immediately after the sterilizer door is opened and can be contaminated by dust or aerosols in the air, by contact with moisture, by improper handling, or by contact with contaminated surfaces.

Packaging involves wrapping cleaned instrument cassettes or organizing cleaned loose instruments in functional sets and wrapping them or placing them in sterilization pouches, bags, trays, or cassettes. One adds biological and chemical indicators (described later) during the packaging procedures.

General Packaging Procedures

One should use only packaging material or open containers that have been designed for use in sterilizers and should use

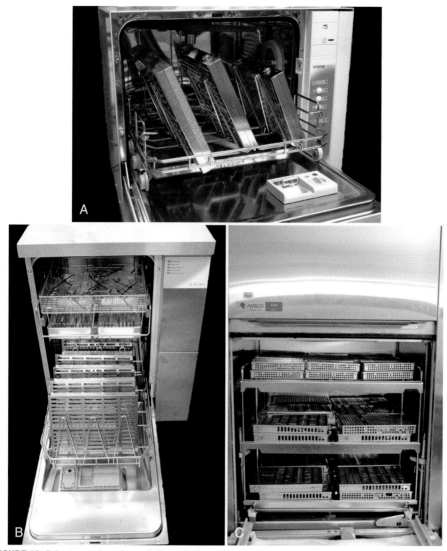

FIGURE 12-4 Instrument washers. **A**, Benchtop model holding 3 cassettes or baskets of instruments. **B**, Floor model holding 6 cassettes and baskets of instruments or 11 cassettes. **C**, Large production model holding 36 cassettes.

the appropriate sterilization packaging materials for the sterilization method being used (Table 12-2). Sterilization packaging materials are medical devices and are to be cleared by the FDA for safety and effectiveness. These materials must be shown to allow penetration of the sterilizing agents and to maintain sterility for at least 6 months before being cleared for sale in the United States. Other general wrap, plastic bags, containers, or paper may melt, prevent the sterilizing agent from penetrating to the instruments inside, or release unwanted chemicals into the sterilizer chamber. Cloth should not be used as a sterilization wrap because it is not a barrier to microbes. Paper sterilization bags should not be used to package heavy or sharp instruments because they will commonly protrude through the paper. Such bags are better used for gauze pads, cotton rolls or pledgets, or paper products. Sterilization pouches, wraps, or bags should never be sealed with metal closures, including staples or anything that can puncture the material and breech sterility.

Closed containers, such as trays or pans with solid tops and bottoms, capped glass vials, or wrap, such as aluminum foil, should never be used to package items for sterilization in steam or unsaturated chemical vapor sterilizers. The steam or hot chemical vapor will not penetrate these containers or materials to reach the items inside. These containers may be appropriate for sterilization in dry heat, however, if sufficient exposure time is used. Sharps containers and biohazard bags containing regulated waste that will be sterilized before disposal must be left open during the sterilization process and then closed after removal from the sterilizer (see Chapter 17). If these containers are closed before heat processing, the steam or chemical vapor will not reach the items inside the containers or bags. Not all sharps containers and biohazard bags can withstand the high temperature in heat sterilization. Those that can are usually marked "sterilizable."

One can test penetration of steam, hot chemical vapor, or heated air through a particular type of packaging material

TABLE 12-2 **Types and Use of Sterilization Packaging Materials**

Sterilization Method	Packaging Materials	Precautions
Steam autoclave*	Paper wrap† Nylon plastic tubing Paper/plastic peel pouches Wrapped perforated cassettes	No closed containers Thick cloth may absorb too much steam Some plastic containers melt Use only material approved for steam
Dry heat sterilizers	Paper wrap† Appropriate nylon plastic tubing Closed containers‡ Wrapped perforated cassettes	Some plastic may char Some plastic containers melt Only use material approved for dry heat
Unsaturated chemical sterilizer	Paper wrap† Paper/plastic peel pouches Wrapped perforated cassettes	No closed containers Cloth absorbs too much chemical vapor Some plastic containers melt Use only material approved for chemical vapor

*Flash (or unwrapped) sterilization cycles that operate at higher temperatures for shorter times indicate that the items being processed are not to be packaged.
†Heavy or sharp items may penetrate paper bags.
‡Biological indicators (spore tests) should be used to confirm that sterilizing conditions are achieved within any closed containers used.

or container by placing spore strips inside and processing through the sterilizer to make sure the spores are killed. This procedure is not recommended for testing filled sharps containers unless one takes special care to avoid injuries when placing and retrieving the spore strips.

Wrapping or Bagging

One can place functional sets of instruments on a small, sterilizable tray and wrap the entire tray with sterilization wrap. Figure 12-5 diagrams the wrapping procedure. One should seal the wrap with tape that will withstand the heat process (e.g., autoclave tape).

One also may place functional sets in see-through paper/plastic pouches that have clear plastic film on one side and heavy sterilization paper on the other side (Figure 12-6). These pouches are available in many different sizes, can be used in steam or unsaturated chemical vapor sterilizers, and have chemical indicators (discussed later) printed directly on the paper side of the pouch. Some pouches have chemical indicators inside the pouch and most are self-sealing; others need to be sealed with tape. The pouches are easy to open after sterilization by peeling the plastic away from the paper. Although less commonly used, a nylon type of clear plastic tubing comes on a roll and may be cut to varying lengths, filled with instruments, and heat sealed or taped. One can use one type in steam and another type in dry heat sterilizers. Paper bags are available, but one must take care because sharp and pointed instruments can puncture the paper easily, and paper becomes wet during steam sterilization and will tear if handled before drying. One should expel as much air as possible from the bags and pouches before sterilization.

Use of Instrument Cassettes

Numerous styles of cassettes are available that contain functional sets of instruments during use at chairside and

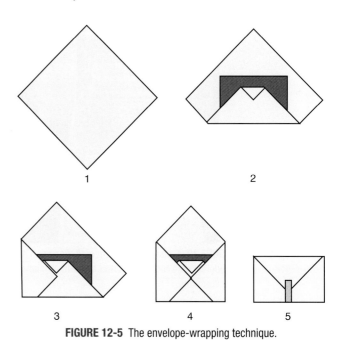

FIGURE 12-5 The envelope-wrapping technique.

during the precleaning, rinsing, and sterilizing processes (Figure 12-7). Use of cassettes reduces direct handling of contaminated instruments and keeps the instruments together through the entire process of cleaning, sterilization, and presentation to the next patient. After ultrasonic cleaning, rinsing, and drying, one may add sterilizable supply-type items to the cassette and wrap, sterilize, and store or use the cassette immediately. Use of an instrument cassette system requires planning to ensure that the proper size of ultrasonic cleaner and sterilizer is available for processing. Cassettes are available in stainless steel, aluminum, and plastic/resin material that can withstand steam, chemical vapor, and dry heat sterilization. One should follow the cassette manufacturer's recommendations for

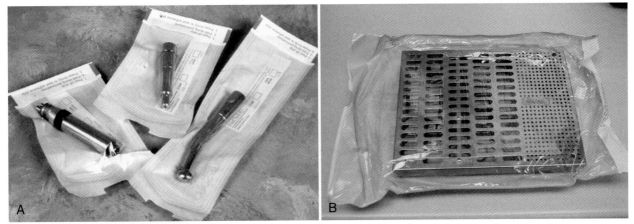

FIGURE 12-6 Instrument packaging using a self-sealing, paper/plastic peel pouch. **A,** Packaged handpieces. **B,** Packaged instrument cassette.

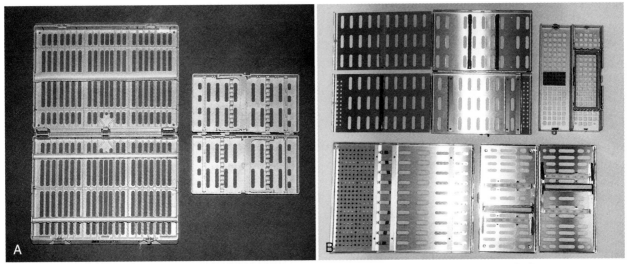

FIGURE 12-7 Examples of opened cassettes used to package functional sets of instruments through ultrasonic cleaning, rinsing, drying, packaging, and sterilizing and for direct use at chairside. **A,** Resin cassettes. **B,** Metal cassettes.

ultrasonic cleaning, wrapping or bagging, and sterilization. One should wrap cassettes before processing them through a sterilizer.

Unwrapped Instruments

Sterilizing unpackaged instruments using the short exposure times (**flash sterilization**) is the least satisfactory approach to patient protection because it allows for unnecessary contamination before the instruments actually are used on the next patient. The CDC recommendations state that flash sterilization should not be used as a routine sterilization procedure for patient care items. If for some reason unwrapped instruments are sterilized (e.g., flash sterilization of an item in short supply that was dropped on the floor during patient care and will be used immediately), the instruments subsequently must be handled with special care to reduce poststerilization contamination as much as possible. If semicritical instruments will be used immediately or in a short time, they can be sterilized

unwrapped and handled aseptically during removal from the sterilizer and transport to the point of use. Critical instruments intended for immediate reuse may be sterilized unwrapped, provided that the instruments are maintained sterile during removal from the sterilizer and transport to the point of use. One may accomplish this using sterile tongs to remove the instruments from the sterilizer and placing them in a sterile covered transport container. A carefully written protocol for minimizing the risk of poststerilization contamination of unpackaged instruments should be prepared and strictly followed. One also should monitor every flash sterilization cycle with mechanical, chemical, and biological monitors using procedures described later in the chapter.

Sterilization

Precleaned, packaged instruments are ready for processing through a heat sterilizer. One should use only FDA-cleared

TABLE 12-3   Comparison of Heat Sterilization Methods Using Small Office Sterilizers

Method	Standard Sterilizing Conditions*	Advantages	Precautions	Spore Testing
STEAM AUTOCLAVE				
Standard cycles	20-30 minutes at 121° C (250° F)	Time efficient Good penetration Sterilizes water-based liquids in standard cycles†	Do not use closed containers Damage to plastic and rubber Non–stainless steel metal items corrode Use of hard water may leave deposits Items may be wet after cycle Unwrapped items quickly contaminate after processing	*Geobacillus stearothermophilus* strips or vials
Flash cycles	3-10 minutes at 133.9° C (273° F)	Quick turn-around	Unwrapped items quickly contaminate after processing	
UNSATURATED CHEMICAL VAPOR	20 minutes at 132.2° C (270° F)	Time efficient No corrosion Items dry quickly after cycle	Do not use closed containers Damage to plastic and rubber Must use special solution Predry instruments Provide adequate ventilation Cannot sterilize liquids Cloth wraps may absorb chemicals Unwrapped items quickly contaminate after processing	*Geobacillus stearothermophilus* strips
DRY HEAT				
Oven-type sterilizer (static-air)	60-120 minutes at 160° C (320° F)	No corrosion Can use closed containers‡ Low cost Items are dry after cycle	Long sterilization time Damage to plastic and rubber Predry instruments Do not open door during cycle Cannot sterilize liquids Unwrapped items quickly contaminate after processing	*Bacillus atrophaeus* strips
Rapid heat transfer (forced-air)	12 minutes at 190.6° C (375° F) (wrapped) 6 minutes at 190.6° C (375° F) (unwrapped)	No corrosion Short cycle Items are dry after cycle	Damage to some plastic and rubber Predry instruments Do not open door during cycle Cannot sterilize liquids Unwrapped items quickly contaminate after processing	*Bacillus atrophaeus* strips

Adapted from Miller CH: Take the safe approach to disease prevention, *RDH* 9:35, 1989; and Miller CH: Sterilization and disinfection: what every dentist should know, *J Am Dent Assoc* 123:26, 1992.

*These conditions do not include warm-up or cool-down time, and they may vary depending on the nature and volume of the load and brand of the sterilizer. Sterilizing conditions actually achieved in the office should be defined by results of spore testing.

†To use, it is best to purchase sterile irrigating fluids with certified sterility for clinical use.

‡Processing in closed containers should be checked carefully by spore testing.

medical devices for sterilization. Although regular cooking ovens or toaster ovens certainly get hot, they are not intended for use as sterilizers and have not gone through the same rigorous testing or quality assurance in manufacturing to show safety and effectiveness, as is true for sterilizers. Table 12-3 compares the three most common types of sterilizers used in dental offices. Most metal hand instruments and equipment can be sterilized in any of these three sterilizers. The most notable exceptions are handpieces, as they cannot be processed through dry heat. If

there is ever a question, check with the manufacturer of the instrument.

Steam Sterilization

Types of steam sterilizers

Steam sterilization involves heating water to generate steam in a closed chamber, producing a moist heat that rapidly kills microorganisms.

Boiling water (100° C [212° F]) is not hot enough to routinely kill all microbes, but steam under pressure can. In the steam sterilizer, it is very important that the steam reach all surfaces of the instruments to be sterilized. Because air can act as a barrier (insulator) around the instruments, it is important to remove the air from the sterilizer chamber or cassette. Any air pockets left there will never be heated to above 100° C (212° F). As the sterilizer heats up, it boils the water and produces steam, which pushes the air out of an escape valve that then closes and allows a buildup of pressure. There are three types of steam sterilizers based on how air is removed from the chamber or sterilizing cassette.

• **Gravity displacement steam sterilizer**

As steam is generated, it forces the air out the bottom of the chamber through a drain. When sterilizing temperatures are reached (e.g., 121° C [250° F]), the drain closes and the temperature is held for the prescribed time.

• **Vacuum pump sterilizer (type B sterilizer)**

A vacuum pump removes air before steam is generated.

• **Positive steam flush/pressure pulse sterilizer**

A positive steam flush/pressure pulse sterilizer uses repeated sequences of steam flushes and pressure pulses to remove the air.

The heat, not the pressure, inside a steam sterilizer is what actually kills the microorganisms. In the absence of air in a closed system, the steam creates higher temperatures than steam coming from an open pan of boiling water, which allows the steam to be mixed with cooler air above the pan. Manufacturers set their sterilizers to reach maximum steam temperatures of approximately 121.1° C (250° F) or 134° C (273° F) with respective pressures of 103 or 206 kilopascals (kPa), which is the same as 15 or 30 pounds per square inch (psi).

• Small office sterilizers

A typical dental office steam sterilizer usually operates through four steps: the heat-up cycle, the sterilizing cycle, the depressurization cycle, and the drying cycle. After adding the water, one loads the chamber, closes the door, and turns on the unit, and the heat-up cycle begins to generate the steam and remove air. Once the sterilizing temperature is reached, the sterilization cycle begins and the temperature is held for the set time, usually ranging from 3 to 30 minutes. Typical preset sterilizing cycles are:

• 121° C (250° F) for 30 minutes
• 121° C (250° F) for 15 minutes
• 134° C (273° F) for 10 minutes
• 134° C (273° F) for 3 minutes

At the end of the sterilizing cycle, the depressurization cycle begins and the steam is slowly released, with a decrease in temperature and pressure. At the end of this cycle, all of the items inside are wet, and the drying cycle (if available) is initiated. Drying packages before removing them from the sterilizer chamber is important (see Drying and Cooling below). Some steam sterilizers pull in fresh air through a microbial filter (e.g., a high-efficiency particulate air filter) at the end of the sterilizing cycle to facilitate drying. Some sterilizers have a poststerilization vacuum cycle to facilitate drying, then pull in fresh air through a filter. Other sterilizers have an automatic open door drying cycle. This cycle maintains heat inside the chamber to evaporate the remaining water, but the chamber is open to the air so that water vapor can escape and the items can dry. With other sterilizers, one opens the door manually approximately 1/2 inch for a time to let the moisture escape.

Small office steam sterilizers usually have chambers of 8 to 12 inches in diameter (Figure 12-8, *A*) or have a closable cassette containing the instruments that is inserted into the sterilizer, serving as the sterilizer chamber (see Figure 12-8, *B*). Some units also have printout devices that record the time, temperature, and pressure for mechanical monitoring of each sterilizing cycle to help maintain sterility assurance records.

• Hospital-type sterilizers

Steam sterilizers used in hospitals, dental schools, and some large clinics have much larger chambers and are connected directly to a steam line, which eliminates the need for the sterilizers to generate their own steam, or are connected to a water line that allows them to generate their own steam (Figure 12-9). Most of these sterilizers have a vacuum system for air removal from the chamber so that when

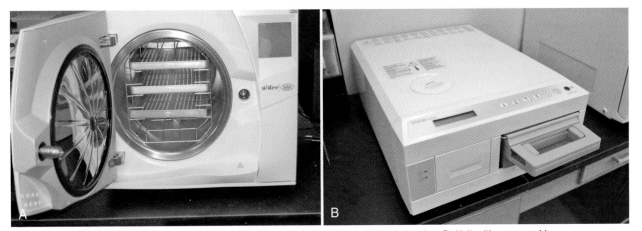

FIGURE 12-8 Examples of steam sterilizers. **A,** Unit with a cylindrical chamber. **B,** Unit with a removable chamber (cassette).

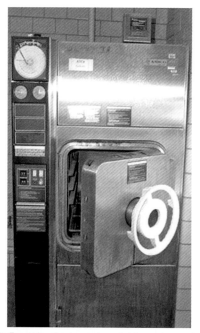

FIGURE 12-9 Example of a large, hospital-type steam sterilizer. (From VanMeter KC, VanMeter WG, Hubert RJ: *Microbiology for the healthcare professional*, St. Louis, 2010, Mosby, pp 80-97.)

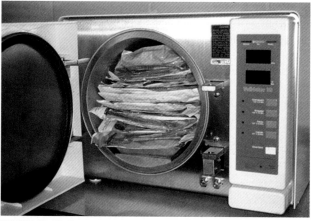

FIGURE 12-10 Do not load a sterilizer like this. Place the items on their edges as shown in Figure 12-11.

the steam enters, it has a better chance of coming into direct contact with everything in the chamber because no air is around the items that can insulate them from the hot steam. These units also have a poststerilization vacuum cycle that removes the steam and water after the sterilizing cycle to dry instrument packs. No matter what type of sterilizer one uses, one must be sure to follow all of the manufacturer's directions for routine maintenance, loading, monitoring, and safe operation.

Loading

Do not stack packages, pouches, or cassettes flat in layers as shown in Figure 12-10; stacking impedes steam circulation and air removal in the chamber. One should load the sterilizer as instructed by the manufacturer and keep packs, pouches, or cassettes separated from each other so that steam has access to all package surfaces. Place items on their edges as shown in Figure 12-11. Some sterilizers come with racks for packages that keep them separated and on their edge.

Sterilizing

One should follow the manufacturer's instructions for the time and temperature of exposure and should remember that the sterilizing cycle does not begin until the chamber reaches a temperature of 121° C (250° F) or 134° C (273° F). The exposure times of approximately 3 to 30 minutes at these temperatures are set to include extra time to ensure microbial killing (safety factor). Thus use of shorter times reduces safety factors. This is of particular concern with flash sterilization cycles (defined previously) that operate

in the range of 3 minutes at the higher temperature. These flash cycles originally were designed for use only in emergency situations, for example, when an expensive instrument in short supply is dropped on the floor while one is caring for a patient and the instrument has to be cleaned and resterilized quickly for continued use. Not only is the time shortened in a flash cycle, but the item to be sterilized also is not wrapped or packaged in any way so that it can have immediate contact with the steam in this short cycle. Because the item is not wrapped, it is open to immediate recontamination on removal from the sterilizer. Thus one should not use flash sterilization of instruments routinely as a substitute for purchasing additional instruments or simply to reduce instrument processing time because this weakens sterility assurance and might jeopardize patient protection.

Unloading

Drying packages inside the steam sterilizer is important to maintain the sterility of the instruments. Handling of wet packages can easily tear the paper, causing contamination of the instruments (Figure 12-12). Exposing wet packages to the environment outside the sterilizer also can cause wicking. **Wicking** is the process that allows bacteria and fungi to penetrate wet sterilization paper (paper/plastic peel pouches, sterilization wrap, or paper pouches). Wicking enables microbes from the air, spatter, dust, fingers, or other contaminated surfaces that contact the outer surface of a wet instrument package to be drawn through to the instruments inside. Thus one should not handle wet packs or expose wet packs to the office environment. One should let these packages dry inside the sterilizer before handling them.

Unsaturated Chemical Vapor Sterilization

Unsaturated chemical vapor sterilization involves heating a special chemical solution in a closed chamber, producing hot chemical vapors that kill microorganisms. The chemical solution contains 0.23% formaldehyde (the active ingredient) and 72.38% ethanol plus acetone, ketone, water, and

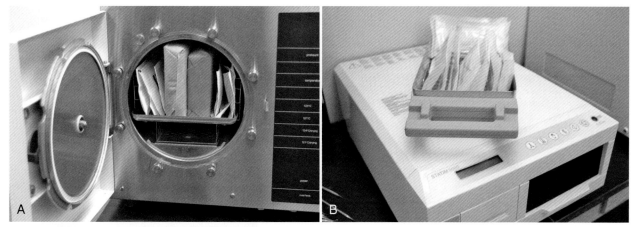

FIGURE 12-11 Proper loading of sterilizers. **A,** Loading a sterilizer with a cylindrical chamber. **B,** Loading a cassette sterilizer.

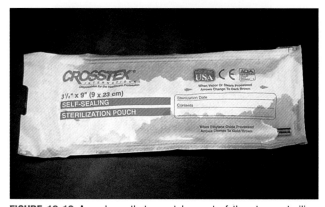

FIGURE 12-12 A package that was taken out of the steam sterilizer before it was dry. Note the tear allowing an instrument to protrude and breach sterility.

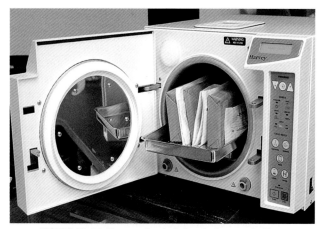

FIGURE 12-13 The unsaturated chemical vapor sterilizer.

other alcohols. One should protect the skin and eyes from contact with the solution and should not breathe its vapors.

The unsaturated chemical vapor sterilizer is called the Thermo Scientific Harvey sterilizer and was formerly known as the Chemiclave (Figure 12-13). This sterilizer operates through four cycles: the heat-up/vaporization cycle, the sterilization cycle, the depressurization cycle, and an optional purge cycle. After one adds the special chemical solution, one loads the chamber by placing items on their edges, closes the door, and turns on the unit. The heat-up cycle causes the chemical solution to vaporize, yielding a pressure of approximately 172 kPa (25 psi), and when the temperature reaches approximately 132° C (270° F), the sterilizing cycle begins. The temperature is maintained for 20 minutes, and the chamber is depressurized, with a decrease in temperature.

A positive feature of chemical vapor sterilization is that it greatly reduces or eliminates corrosion of carbon steel instruments. The amount of water in the chemical solution used is below the level that causes corrosion. For this reason, drying of the instruments before processing them in this sterilizer is important. Residual water remaining on wet instruments could override the rust-free process. Because the chemical solution used rapidly vaporizes in heat, items

processed through this sterilizer are essentially dry at the end of the depressurization cycle. So there is no need for an additional drying cycle.

One should follow the manufacturer's directions for packaging, loading, and operating and should wear gloves and protective eyewear when handling the special chemical solution. As with the steam sterilizer, leaving space around the packages being processed through the chemical vapor sterilizer is important to ensure adequate contact with the chemical vapors. One can achieve this best by placing packages or cassettes on their edges. One should not use closed containers; however, paper/plastic peel pouches, paper bags, or paper sterilization wrap indicated for this use in these units is appropriate for packaging. One should not use as packaging or attempt to sterilize linens, textiles, fabrics, or other absorbent materials such as paper towels. These materials may absorb the chemicals and reduce vaporization.

One should operate the sterilizer in a room that has at least normal ventilation. A purge system that collects chemicals from the vapors in the chamber at the end of the process can be purchased as an attachment to the sterilizer. This system greatly reduces the smell from the chemicals when one opens the door. In California, the chamber vapors are to be vented outside the office.

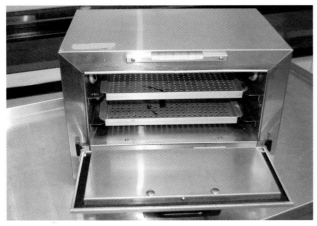

FIGURE 12-14 Example of a static-air dry heat sterilizer.

Dry Heat Sterilization

Dry heat sterilization involves heating air with transfer of heat energy from the air to the instruments. This form of killing requires higher temperatures than steam or unsaturated chemical vapor sterilization. Dry heat sterilizers operate at 160° C to 190° C (320° F to 375° F), depending on the type of sterilizer. The main advantage of dry heat sterilization is that carbon steel items do not corrode as they do during steam sterilization. Thus instruments need to be pre-dried before processing to keep residual water from promoting rusting.

Static-air type of dry heat sterilizer

This type of dry heat sterilizer is sometimes referred to as the oven type of dry heat sterilizer. The heating coils in the bottom or on the sides of these sterilizers cause the hot air to rise inside the chamber through natural convection (Figure 12-14). Heat energy from the static air is transferred to the instruments, and sterilization is reported to occur after 1 to 2 hours at 160° C (320° F). Because sterilization time may vary depending on the load, spore testing of these units is important (as is true for all types of sterilizers) to determine the proper exposure time under the conditions of actual use.

The heat-up time for this type of sterilizer may be 15 to 30 minutes from a cold start. Thus the sterilization cycle is not started until the proper temperature (e.g., 160° C [320° F]) is reached. The instruments then are held at this "sterilizing temperature" for the proper time. Because many of these units do not have automatic timers, one must include sufficient time for heat-up in the timer setting. After the sterilizing temperature is reached, one must not open the chamber door (e.g., to add forgotten items) until the scheduled time. If opened during the cycle, the temperature drops greatly and the cycle must be started again from time zero. One should follow the sterilizer manufacturer's directions carefully for loading and operating these sterilizers. Again, one should not layer or stack items in the chamber, but should place them on their edges.

The type of packaging or wrapping material used must be able to withstand the high temperatures of dry heat

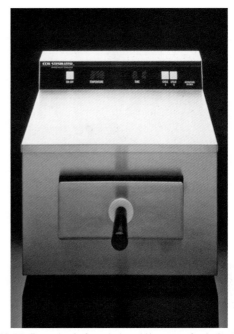

FIGURE 12-15 Example of a forced-air rapid heat transfer dry heat sterilizer.

sterilizers. Some wraps appropriate for steam or chemical vapor sterilization may melt in dry heat units. One can use closed containers in dry heat sterilizers if sterilization inside the containers is confirmed routinely by biological monitoring (spore testing). Although the static-air type of dry heat sterilizer requires longer sterilization times than the forced-air type described next, it is the least expensive.

Forced-air type of dry heat sterilizer

This type of dry heat sterilizer is sometimes referred to as a rapid heat transfer sterilizer. The sterilizer circulates the heated air throughout the chamber at a high velocity (Figure 12-15). This circulation permits a more rapid transfer of heat energy from the air to the instruments, reducing the time needed for sterilization.

One type of forced-air unit is a continuous heating type. One places the instruments into a preheated chamber and, when the unit reaches the factory-set temperature of 190° C (375° F), the selected exposure time for the sterilizing cycle automatically begins. One removes the instruments from the chamber at the end of the exposure period and allows them to cool. A second type of forced-air dry heat sterilizer begins from a cold (room temperature) start. After the chamber is loaded and the unit activated, the sterilizing cycle automatically begins when the unit reaches the factory-set temperature and continues for the selected exposure time. At the end of the exposure period, the heating elements automatically turn off and the unit circulates air in the chamber to cool the instruments.

Exposure time after the sterilizing temperature has been reached in these forced-air units ranges from 12 minutes for packaged items to 6 minutes for unpackaged items. As with the static-air dry heat sterilizers, important procedures to achieve successful sterilization are to keep the chamber door closed, use proper packaging material and routine spore testing, and follow manufacturer's directions for loading and operating forced-air dry heat sterilizers.

Sterilization Monitoring

The goal of sterilization is the complete killing of all forms of microbial life on the items being processed. The only way to determine if all items processed through a sterilizer are truly sterile is to test each item for all living microorganisms. This is impossible because such tested items then could not be used for patient care. Thus no procedures or products can be used to prove sterility of the items absolutely. Therefore a degree of risk that a nonsterile item exists in a processed load is always present. The object is to keep this risk as low as possible by using properly designed sterilization equipment in a carefully controlled manner. With such efforts, achieving a 99.9999% or better probability of success is possible, which means the possibility of the presence of a nonsterile item is only 1 in 1,000,000. Sterilization monitoring is part of the overall controlled sterilization process needed to achieve this sterility assurance level.

Heat sterilization failures result when direct contact between the sterilizing agent and all surfaces of items being processed does not occur for the appropriate length of time. Several things can cause sterilization failures, including improper instrument cleaning and packaging and improper use and functioning of the sterilizer (Table 12-4). In many instances, one does not detect these failures unless one performs proper sterilization monitoring. Three forms of sterilization monitoring, all of which must be used to achieve sterility assurance, are biological, chemical, and mechanical monitoring.

Biological Monitoring

Biological monitoring (also called spore testing) provides the main guarantee of sterilization. It evaluates the

TABLE 12-4   **Some Causes of Sterilization Failure**

Causes	Potential Problem
IMPROPER CLEANING OF INSTRUMENTS	Debris may insulate organisms from direct contact with the sterilizing agent
IMPROPER PACKAGING	
Wrong packaging material for method of sterilization	Prevents penetration of the sterilizing agent; packaging material may melt
Excessive packaging material	Retards penetration of the sterilizing agent
Cloth wrap in chemical vapor sterilizer	Cloth may absorb chemicals, preventing sufficient vaporization needed for sterilization
Closed container in steam or chemical vapor sterilizer	Prevents direct contact with the sterilizing agent
IMPROPER LOADING OF STERILIZER	
Overloading	Increases heat-up time and retards penetration of the sterilizing agent to the center of the sterilizer load
No separation between packages or cassettes even without overloading	May prevent or retard thorough contact of sterilizing agent with all items in the chamber
IMPROPER TIMING	
Incorrect operation of the sterilizer	Insufficient time at proper temperature to achieve kill
Timing for sterilization started before proper temperature is reached in units with nonautomatic timers	Insufficient time at proper temperature to achieve kill
Dry heat sterilizer door opened during sterilizing cycle without starting cycle over	Insufficient time at proper temperature to achieve kill
Sterilizer timer malfunction	Insufficient time at proper temperature to achieve kill
IMPROPER TEMPERATURE	
Incorrect operation of the sterilizer	Insufficient heat for proper time to achieve kill
Sterilizer malfunction	Insufficient heat for proper time to achieve kill
IMPROPER METHOD OF STERILIZATION	
Solutions or water processed in a chemical vapor sterilizer	Sterilizing agent will not penetrate the solution
Solutions or water processed in a dry heat sterilizer	Will boil over and evaporate
Processing of heat-sensitive item (e.g., some plastics)	Items will melt or be distorted

procedure's effectiveness. Since we cannot test for the death of all microorganisms on all processed items, we select the most difficult microbe to kill and test for its death. Thus biological monitoring involves processing highly resistant bacterial spores (see Figure 12-1) through the sterilizer and then culturing the spores to determine whether they have been killed.

Types of biological indicators

Biological indicators (BIs) contain the bacterial endospores used for monitoring. The spores used are *Geobacillus stearothermophilus*, previously known as *Bacillus stearothermophilus* (for testing steam or chemical vapor sterilization), or *Bacillus atrophaeus*, previously known as *Bacillus subtilis* (for testing dry heat or ethylene oxide gas sterilization). No BIs are available to test liquid chemical sterilants or disinfectants routinely during use in the office.

BIs are packaged in different forms (Figure 12-16). Spore strips are paper strips approximately 1 inch long that contain one type of spore or may contain both types of spores (dual-species BIs) that can be used to test all four types of sterilizers. Spore strips are enclosed in a protective glassine envelope, and after processing through the sterilizer, one removes the internal spore strip aseptically and places it in a tube of appropriate culture medium for incubation for 2 to 7 days at 55° C (131° F) (for *G. stearothermophilus*) or at 37° C (98.6° F) (for *B. atrophaeus*). If live spores are still present, they will grow and produce cloudiness or change the color of the growth medium, indicating sterilization failure. One can use spore strips to monitor all forms of heat sterilization.

Another form of BI is called a self-contained vial and contains a spore strip or disk with an ampule of growth medium in a plastic vial with a vented cap to permit entrance of the sterilizing agent into the vial (see Figure 12-16). After processing through the sterilizer, one squeezes the vial or pushes down the cap to break the internal ampule, mixing the growth medium with the spores.

One then incubates the vial at 55° C (131° F), and if live spores are still present, they will grow and change the color of the growth medium, indicating sterilization failure. One can use currently available self-contained vials to monitor steam sterilization.

Use of biological indicators

In hospital-type steam sterilizers, BIs are placed inside of a standardized test pack of towels, processed through the sterilizer, and analyzed. Test packs are still under development for use with small office steam, chemical vapor, and dry heat sterilizers. Until such test packs are developed and verified, routine biological monitoring of small office sterilizers should involve placement of the BI inside one of each type of package (pouch, bags, pack, cassette) processed through the sterilizer (Figure 12-17). A control BI that is not processed through the sterilizer but is otherwise handled the same way as the test BI must be analyzed along with the test BI that is processed through the sterilizer. The control BI should yield growth of the spores, confirming that if live spores are present, they can grow and be detected.

The CDC, American Dental Association, Organization for Safety and Asepsis Procedures, and Association for the Advancement of Medical Instrumentation recommend at least weekly spore testing of each sterilizer in the office. Spore tests also should be performed with every flash sterilization cycle. Some states have passed laws requiring routine spore testing of dental office sterilizers, including California, Florida, Indiana, Ohio, Oregon, and Washington. Nonroutine use of biological monitoring is also important, as described in Table 12-5.

Analysis of biological indicators

Proper analysis of a microbiological test such as use of a BI involves confirming that the test organisms were alive before the test (by using a control BI that is not processed through the sterilizer but is handled like the test BI in every other way) and confirming that organisms that grow after the test BI has been processed through the sterilizer are indeed the

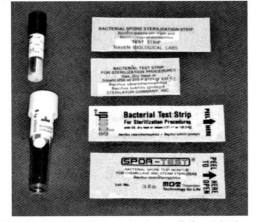

FIGURE 12-16 Examples of biological indicators. Self-contained spore vials used in steam sterilizers (*left*); spore strips in protective glassine envelopes used in steam, unsaturated chemical vapor, or dry heat sterilizers (*right*).

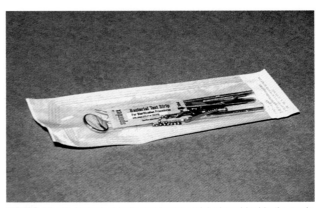

FIGURE 12-17 Biological indicator (spore strip) placed inside the package along with the instruments.

TABLE 12-5   Spore Testing of Small Office Sterilizers

When	Why
Once per week	To verify proper use and functioning
Whenever a new type of packaging material or tray is used	To ensure that the sterilizing agent is getting inside to the surface of the instruments
After training of new sterilization personnel	To verify proper use of the sterilizer
During initial uses of a new sterilizer	To make sure unfamiliar operating instructions are being followed
First run after repair of a sterilizer	To make sure that the sterilizer is functioning properly
With every implantable device and hold device until results of test are known	To take extra precaution for sterilization of item to be implanted into tissues
After any other change in the sterilizing procedure	To make sure change does not prevent sterilization

Reprinted with permission from Miller CH, Palenik CJ: Sterilization, disinfection and asepsis in dentistry. In Block SS, editor: *Sterilization, disinfection and preservation*, Philadelphia, p. 1054, Philadelphia, 2001, Lea & Febiger.

actual test microorganisms and not just a contaminant from hands or the air that accidentally entered the growth medium before incubation. Thus, control BIs should always yield growth of the spores, and growth from test BIs should be gram-positive bacilli when a sample of the growth medium is smeared on a glass slide, Gram stained, and observed at a magnification of approximately 1000 times under the microscope. These techniques, with use of a growth medium that has been verified as being sterile to begin with and able to support growth of the test spores, confirm the reliability of each biological monitoring test. The equipment and supplies necessary to perform these verification techniques are not commonly found in dental offices. Self-contained vials also do not lend themselves easily to microbiological analysis of a positive test BI through sampling of the growth medium inside the capped vial.

Management of biological monitoring

Two acceptable approaches to biological monitoring are in-office monitoring and mail-in monitoring (Procedure 12-2). In-office monitoring involves purchasing the appropriate supplies and equipment, analyzing the test and control BIs in the office, and preparing appropriate records. One can monitor steam sterilizers in the office by purchasing a self-contained vial type of BI of *G. stearothermophilus* and a 55° C (131° F) incubator available from the BI supplier. One must take care to handle the BIs aseptically and to perform the incubation and analysis as described in the manufacturer's directions. Records of the testing should include the date of the test, type of sterilizer, time and temperature of the sterilizing conditions, type of packaging material (packs, pouches, cassettes), location in the sterilizer, results of the test and of the control BI, and name of whoever conducted the test. Microbiological confirmation of growth in the self-contained vial should not be attempted in the office unless specific training to do so has been provided. Self-contained plastic vial BIs are not currently available for in-office testing of chemical vapor or dry heat sterilizers. One can use

spore strip types of BIs to test these sterilizers and the steam sterilizer, but this requires the purchase of separate tubes of growth medium plus the incubator and even greater care to avoid contamination of the growth medium used for analysis.

Mail-in monitoring involves the office subscribing to a mail-in sterilization monitoring service available from private companies or through some dental schools. These services can monitor any type of sterilizer and provide the office with the appropriate BIs (usually spore strips) and instructions for their use. After processing through the sterilizer, one mails the BIs to the service where they are analyzed, and a report of the results is sent to the office for recordkeeping. If the service detects a sterilization failure, the service usually notifies the office by phone. The most complete mail-in services provide a control BI and two test BIs for each test. Some also provide newsletters on asepsis, a certificate of participation, and a phone number to call with questions about spore testing or any aspect of office infection control. Mail-in services should use FDA-cleared BIs, perform microbiological confirmation of results, and use a growth medium that has been verified for sterility and growth promotion.

What to do after a sterilization failure

The desired outcome of biological monitoring is the killing of test spores. Failure to kill the spores (i.e., having a positive spore test) is a significant event that requires immediate action so as not to compromise patient safety. However, before one can put this action program in place, the office has to develop confidence in the biological monitoring procedure used, so that when a positive spore test result occurs, the validity of the test itself is not questioned. One can elicit confidence in the spore-testing procedures by using the same four steps described previously to achieve sterility assurance (p. 123). One should ask the following questions and act accordingly to ensure the correctness of the spore testing procedure:

- Were the proper BIs used and were they stored properly as described on their labels?

PROCEDURE 12-2

Biological Monitoring

GOAL: To determine whether the sterilization process is achieving the desired result of providing instruments safe for use on patients; it evaluates the procedure's effectiveness

Materials Needed
For mail-in monitoring: Spore test kits from mail-in monitoring service
For in-office monitoring: Biological indicators, culture broth, incubator, and record book

1. Use biological indicators containing *Geobacillus stearothermophilus* spores for monitoring steam and chemical vapor sterilizers and *Bacillus atrophaeus* for monitoring dry heat or ethylene oxide gas sterilizers.
   Rationale: If the death of these highly resistant bacterial spores can be determined, then one is assured that all other important microorganisms are killed.

2. Insert biological indicator inside of a pack, pouch, or cassette and complete the packaging procedure. If a spore strip biological indicator is used, do not remove the strip from the blue glassine envelope. If appropriate, identify the pack, pouch, or cassette containing the biological indicator.
   Rationale: Placing the spores inside the packages confirms that the sterilizing agent (steam, hot chemical vapor, hot air, or ethylene oxide gas) has penetrated the packaging material and contacted the instruments inside.

3. Place the pack, pouch, or cassette in the center of the load and process as part of a normal load through a normal sterilizer cycle.
   Rationale: The center of the load may be the most challenging part of the load. If the sterilizer manufacturer identifies another spot in the chamber where spore tests should be placed, follow those directions.

4. Record the date of the test, type of sterilizer, temperature and time of the sterilization cycle, nature of the package containing the biological indicator, and the name of the sterilizer operator.
   Rationale: This information documents the test so that one can identify the load and conditions if a sterilization failure occurs.

5. Retrieve the test biological indicators and, with the control biological indicator, mail back to the sterilization monitoring service. If analyzed in the office, follow the biological indicator manufacturer's directions carefully and monitor the temperature of the incubator.
   Rationale: This step helps ensure the reliability of the test.

6. Receive and maintain records of results from the monitoring service or record the proper results for the test and control biological indicators analyzed in the office.
   Rationale: These records may be needed should questions about the sterility of instruments ever arise. Some states also require documentation that biological monitoring has been performed.

7. If a positive biological indicator occurs (sterilization failure), take the sterilizer out of service and repeat the test under carefully controlled conditions (see Procedure 12-3). Do not use instruments processed through that sterilizer until the nature of the problem has been identified.
   Rationale: A sterilization failure suggests that a problem exists with the sterilizer or the procedures used and that the instruments may not be safe to use.

- Did all of the BIs used in the testing have the same manufacturer's lot number?
- Were the BIs used before their expiration date?
- Were the BIs handled properly before and after processing through the sterilizer?
- Were all the BIs mailed back to the service together or analyzed in the office together?
- Were the BIs incubated for the correct time at the correct temperature?
- Did the unprocessed control BI from the same lot number show growth (yield a positive result) after culturing?
- If a mail-in service is used, did the service confirm the positive result by microbiological means?

When a spore test is positive, indicating a sterilization failure, one should follow the steps given in Procedure 12-3.

Chemical Monitoring

Chemical monitoring uses heat-sensitive chemicals (rather than live spores as in biological monitoring) to assess the physical conditions during the sterilization process. Chemical monitoring involves the use of indicators that change color or physical form when exposed to high temperatures or to certain combinations of time, temperature, and the presence of steam. Examples include autoclave tape; special markings on pouches and bags; chemical indicator strips; and tabs, packets, or tubes of colored liquid (Figure 12-18).

PROCEDURE 12-3

Follow-up on a Sterilization Failure

GOAL: To identify and correct the cause of a sterilization failure

Materials Needed
Biological and chemical indicators
Items necessary to analyze spore tests (see Procedure 12-2)
Copy of sterilizer operating procedures
Backup sterilizer

1. Take the sterilizer out of service.

Immediately stop using the sterilizer for patient care items until the cause of failure is determined and appropriate changes are made. Items processed in the sterilizer since the last spore test may not have been sterilized and, if still unused, need to be collected, repackaged, and reprocessed through a properly operating sterilizer. A second properly monitored sterilizer in the office may be used, or a loaner from the sales/repair company may be obtained so that patient flow is not interrupted.
Rationale: Once a failure is detected, the sterilizer cannot be considered safe to use until the problem is identified and resolved.

2. Review sterilization procedures.

Review all past chemical monitoring records since the last negative spore test. Review the proper sterilizer loading and operating procedures and determine whether the instrument processing staff actually followed procedure. Were any changes made in the packaging or loading procedures? Was sufficient fluid added to the sterilizer before the cycle? Were the times and temperatures set correctly? Was anything different about the cycle that yielded a failure? Was a new staff person involved with instrument processing?
Rationale: Some sterilization failures are a result of improper procedures being performed and not because of a malfunction of the sterilizer itself.

3. Retest and observe the cycle.

If problems were detected in step 2, make the necessary changes. Retest the sterilizer using the same cycle and approximate load that yielded the sterilization failure. Place a chemical indicator next to the biological indicator on the inside of a package. Observe the sterilizer gauges, lights, and dials or digital readouts during this repeat cycle to determine whether they indicate the proper sterilizing conditions.
Rationale: This mechanical, chemical, and biological monitoring retest after the proper operating procedures have been confirmed will determine whether the problem has been corrected or whether the sterilizer has malfunctioned.

4. Determine the fate of the sterilizer.

If the spore test results are negative and if the chemical indicator had changed to an appropriate color, the sterilizer may be placed back into service. If the spore test is positive, and one has confirmed that the packaging, loading, and operating procedures were performed correctly, contact the sterilizer service representative for repair or replacement.
Rationale: This step will determine whether a procedural problem is solved or the sterilizer itself needs to be repaired.

5. Test the repair or replacement sterilizer.

Before a repaired or a new sterilizer is placed into service, it should be spore tested in three consecutive empty-chamber sterilization cycles and achieve a negative result.
Rationale: Any sterilizer (new or used) placed into service needs to be monitored for proper operation before being used to process patient care items. Empty chambers allow a more rapid heat-up time producing a shorter overall heating time, which means a greater challenge to the spores.

Two types of **chemical indicators** exist. One indicator changes color after a certain temperature has been reached (e.g., autoclave tape and special markings on pouches and bags). This type of indicator is used commonly as an external indicator on the outside of every pack, pouch, or cassette to indicate that the item has at least been processed through a heat sterilizer. This identifies items that have been heat processed and items that have not, for otherwise they may look identical. This differentiation prevents the accidental clinical use of unprocessed items. These indicators do not indicate that sterilization has been achieved or even that a complete sterilization cycle has occurred. A sterilizer could heat up to the proper temperature, causing a change in the chemical indicator, and then immediately malfunction,

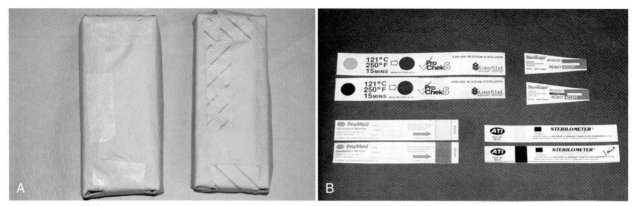

FIGURE 12-18 Examples of chemical indicators. **A,** Autoclave tape before being heat processed (*left*), and autoclave tape after being heat processed (*right*). **B,** Other chemical indicators. The top of each pair shows appearance before heat processing, and the bottom shows the color change after heat processing.

preventing sterilization, but the indicator already would have changed color. Thus these indicators demonstrate only that an item has been exposed to a certain temperature for some unknown length of time.

The second type of chemical indicator is called an integrated indicator that changes color or form slowly, responding to a combination of time and temperature or time, temperature, and the presence of steam. These indicators are used commonly on the inside of every pack, pouch, or cassette to assess whether the instruments have been exposed to sterilizing conditions.

Procedure 12-4 summarizes use of chemical indicators. The CDC recommends that a chemical indicator be placed inside every package that is processed through a sterilizer (Figure 12-19), and if that indicator can't be seen from the outside of the package, another chemical indicator is to be placed inside the package.

Mechanical Monitoring

Mechanical monitoring of the sterilization process involves observation of the gauges and displays on the sterilizer and recording of the sterilizing temperature, pressure, and exposure time. Although correct readings do not guarantee sterilization, incorrect readings can give the first indication that a problem likely has occurred. Many small office sterilizers now have recording devices that print out these parameters, providing a mechanical monitoring record for each run (Figure 12-20). One must remember that sterilizer gauges and displays indicate the conditions in the sterilizer chamber rather than conditions within the packs, pouches, or cassettes being processed. Thus mechanical monitoring may not detect problems resulting from overloading, improper packaging material, or use of closed containers.

Complete Monitoring Program

Appropriate sterilization monitoring (as recommended for dentistry by the CDC) involves use of a chemical indicator on the inside and outside (if the internal indicator cannot be seen from the outside) of each pack, pouch, and cassette. Each load should undergo mechanical monitoring, and biological monitoring of each type of pack, pouch, or cassette should be performed at least once a week. One should maintain records of all three types of monitoring to document sterility assurance. Those who may investigate the infection control practices in the office may request such information, which one also can use to demonstrate the use of safe practices to curious patients. Mechanical monitoring alone will not detect all of the potential problems that may cause sterilization failure. Spore testing provides the main guarantee of sterilization but is performed only periodically and takes 2 to 7 days before the results are available. Use of internal chemical indicators in every pack, pouch, and cassette provides an immediate indication as to whether the sterilizing agent has penetrated the packaging material and actually reached the instruments inside. If the internal chemical indicator displays the appropriate color or form, and mechanical and biological monitoring has not indicated any problems, the instruments are considered safe to use. Use of external chemical indicators (or internal chemical indicators that can be seen from the outside) on every pack, pouch, and cassette helps manage and maintain clear separation of processed and nonprocessed items, eliminating the possibility of using nonsterilized instruments.

Handling of Processed Instruments

One should maintain instrument sterility until the sterilized packs, pouches, or cassettes are opened for use at chairside. Thus proper handling of processed items is an important part of the sterility assurance program for the office. Be careful when handling bags or pouches containing sharp or pointed instruments, for injuries can occur if the instruments protrude (Figure 12-21).

Drying and Cooling

Packs, pouches, or cassettes processed through small office steam sterilizers will be wet at the end of the sterilizing portion of the cycle and must be allowed to dry before handling. This is particularly true when paper or paper/plastic pouches are used because the wet paper may "draw" microorganisms through the wrap or be torn easily when handled.

PROCEDURE 12-4

Chemical Monitoring

GOAL: To determine whether instrument packages and the instruments inside have been exposed to sterilizing conditions such as heat

Materials Needed
Chemical indicators to be placed inside of packages
Packaging with chemical indicators on the outside (if internal indicators are not visible from the outside)

1. Place the appropriate integrated chemical indicator on the inside of every pack, pouch, or cassette to be processed.
   Rationale: This indicator will confirm that the sterilizing agent has penetrated the packaging material and reached the instruments inside.

2. If the internal indicator cannot be seen from the outside of the package, place a chemical indicator on the outside of every pack, pouch, or cassette. Some pouches have a chemical indicator already printed on the pouch. If the internal indicator can be seen through the packaging material, an external indicator is not necessary.
   Rationale: This step ensures that a chemical indicator can be seen on or in each package.

3. After packs, pouches, or cassettes have been processed through the sterilizer, observe the external indicators. If the appropriate color change has not occurred, do not use the processed items. Immediately spore test the sterilizer process to verify and ultimately correct any problem with the use or functioning of the sterilizer (see Procedure 12-2). Do not use the sterilizer until the problem has been corrected. If the indicator has changed appropriately, distribute the packages for clinical use.
   Rationale: An external indicator that has not changed to the proper color suggests a sterilization failure or that the package has not been processed through a sterilizer.

4. After opening a processed pack, pouch, or cassette, immediately observe the internal indicator. If the appropriate change has not occurred, do not use the items, and verify and correct any problem with the use or functioning of the sterilizer as described in step 3. If the appropriate change has occurred, use the instruments as long as the periodic spore testing has verified the sterilization process routinely.
   Rationale: An internal indicator that has not changed suggests that the sterilizing agent did not penetrate the packaging material or that the package has not been processed through a sterilizer.

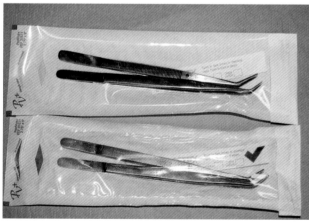

FIGURE 12-19 Chemical indicators used inside of packages. This paper/plastic peel pouch has an internal, diamond-shaped, chemical indicator printed on the inside of the package (left side of package). For demonstration purposes a chemical indicator strip has also been placed inside the package. The top package shows the appearance of the indicators before heat processing, and the bottom shows their color change after heat processing.

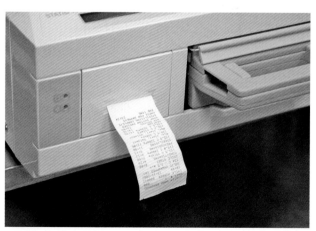

FIGURE 12-20 A printout on a steam sterilizer for documentation of mechanical monitoring.

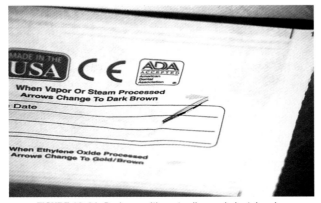

FIGURE 12-21 Package with protruding periodontal probe.

Most steam sterilizer manufacturers provide drying instructions, and some even may have a programmed closed-door or open-door drying cycle, as described earlier.

Hospital-type and some small office steam sterilizers have a poststerilization vacuum cycle that removes the moisture by evacuating the chamber at the end of the cycle. Unsaturated chemical vapor and dry heat sterilizers yield dry packs after the sterilization cycle.

Cooling of warm packs should be done slowly to avoid the formation of condensation on the instruments. One should not place warm packs under air-conditioning or cool-air vents or transfer them to cold surfaces. Use of a fan or blower in the sterilizing room to dry or cool down instruments is not recommended; this causes undue circulation of potentially contaminated room air around the packs.

If one processes unpackaged instruments through the sterilizer (e.g., in an emergency "flash" sterilization cycle), they must be covered immediately or otherwise be protected from the air and from coming into contact with contaminated surfaces before presentation at chairside.

Storage

One should keep handling of sterile packages to a minimum, and those that are dropped on the floor, are torn, are compressed, or have become wet must be considered as contaminated. One also must act to prevent the mingling of sterile packs with nonsterile packs. External chemical indicators serve as the primary control measure to identify items that already have been processed through the sterilizer.

Storage of sterile packs for more than a few days at the most is uncommon in dentistry because a short turnaround time reduces the total number (and expense) of instrument sets needed. Nevertheless, proper sterility assurance dictates the need for protection of sterile instruments from recontamination, regardless of the time between sterilization and reuse at chairside.

One should store sterile packages in covered or closed cabinets in dry, enclosed, low-dust areas protected from obvious sources of contamination. One should store sterile packages away from sinks and sewer and water pipes and a few inches away from ceilings, floors, and outside walls.

This prevents packages from becoming wet with splashed water, floor-cleaning products, and condensation on pipes or walls. One also should store the packages away from heat sources that may make the packaging material brittle and more susceptible to tearing or puncture.

Shelf life of sterile packages is the period of time during which sterility is assumed to be maintained. If sterile packages become wet or are torn or punctured, sterility is compromised. Unwrapped instruments have no shelf life. Because shelf life primarily depends on maintaining the integrity of the packaging material, no exact time exists for which all instrument packages may be stored safely. Thus shelf life is mainly a function of how carefully the packages are handled and stored. This concept is referred to as event-related storage. One should use the "oldest" sterile packs first, as long as the packaging material is intact. This is referred to as the "first in, first out" system of stock rotation. FDA-cleared packaging materials maintain sterility of the contents for a minimum of 6 months under ideal storage conditions. But a maximum storage time in the office might be considered as 1 month, at which time all unused items would be unpackaged, repackaged with new packaging material, and reprocessed through the sterilizer.

A key point in sterility assurance and event-related storage is to examine each pack, pouch, and cassette carefully before opening it to ensure that the barrier wrap has not been compromised during storage.

Distribution

One can place instruments from sterile packs or pouches on sterile, disposable, or at least cleaned and disinfected trays at chairside. Sterilized instrument cassettes are distributed to and opened at chairside. Placement of unwrapped or wrapped instruments in drawers or cabinets for direct use at chairside during patient care is not recommended. The drawers or cabinets and their contents are contaminated too easily from retrieval of items with saliva-coated fingers and from contaminated aerosols. This type of storage/distribution system at chairside for instruments or supplies is fraught with great potential for cross-contamination.

Opening of Instrument Packages

For routine dentistry, one should check instrument packages at chairside for tears or punctures and, if intact, should open the packages without touching the instruments inside. As described in Chapter 11, one should open the packages with clean, ungloved hands after the patient is seated and then put on gloves just before first contact with the patient's mouth. Alternatively, one may open the packages with ungloved hands and immediately cover the instruments with a sterile drape before seating the patient. If one opens instrument packages with gloved hands, the gloves will become contaminated with any microorganisms on the outside of the packaging. If one must manipulate instruments just before patient treatment begins (e.g., arranging bagged instruments on the bracket table), one should handle them with sterile tongs. Prearranging instruments on packaged trays or in cassettes before placing them into the sterilizer eliminates the need to manipulate the instruments after sterilization. The trays or cassettes hold the instruments at chairside.

For surgery, the instruments commonly are double wrapped to enhance sterility maintenance. Any contamination of the packaging during storage and transport to the surgical operatory can be removed by removing the outer packaging. On removing the outer packaging, one may touch and open the protected inner packaging with gloved hands.

DESIGN OF THE INSTRUMENT PROCESSING AREA

One should accomplish three goals when designing or organizing an instrument processing area in a dental office.

- Locate in a low-contamination low-traffic environment.
- Base the physical design on workflow.
- Separate "clean" instruments from "dirty" instruments (sterile from contaminated).

General Location and Utilities

The instrument processing area should be located centrally, if possible, for easy access from all operatories, but it should be away from traffic flow. That is, the area should be a facility dedicated only to instrument processing, be physically separated from the operatories and dental laboratory, and not be part of a common walkway. The processing area should not have a door that opens to the outside and should not have open windows because these enhance entrance of dust. The processing area should have good ventilation to control the heat generated by the sterilizers and should allow good access to the room air filters for frequent changing. The size of the facility must accommodate all the equipment and supplies needed to perform instrument processing, such as those listed in Table 12-6. Utilities should include multiple outlets and proper lighting, water, and an air line and vacuum line for lubricating and flushing high-speed handpieces. The cabinetry should include chemical- and heat-resistant countertops wide enough for sterilizers and other equipment, a deep sink with hands-free controls for instrument rinsing, closed storage areas, and (if space permits) a separate handwashing sink with hands-free controls. Accessories should include a hands-free soap dispenser and foot-operated or other hands-free trash receptacle. The flooring should be an uncarpeted, seamless hard surface.

If the instrument processing area is not located in a room separate from the clinical area, then consider the following:

- The instrument processing area should be as far away as possible from the dental chairs.
- Use surface covers to protect the processing area when not in use and when patients are being treated.
- Store sterile packages, trays, and cassettes in closed cabinets or drawers.
- Do not process instruments or handle sterile packages when patients are being treated.

Workflow Design

Just about any room or group of adjacent rooms can be used for instrument processing if space is sufficient; the utilities, flooring, and ventilation are appropriate; and the placement of the equipment in the room or rooms is based on the workflow pattern. One approach to the general layout of the instrument processing area is to have a long, narrow room with doors at each end and a linear workflow proceeding from one end to the other. Figure 12-22 shows a U-shaped workflow pattern in a room with a single door.

A key aspect in design of the processing area is to separate the three main areas of activity.

- Decontamination area
- Packaging area
- Sterilizing and storage area

Ideally, three adjoining rooms should be separated physically, but such space seldom is available in a dental office. Usually a single room is involved and the separation is by space designation, using signs rather than walls or partitions. Proper placement of signs (e.g., "Contaminated Items Only," "Cleaned Items Only," "Sterile Items Only," "Decontamination Area," "Clean Packaging Area," "Sterilization Area"), with training on the exact meaning of the signs used, can work well in preventing the intermingling of contaminated and sterile items.

As shown in Table 12-6, the decontamination area contains the items needed for personal protection, waste disposal, and cleaning and rinsing of instruments and handpieces. The packaging area contains the materials and space for rust inhibition, wrapping and bagging, addition of spore tests and chemical indicators, and addition of replacement instruments, burs, and supplies. The sterilizing area contains the sterilizers and related supplies and incubators for analyzing spore tests in the office and can contain enclosed storage for sterile items and disposable (single-use) items.

If one uses carts for distribution and collection of instruments to and from the operatories, one also should identify the carts for "Contaminated" or "Sterile" items, and should clean them properly and disinfect or cover them with barriers between uses.

INSTRUMENT SHARPENING

Instrument sharpening is difficult to manage from an infection control point of view. Sharpening of contaminated instruments presents a risk for disease spread through accidental cuts or punctures. The greatest safety is achieved by cleaning, sterilizing, sharpening, and resterilizing the instruments. If instruments (e.g., scalers) need to be resharpened while being used on a patient, the best (and safest) option is to provide several scalers in each instrument setup rather than to sharpen contaminated scalers. If one must sharpen instruments at chairside, one should provide cleaned and sterilized sharpening stones for each patient. One must take great care when sharpening a contaminated instrument and

TABLE 12-6   **Equipment and Supplies Used in the Instrument Processing Facility**

Item	Use
DECONTAMINATION AREA	
Gloves, mask, eyewear, clothing	Prevent exposure to contaminated materials
Sharps container	Receive any sharps not discarded in the operatory
Tongs	Pick up sharps
Biohazard bags	Receive nonsharp, solid, regulated waste
Trash receptacle	Receive nonregulated waste
Instrument cleaner	Ultrasonically clean or wash instrument
Instrument detergent	Use in instrument cleaner
Cleaners/lubricants	Clean/lubricate handpieces
Air line and vacuum line	Flush materials out of handpieces into vacuum line
Sink with hands-free faucets	Handwashing and instrument rinsing
Disinfectant and towels	Disinfect countertops and ultrasonic cleaner chamber
Instrument scrub brush	Clean occasional item still soiled after mechanical cleaning
Handwashing dispenser and detergent	Wash hands
Drainer	Dry instruments/cassettes after cleaning and rinsing
Signs identifying decontamination area	Prevent intermingling of sterile and contaminated items
PACKAGING AREA	
Rust inhibitor	Retard corrosion of non–stainless steel items in steam
Replacement instruments and burs	Replace damaged items in instrument setups
Instrument cassettes	Hold instruments during processing and use
Gauze pads	Place in cassettes or packages before heat processing
Biological indicators (spore tests)	Monitor the use and functioning of the sterilizers
Chemical indicators	Monitor the sterilization process
Instrument packaging materials	Protect instruments from contamination after sterilization
Heat sealer	Seal nylon plastic instrument packaging tubing
Heat-resistant (e.g., autoclave) tape	Seal wrapped cassettes or other instrument packages
Signs identifying packaging area	Prevent intermingling of sterile and contaminated items
STERILIZING AREA	
Sterilizers	Heat process cleaned and packaged instruments
Distilled water or special solution	Use with sterilizer
Liquid sterilant (e.g., glutaraldehyde)	Kill microorganisms on items that cannot be heat processed
Covered container for liquid sterilant	Use with liquid sterilant
Glutaraldehyde monitor	Estimate the potency of the glutaraldehyde sterilant
Handpiece lubricant	Lubricate sterilized handpieces
Air line and vacuum line	Flush excess lubricant from handpieces into vacuum line
Incubator	Culture spore tests for in-office analysis
Enclosed storage	Store sterile instruments and clean disposable items
Signs identifying sterilizing area	Prevent intermingling of sterile and contaminated items

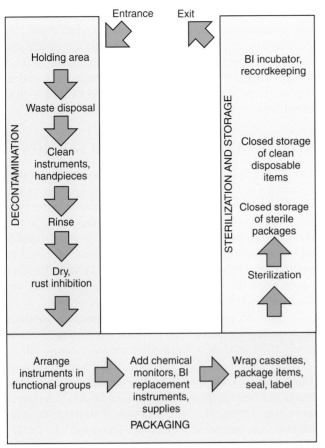

FIGURE 12-22 U-shaped sterilization room work flow pattern. Work flow proceeds through the area from decontamination to packaging to sterilization and storage.

should consider taping the sharpening stone to the countertop and using one hand to sharpen the instrument.

INSTRUMENT PROTECTION

Instrument processing can cause damage to instruments, but one can take several steps to keep damage at a minimum (Box 12-2).

Stainless steel instruments are least affected by corrosion from moisture and heat, but some dentists prefer instruments with carbon steel rather than stainless steel because carbon steel cutting surfaces may retain a sharp edge longer. Unfortunately, carbon steel items corrode and lose sharpness during steam sterilization. For example, tungsten carbide burs lose approximately 64% of their cutting efficiency after steam sterilization. Use of dip or spray rust inhibitors usually reduces corrosion, but with repeated steam sterilization cycles, the items will be damaged. Carbon steel items are sterilized best in a non–corrosion-producing environment such as dry heat or unsaturated chemical vapor sterilizer. One should make every effort to rinse away or remove biological debris, disinfecting or sterilizing solutions, chloride salts, and highly alkaline detergents before heat-processing instruments. These substances may cause pitting or staining

---

BOX 12-2

Tips for Protecting Dental Instruments

1. Clean as soon as possible after use. Cleaning removes corrosive materials such as blood and salts and may counteract the drying of the bioburden that will make cleaning more difficult.
2. Keep instruments from knocking against each other as much as possible during the cleaning process. This practice reduces damage to instruments.
3. Do not store instruments for long periods of time in water or chloride solutions. Corrosion requires water, and extended exposure to chlorine can damage some metals.
4. Use only cleaning solutions that are recommended for dental or medical instruments. Cleaning solutions designed for medical and dental instruments have special properties that are gentle to metal surfaces, that facilitate rinsing, and that interfere with corrosion.
5. Rinse well after cleaning. Residual cleaning solution on the instruments contains microbes that need to be rinsed away. If necessary, rust inhibitors from the cleaning solution that are rinsed away can be replaced before steam sterilization.
6. Use distilled or deionized water in steam sterilizers. Water spots on instruments give the impression that the instruments are not clean, and hard-water deposits can build up in the sterilizer and cause malfunctions.
7. Use rust inhibitors for carbon steel items to be processed through steam, or process these items through a dry heat or unsaturated chemical vapor sterilizer to prevent corrosion. Corrosion can interfere with the sharpness and functioning of some instruments.
8. Dry items before processing through dry heat or chemical vapor sterilizers. Excess water on instruments interferes with the anticorrosion aspects in these types of sterilizers.

---

of metal surfaces, which can be aggravated with heat. Packaging together of items of widely dissimilar metals during heat processing is not prudent because of a potential for electrolytic damage to instrument surfaces. However, this procedure is difficult to accomplish practically because of the wide variety of instruments needed for single procedures.

HANDPIECE ASEPSIS

Clean, package, and sterilize high-speed handpieces, reusable prophylaxis angles, contra-angles, nose cones, and slow-speed handpiece motors by heat processing between patients. Patient material possibly may enter the internal portions of handpieces and their attachments during use. Likewise, these materials may exit into the mouth of the next patient if this equipment has not been decontaminated properly. Thus decontamination procedures must address the outside *and the inside* of handpieces and other intraoral devices that can be removed from the air and water lines of the dental unit. Procedure 12-5 presents guidelines for processing handpieces.

Although some dental units contain antiretraction valves in their water lines that prevent retraction of fluids back into the high-speed water spray handpieces and air/water syringe when they are turned off, these valves periodically fail. Consequently, one should flush the high-speed handpiece, air/water syringe, and ultrasonic scalers for approximately 25 seconds at the completion of each appointment. This helps flush out any foreign materials and brings fresh water (and chlorine if city water) into the system. One also should check the functioning of the antiretraction valves at least every month.

One should carefully follow the handpiece manufacturer's directions for cleaning, lubricating, and heat processing, which is essential to achieve maximum longevity of the working parts. As with any decontamination process, one should wear personal protective equipment such as gloves, mask, protective eyewear or face shield, and protective clothing during these procedures. Also, when flushing out cleaner or lubricant, one should spray into a vacuum line or container to avoid spread of potentially contaminated aerosols. Handpiece cleaning equipment that automatically cleans, flushes, and captures the flushed aerosols is available.

STERILIZATION OF HEAT-LABILE ITEMS

Although most reusable instruments can withstand heat processing, a few plastic-type items such as certain rubber dam frames, shade guides, rulers, and x-ray collimating devices will be damaged by the heat. Thus one can use a liquid sterilant/high-level disinfectant (e.g., 2.0% to 3.4% glutaraldehyde; a special 7.0% hydrogen peroxide) to sterilize these items. Sterilization in a liquid sterilant/high-level disinfectant requires an extended contact time that ranges from 3 to 12 hours, depending on the product (e.g., glutaraldehyde requires a 10-hour contact time, anything less than 10 hours is disinfection, not sterilization). Use of a liquid sterilant/ high-level disinfectant or other liquid germicide to disinfect heat-tolerant instruments is not recommended. Procedure 12-6 gives step-by-step procedures for the use of a liquid sterilant. A major problem with liquid sterilants/high-level disinfectants is that their effectiveness cannot be tested as they are being used, There is no way to perform biological monitoring on these solution in the office.

OTHER METHODS OF STERILIZATION

The use of ethylene oxide gas is a recognized method of sterilization. The advantage is that the method operates at low temperatures, permitting sterilization of plastic and rubber items that melt in heat sterilizers. Disadvantages are that this method requires from 4 to 12 hours for sterilization, depending on the sterilizer model; requires at least 16 hours of poststerilization aeration to remove gas molecules that have bound to plastic and rubber surfaces; is ineffective on wet items; and is potentially toxic if not handled properly.

A more recently developed low-temperature sterilizer involves vaporized hydrogen peroxide gas plasma. Unfortunately, these units are still expensive for use in dental offices.

Bead "sterilizers" provide a form of dry heat processing. These small, flower pot–shaped units contain an electric heater that heats up glass beads (or sand or salt) to temperatures near 218° C (425° F). The tips of instruments, endodontic files, and broaches then are immersed into the hot beads for 25 to 30 seconds. However, the temperature varies at different levels in the beads, and biological indicators are not available for monitoring these units. Thus one should not use bead sterilizers as a means of sterilizing instruments for reuse on another patient.

Hot oil sterilizers are not commonly used today, but consist of a pan of mineral oil and a heater. As with bead sterilizers, uneven temperatures occur in the oil, and no method exists for routinely verifying effectiveness. Consequently, one should not use the hot oil bath as a means of sterilizing instruments for reuse on another patient.

PROPERTIES OF DECONTAMINATION AND STERILIZATION EQUIPMENT AND PRODUCTS

Boxes 12-3 and 12-4 give properties to consider when selecting cleaners, sterilizers, instrument cassettes, packaging materials, spore testing services, and in-office monitoring.

PROCEDURE 12-5

Handpiece Asepsis

GOAL: To sterilize handpieces while causing minimal damage

Materials Needed
Handpiece manufacturer's directions for cleaning and sterilizing handpieces
Appropriate cleaning solution
Appropriate lubricant when needed
Alcohol
Cotton swabs
Packaging material
Biological and chemical indicators
Sterilizer
Follow carefully the handpiece manufacturer's directions for cleaning, lubricating, and sterilizing. Automatic equipment designed to clean handpieces may be available.

1. Leave the handpiece attached to the hose after treatment, and wipe away visible debris from the handpiece. For high-speed handpieces, operate the air/water system for 20 to 30 seconds to flush the water and air lines into the vacuum line or a sink, container, or absorbent material.
   Rationale: This step gives preliminary cleaning and aids in flushing out materials that may have been drawn back into the water lines.

2. Remove the handpiece from the hose and clean the outside thoroughly, rinse, and dry. Do not soak unless recommended by the manufacturer. Use ultrasonic cleaning only when recommended by the handpiece manufacturer.
   Rationale: This step removes debris on the outside of the handpiece to facilitate sterilization.

3. Clean/lubricate internal portions as directed by the manufacturer. Reattach to the air/water system and blow out excess cleaner/lubricant into a vacuum line or sink, container, or absorbent material. Depending on the handpiece, some must be lubricated before, after, or before and after sterilization, or not at all. Use separate cans of lubricant for presterilization and poststerilization lubrication. Most handpiece brands should be operated only with a bur or blank in place. Check manufacturer's instructions.
   Rationale: The internal portions of handpieces may become contaminated with patient material, and if not decontaminated, this material may contaminate the next patient.

4. Wipe away excess lubricant from the outside. If using fiber-optic handpieces, clean away lubricant from the fiber-optic connecting interface as directed by the manufacturer.
   Rationale: Excess lubricant can build up on handpieces and interfere with the functioning of the handpiece and fiber-optic system.

5. Follow the handpiece manufacturer's instructions for the type of heat sterilizer (e.g., steam autoclave or chemical vapor) and maximum temperature that can be used. Package the handpiece in the proper bag for the type of sterilizer being used, and heat process following the sterilizer operating instructions.
   Rationale: Some handpiece brands will be damaged at certain high temperatures. The packaging prevents recontamination after removal from the sterilizer.

6. Following heat processing, allow time for the handpiece to dry and cool and keep it packaged until ready to prepare it for patient use.
   Rationale: Removing packages from a steam sterilizer before they are dry can tear the packaging material and permit contamination of the contents through wicking.

7. If poststerilization lubrication is required, handle the heat-processed handpiece aseptically. Open the bag, spray the lubricant into the handpiece (use a separate can reserved only for poststerilization lubrication), attach to the hose, and blow out excess lubricant.
   Rationale: This reduces chances for recontamination before the handpiece is used on the next patient.

Adapted from Miller CH: Cleaning, sterilization and disinfection: the basics of microbial killing for infection control, *J Am Dent Assoc* 124:(1):48-56, 1993; and *Universal precautions rule clarification: dental handpiece sterilization*, Indianapolis, Indiana State Department of Health, 1992; with additional information provided by John Young (personal communication), 1993.

PROCEDURE 12-6

Use of a Liquid Sterilant/High-level Disinfection for Heat-sensitive Items

GOAL: To sterilize items safely that cannot be heat sterilized

Materials Needed

Appropriate material safety data sheet (MSDS)
Personal protective barriers
Liquid sterilant/high-level disinfectant properly activated (if needed) and labeled with an expiration date based on use life
Closable container for the sterilant
Instrument cleaning equipment and supplies
Sterile tongs to retrieve processed items
Sterile water if a sterile rinse is necessary
Clean or sterile packaging material
Chemical test kit to measure sterilant potency, if available

1. Make sure an MSDS for the liquid sterilant (e.g., glutaraldehyde) is on file in the office and that employees have been trained properly on how to handle the product.
   Rationale: The MSDS provides information on how to protect against exposure to a chemical and what to do if exposure occurs. Training will help prevent exposure to chemicals.

2. Use gloves, mask, protective eyewear, and protective clothing when preparing, using, and discarding the solution.
   Rationale: This step protects against exposure to the chemical from splashing.

3. Follow the manufacturer's directions for preparing/activating, using, and disposing of the solution.
   Rationale: This step helps ensure effectiveness of the solution and reduces exposure to the chemical.

4. Prepare the solution for use as a sterilant, and label the containers with the appropriate date to indicate the length of the shelf life.
   Rationale: Some solutions must be mixed before use, and they may have a use life.

5. Use a cover on the use-container, and label this container with the name of the chemical, the date to indicate the length of the use life, and any other information that relates to the office hazard communication program for the safe use of chemicals.
   Rationale: Covers keep out dust and other debris, and the labeling identifies the chemical for proper handling.

6. Use the solution to sterilize only items that are not heat-tolerant and are not intended to penetrate tissue but can be submerged.
   Rationale: Heat-tolerant items and all critical items need to be heat-sterilized.

7. Preclean, rinse, and dry all items to be processed.
   Rationale: Bioburden on the items interferes with the sterilization process.

8. Place the items in a perforated tray or pan, place the pan in the solution, and cover the container. Alternatively, place the items in the solution using tongs and avoid splashing.
   Rationale: This step allows for easy removal of the items from the solution and avoids direct contact with the chemical.

9. Make sure items being sterilized are submerged completely for the entire contact time needed for sterilization as indicated on the product label.
   Rationale: Items must have direct contact with the chemical for effective sterilization.

10. Rinse processed items thoroughly with water and dry.
    Rationale: Rinsing removes the residual chemical and debris from the items, so they will not contact the patient during use of the item.

11. Handle processed items with aseptic techniques (e.g., sterile tongs).
    Rationale: This step helps ensure sterility maintenance of the items.

12. Place items in clean packaging material. (Note: Sterility is maintained best by rinsing with sterile water, drying, and placing in a sterile container.)
    Rationale: This step helps prevent recontamination before use on the next patient.

PROCEDURE 12-6

Use of a Liquid Sterilant/High-level Disinfection for Heat-sensitive Items—cont'd

13. Periodically test the concentration of the use solution with a chemical test kit (contact the manufacturer/distributor for the proper test kit). Replace the used solution when indicated based on label instructions, concentration test results, or when the level of the solution is low, or the solution becomes visibly dirty. *Rationale:* These solutions lose their potency and effectiveness over time.

14. When replacing the use-solution, discard all of the solution in the use-container, clean with a detergent, rinse with water, dry, and fill the container with fresh solution. *Rationale:* This step ensures that no resistant microbes and debris are left to contaminate the fresh solution.

BOX 12-3

Some Properties of Instrument Cassettes, Cleaning Equipment, and Packaging Material

One should consider these properties before making a selection.

Instrument Cassettes
- Closing mechanism
- Sharpness of edges
- Size to fit ultrasonic cleaner or washer
- Instrument holding mechanism
- Compatibility with sterilization method
- Number of instrument slots
- Size to fit sterilizer chamber
- Stability of the cassette

Ultrasonic Cleaner and Instrument Washer
- Requirements for power, water, drain
- Chamber size to fit cassettes
- Basket or cassette rack available
- Cycle time
- Recommended detergent
- Space requirements

Packaging Materials
- Compatibility with sterilization method
- Sealing mechanism
- Presence of chemical indicator
- Stability of the material
- Size
- Intensity of indicator color change

BOX 12-4

Some Properties of Sterilizers, Spore-testing Services, and In-office Monitoring Systems

One should consider these properties before making a selection.

Sterilizers
- Method of sterilization
- Total cycle time
- Chamber size to fit cassettes
- Water reservoir system, if steam
- Electric requirements
- Corrosive nature of instruments to be processed
- Type of dry cycle, if steam
- Tray or rack availability
- Ease of operation
- Space requirements

Spore-testing Services
- Number of spore strips per test
- Notification of sterilization failures
- Availability for questions
- Internal verification of results
- Adequate instructions provided
- Use of control strips
- Method of reporting final results
- Associated newsletters or other information
- Use of appropriate materials
- Expiration date of the spores

In-office Monitoring Systems
- Self-contained versus spore strips system
- Type of incubator required
- Adequate instructions provided
- Recordkeeping system provided
- Method of sterilization that can be tested
- Clear determination of sterilization failure
- Expiration date of the spores
- Ease of use

SELECTED READINGS

American Dental Association: Councils on Scientific Affairs and Dental Practice: Infection control recommendations for the dental office and the dental laboratory, *J Am Dent Assoc* 127:972, 1996.

Chin JR, Miller CH, Palenik CJ: Internal contamination of air driven low-speed handpieces and attached prophy angles, *J Am Dent Assoc* 137:1275–1280, 2006.

Herd S, Chin J, Palenik CJ, Ofner S: The in vivo contamination of air-driven low-speed handpieces with prophylaxis angles, *J Am Dent Assoc* 138:1360–1365, 2007.

Kohn WG, Collins AS, Cleveland JL, et al: Centers for Disease Control and Prevention: Guidelines for infection control in dental health-care settings–2003, *MMWR Morb Mortal Wkly Rep* 52(RR-17):1–61, 2003.

Miller CH: Cleaning, sterilization and disinfection: the basics of microbial killing for infection control, *J Am Dent Assoc* 124:48–56, 1993.

Miller CH: Make clean routine, *Dent Prod Rpt* 42:84–87, 2008.

Miller CH: Select and protect: Part II, *Dent Prod Rpt* 41:132–136, 2007.

Miller CH: Instrumentally clean, part 1, *Dent Prod Rpt* 42:120–124, 2008.

Miller CH: Strategies for infection control in dentistry. *ADA guide to dental therapeutics*, ed 3, Chicago, 2003, ADA Publishing, pp 551–566.

Miller CH, Hardwick LM: Ultrasonic cleaning of dental instruments in cassettes, *Gen Dent* 36:31–36, 1988.

Miller CH, Palenik CJ: Sterilization, disinfection, and asepsis in dentistry. In Block SS, editor: *Sterilization, disinfection, and preservation*, ed 5, Philadelphia, 2001, Lea & Febiger, pp 1049–1068.

Miller CH, Riggen SD, Sheldrake MA, Neeb JM: Presence of microorganisms in used ultrasonic cleaning solutions, *Am J Dent* 6:27–31, 1993.

Rutala WA, Weber DJ: Sterilization, high-level disinfection and environmental cleaning, *Infect Dis Clin N Am* 25:45–76, 2011.

Spaulding EH: Chemical disinfection of medical and surgical materials. In Lawrence CA, Block SS, editors: *Disinfection, sterilization, and preservation*, Philadelphia, 1968, Lea & Febiger, pp 517–531.

REVIEW QUESTIONS

Multiple Choice

1. How should one load a sterilizer?
   a. Place the packages on their edges.
   b. Pack the packages tight to eliminate as much air as possible.
   c. Stack the packages one on top of the other.
   d. Put only one package at a time in the sterilizer.

2. The rationale for packaging instruments before placing them into a sterilizer is to:
   a. eliminate water spots
   b. maintain their sterility after sterilization
   c. prevent rusting of carbon steel items
   d. reduce by half the time needed at the sterilizing temperature

3. Spores of *Geobacillus stearothermophilus* are used to monitor what types of sterilizers?
   a. Steam and dry heat
   b. Unsaturated chemical vapor and dry heat
   c. Unsaturated chemical vapor and steam

4. What type of sterilization causes carbon steel instruments to rust?
   a. Steam
   b. Dry heat
   c. Unsaturated chemical vapor
   d. Ethylene oxide gas

5. How should one sterilize a plastic rubber dam frame?
   a. Steam
   b. Dry heat
   c. Unsaturated chemical vapor
   d. Liquid sterilant such as glutaraldehyde

6. Spores of *Bacillus atrophaeus* are used to monitor what type of sterilizer?
   a. Steam
   b. Dry heat
   c. Unsaturated chemical vapor

7. A chemical indicator provides that an item
   a. is sterile
   b. is clean
   c. has been packaged properly
   d. has been processed through a heat sterilizer

8. The leading cause of sterilization failure is:
   a. not pushing the correct buttons to operate the sterilizer
   b. using the wrong type of sterilizer for heat-sensitive items
   c. overloading the sterilizer
   d. opening the sterilizer door before the end of the cycle

9. The purpose of an aluminum foil test is to:
   a. see if the steam in a sterilizer is at the proper temperature
   b. measure the strength of a liquid sterilant/high-level disinfectant
   c. assess the kill of bacterial spores in a sterilizer
   d. determine whether an ultrasonic cleaner chamber has an even distribution of sonic energy

10. The main rationale for cleaning instruments before sterilization is to:
    a. give the sterilization procedure the best chance to work
    b. prevent the formation of water spots on the instruments
    c. reduce rusting of instruments
    d. eliminate the need for packaging the instruments

11. Placing wet instruments into a dry heat sterilizer or an unsaturated chemical vapor sterilize can:
    a. prevent sterilization
    b. reduce the sterilization time by half
    c. counteract the antirusting nature of these sterilizers

12. Instrument packages are wet after the sterilization portion of which of the following sterilizer cycles?
    a. Dry heat
    b. Steam
    c. Unsaturated chemical vapor

13. Wet packages should be allowed to dry inside the sterilizer because paper packaging material may tear on handling and because:
    a. the instruments will have water spots
    b. the chemical indicators will not have changed color yet
    c. of wicking

14. A high-speed handpiece that is destroyed at 149° C (300° F) cannot be sterilized in:
    a. a steam sterilizer
    b. a dry heat sterilizer
    c. an unsaturated chemical vapor sterilizer

15. The active ingredient in the unsaturated chemical vapor sterilization process is:
    a. glutaraldehyde
    b. peracetic acid
    c. formaldehyde
    d. hydrogen peroxide

16. The first thing to do after a sterilization failure is to:
    a. retest the sterilizer with biological indicators
    b. take the sterilizer out of service for processing patient care items
    c. review the sterilizer operating instructions
    d. inform the Occupational Safety and Health Administration

17. The sterilization process is described best as being:
    a. virucidal
    b. tuberculocidal
    c. sporicidal
    d. bactericidal

18. When analyzing spore tests, *Geobacillus stearothermophilus* is incubated at what temperature?
    a. 100° C (212° F)
    b. 55° C (131° F)
    c. 37° C (98.6° F)
    d. 7° C (44.6° F)

19. What sterility assurance procedure should be performed while setting up for the next patient?
    a. The instrument packages should be opened and the instruments should be wiped with alcohol.
    b. The instrument packages should be observed for tears or punctures before being opened.
    c. The outside of the instrument packages should be wiped with alcohol to remove dust.

20. Critical patient care items are to be cleaned and _____ for reuse.
    a. low-level disinfected
    b. intermediate-level disinfected
    c. sterilized

Please visit http://evolve.elsevier.com/Miller/infectioncontrol/ for additional practice and study support tools.

Surface and Equipment Asepsis

OUTLINE

LEARNING OBJECTIVES

After completing this chapter, the student should be able to do the following:

1. Differentiate between clinical contact surfaces and housekeeping surfaces and determine which operatory surfaces may be involved in the patient-to-patient spread of microbes.
2. List the operatory surfaces that should be covered with barriers before patient care and describe how to place and remove surface covers properly.
3. Describe the importance of precleaning before surface disinfection and describe how to preclean and disinfect contaminated surfaces and equipment.
4. Do the following regarding the characteristics of disinfectants:
   - List the types of surface disinfectants and describe their properties.

- Differentiate between low-, intermediate-, and high-level disinfectants, and give examples when each should be used.
- Read with understanding the labels on disinfectants.
5. List general considerations for dental equipment decontamination and management of high-tech equipment in the dental office.
6. Describe how aseptically to retrieve and distribute clinical supply items.

KEY TERMS

Antibiotics
Antiseptics
Bactericidal
Bioburden
Chlorine
Clinical Content Surfaces
Disinfectants
Disinfection
Fungicidal

High-level Disinfectant
Hospital Disinfectant
Housekeeping Surfaces
Intermediate-level Disinfectant
Iodophors
Low-level Disinfectant
Phenolics
Precleaning
Quaternary Ammonium Compounds

Sodium Hypochlorite
Sporicidal
Spray-Wipe-Spray
Sterilants
Surface Covers
Tuberculocidal
Virucidal
Wipe-Discard-Wipe

TYPES OF ENVIRONMENTAL SURFACES

Two types of dental environmental surfaces are related to disease spread: clinical contact surfaces and housekeeping surfaces. Clinical contact surfaces are surfaces that may be touched frequently with gloved hands during patient care or that may become contaminated with blood, saliva, or other potentially infectious material and subsequently contact instruments, devices, hands, or gloves. Box 13-1 gives examples of such surfaces. Housekeeping surfaces are surfaces that do not come into contact with hands or devices used in dental procedures (e.g., floors, walls, and sinks). The clinical contact surfaces need to be treated properly before they become involved in the care of the next patient. Housekeeping surfaces can be treated at the end of the day.

Different microorganisms may survive on environmental surfaces for different periods, as determined in laboratory studies. For example, *Mycobacterium tuberculosis* may survive for weeks, whereas the herpes simplex virus dies in a matter of seconds to minutes. Various conditions influence the survival time of microorganisms in the environment, including humidity, temperature, the presence of nutrients and blood or saliva, and the general surface properties of the microorganism. Accurately predicting how long any microorganism actually may survive on a dental office surface is impossible because of these unknown variables. Consequently, if a surface becomes contaminated with saliva, blood, or other potentially infectious material, the safest approach is to assume that it, indeed, contains live microorganisms that must be removed or killed before the surface is involved in the treatment of the next patient.

Two general approaches to surface asepsis are these: one is to prevent the surface or item from becoming contaminated by use of a surface cover, and the other is to preclean and disinfect the surface after contamination and before reuse. Each approach has advantages and disadvantages, and usually an office will use a combination of both approaches (Table 13-1).

SURFACE COVERS

The best way to manage surface asepsis from an infection control point of view is to prevent contamination of the surface so that it will not have to be precleaned and disinfected before reuse.

Types of Surface Covers

Contamination can be prevented by proper placement of a surface cover before an opportunity for contamination exists. Surface covers should be impervious to fluids to keep microorganisms in saliva, blood, or other liquids from soaking through to contact the surface. Examples of appropriate material for surface covers include clear plastic wrap, bags, or tubes, and plastic-backed paper. Some plastics are designed specifically for use as surface covers

---

BOX 13-1

Examples of Surfaces Susceptible to Contamination During Patient Care Activities

Air/water syringe handle*
Air/water syringe hoses*
Bracket table
Chair control buttons*
Countertops
Dental team chair backs
Drawer handles
Evacuator control*
Evacuator hoses*
Faucet handles*
Handpiece control switches*
Handpiece hoses*
Headrest on chair*
Light curing handle and tip*
Light handles*
Light switch*
Mirror handles
Shade guides
Supply containers and bottles
X-ray unit controls*
X-ray unit handle and cone
X-ray view box switch*

*Usually more easily covered than precleaned and disinfected, although all surfaces lend themselves to covering.

---

in the office in that they have the shape of the item to be covered (e.g., air/water syringe handle covers, hose covers, and pen covers). Some sheets of plastic also have a slightly sticky substance on one side to hold them on the surface. Other plastics (e.g., some food wraps) have a natural clinging ability on contact with a smooth surface. Some plastic bags are available with drawstrings that hold the bag around an item to be protected. To reduce costs, one can use thin rather than thick plastic sheets or bags as long as they are not punctured by the surface being covered. Patient bibs are made of plastic-backed paper and also can be used to cover flat operatory surfaces, although thin plastic sheets may be less expensive.

Use of Surface Covers

Since surface covers are touched with contaminated hands or are spattered with patient materials, fresh surface covers need to be used for each patient. Dental units come in several shapes and sizes with different positioning of the handpiece control system and light and other accessories. Thus, the sizes and shapes of surfaces to be covered vary from one office to the next, but general procedures for use of surface covers are the same (Procedure 13-1).

TABLE 13-1 Surface Covers Versus Precleaning and Disinfection

Advantages	Disadvantages
SURFACE COVERS	
Prevents contamination	A variety of appropriate sizes and types may be needed
Protects surfaces that are difficult to preclean adequately	Adds nonbiodegradable plastic to the environment on disposal
May be less time-consuming to perform	May be esthetically unattractive
Reduces handling and storing of disinfecting chemicals	May be more expensive than precleaning and disinfection
PRECLEANING AND DISINFECTION	
Requires purchase of fewer items to accomplish surface asepsis	Time-consuming when performed properly
May be less expensive than using surface covers	Must use personal protective barriers to protect against contact with the chemicals
Does not change the esthetic appearance of the office	Cannot verify whether the microbes have been removed or killed
Does not add plastic to the environment	Some surfaces cannot be precleaned adequately
	Some chemicals may damage some surfaces
	Use of the chemicals requires proper material safety data sheets to be on file in office
	Use-containers must be labeled properly
	Some disinfectants must be prepared fresh daily
	Chemicals are added to the environment on disposal

Clear plastic bags are available in various sizes and are easy to use. For example, if a chair has control buttons on the side, one can use one bag to cover the headrest and the buttons. It's really not necessary to cover the entire dental chair for most of chair (save the arm rests) is covered with the patient's body. Wraparound backs of side chairs used by the dental team may be touched during patient care and can be covered with a large plastic bag. The bracket table is easily covered, and the handpiece and air/water syringe connectors and hoses can be covered and secured with rubber bands (Figure 13-1). Covering the air/water syringe handle with plastic wrap to prevent contamination is better than trying to preclean and disinfect properly around the buttons that tend to retain debris. If units are set up the night before, a large bag can give overnight dust protection to the bracket table and handpiece unit (Figure 13-2).

Light handles and light switches commonly are touched during patient care and can be covered with plastic wrap or bags, depending on their shape. Some lights have removable handles that can be cleaned and heat sterilized before reuse. One can cover the heads of x-ray units and the control panels (Figures 13-3 and 13-4), and if the water at sinks is not controlled by elbow levers, foot pedals, or automatic devices, one can cover faucet handles with plastic bags (Figure 13-5).

PRECLEANING AND DISINFECTION

Precleaning and disinfection best lend themselves to nonelectric surfaces that are smooth and easily accessible for facilitating good contact with the decontaminating chemicals. Procedure 13-2 describes general procedures for precleaning and disinfecting surfaces.

Approaches to Precleaning and Disinfection

Surfaces to be disinfected first must be precleaned. Precleaning reduces the number of contaminating microorganisms and the blood or saliva present (referred to as bioburden) and facilitates action of the disinfecting chemical. Precleaning is an important step that one must not slight. The organic material in blood and saliva insulates microorganisms from contact with a disinfecting chemical and also may inactivate a portion of the active chemical in the disinfectant.

Use a disinfectant for both the precleaning step and the disinfecting step. Using a disinfectant for the precleaning step starts the killing process early and reduces the chances of spreading the contamination to adjacent surfaces. This (along with wearing heavy utility gloves, a mask, protective eyewear, and protective clothing) provides a little more protection to the person cleaning the surface. Water-based disinfectant-detergents (e.g., some synthetic phenolics, iodophors, and quaternary ammonium compounds—alcohols) solubilize organic materials, such as blood and saliva, and facilitate their removal. One also can use these same products in the disinfection step.

There are two approaches to precleaning and disinfection (see Procedure 13-2). One (using a liquid disinfectant/cleaner) is spray-wipe-spray, and the other (using a disinfectant towelette) is wipe-discard-wipe. For spray-wipe-spray (Figure 13-6), spray the cleaner/disinfectant on the surface

PROCEDURE 13-1

Use of Surface Covers

GOAL: To prevent contamination of surfaces

Materials Needed

Appropriate surface covers
Gloves
Cleaner/disinfectant (when used, will need gloves, mask, clothing, and eye protection)
Material safety data sheet for cleaner/disinfectant

1. Apply appropriate surface covers before the surfaces have a chance to become contaminated with patient material.
   Rationale: Applying the covers after the surfaces become contaminated is a waste of money and time because the contaminated surfaces will have to be precleaned and disinfected anyway when the patient leaves. The covers also may become contaminated themselves when they are applied to a contaminated surface and could contribute to cross-contamination of the next patient.

2. If the surfaces to be covered have been contaminated previously with patient materials, preclean and disinfect the surface and then remove gloves and wash hands before applying the surface covers.
   Rationale: Covers need to be placed on cleaned and disinfected surfaces as explained in step 1. Because the surfaces and the covers are not contaminated, one may use bare hands to place the covers.

3. Place each surface cover so that it protects the entire surface and will not come off when the surface is touched.
   Rationale: Not covering the entire surface defeats the purpose of using surface covers: to prevent contamination. Also, if the covers come off before the end of the appointment, the surfaces will become contaminated.

4. Wear gloves during removal of surface covers after patient care or other activities are completed.
   Rationale: The surface covers are contaminated with patient materials.

5. Carefully remove each cover without touching the underlying surface.
   Rationale: This step prevents the underlying surface from becoming contaminated. Covering surfaces is intended to replace precleaning and disinfecting between patients. If the previously covered surface becomes contaminated, then one must perform extra work.

6. If a surface is touched during removal of the cover, preclean and disinfect the surface.
   Rationale: Covered surfaces must be free of contamination as explained in step 1.

7. Discard used covers into the regular trash unless local laws consider these items as regulated waste; then dispose of them as indicated by the law.*
   Rationale: Federal law (Occupational Safety and Health Administration) states that solid nonsharp waste must be dripping wet or caked with body fluid or partially dried body fluid for it to be handled as regulated waste. Surface covers are never caked or saturated with body fluids unless a blood or saliva spill occurs.

8. Remove and discard contaminated gloves, wash hands, and apply fresh surface covers for care of the next patient.
   Rationale: The gloves become contaminated from contact with the used surface covers. Washing hands after removal of gloves is standard procedure.

---

*In most states, nonsharp contaminated waste such as surface covers is not considered as regulated waste unless an item is soaked or caked with blood or saliva that would be released if the item is compressed.

and wipe (preclean) the surface vigorously with a paper towel or gauze pad. Then respray the disinfectant/cleaner on the precleaned surface and let it remain moist for the longest contact time indicated on the disinfectant label (usually 10 minutes). If moisture remains, one should wipe it away with a paper towel. Some disinfectants are promoted as "one-step" products (i.e., spray and wipe). Although it is usually best to follow manufacturer's directions on all products, it won't hurt to use the one-step products in the two-step procedures (spray-wipe-spray). The two-step procedure becomes even more important should the postcleaning disinfecting contact time stated on the product label be shortened for some reason. If this is the case, at least the precleaning step will have removed/killed some of the microbes in the bioburden on the surface.

Do not store paper towels or gauze pads in a disinfectant and use as wipes to avoid spraying. Wet the towels or pads

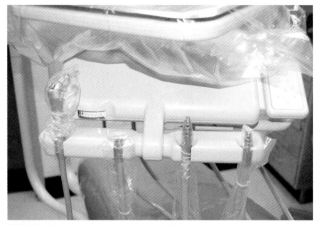

FIGURE 13-1 Surface covers for handpieces and air/water connectors and hoses.

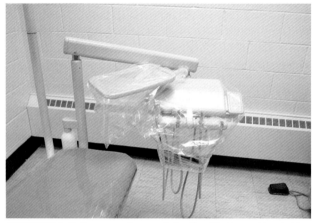

FIGURE 13-2 Surface cover for a control unit and instrument tray holder.

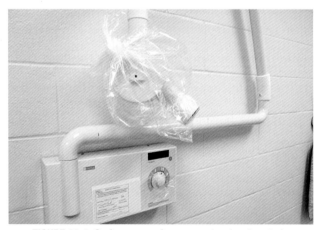

FIGURE 13-3 Surface covers for an x-ray head and controls.

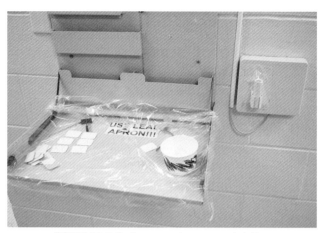

FIGURE 13-4 Surface cover for x-ray workstation.

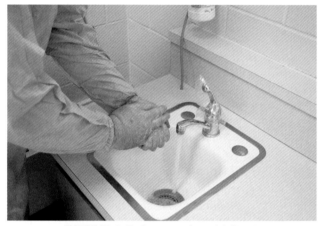

FIGURE 13-5 Surface cover for a sink faucet.

just before use. Paper towels may be held behind some surfaces to catch overspray, if desired.

An alternative to spray-wipe-spray is the wipe-discard-wipe procedure (Figure 13-7) using disinfectant towelettes. Pull a towelette from its container and wipe (preclean) the surface. Then discard that towelette. Obtain another towelette and wipe (disinfect) the surface, let the surface remain wet for the prescribed time, and discard the towelette. Dry off the surface if necessary. As with hand hygiene the physical action of wiping is very important. When using containers of disinfectant towelettes, keep the lid closed when not in use to prevent evaporation of the alcohol. Also, periodically invert the container to redistribute any settled liquid.

If it is difficult to remove all of the bioburden from a given surface, then consider protecting it with a surface cover during future use. This is usually better than attempting to brush it clean and risk spreading contaminants to nearby surfaces.

Unfortunately, one cannot determine the effectiveness of surface disinfection. Thus performing the procedures carefully and using the disinfectant as described on the product label is important.

Characteristics of Disinfectants

There are four general types of antimicrobial chemicals.
- **Antibiotics** (for killing microorganisms in or on the body)
- **Antiseptics** (for killing microorganisms on the skin or other body surfaces)
- **Disinfectants** (for killing microorganisms on environmental/inanimate surfaces or objects)

PROCEDURE

PROCEDURE 13-2

Precleaning and Disinfecting Surfaces

GOAL: To clean and disinfect contaminated surfaces and equipment

Materials Needed
Liquid cleaner/disinfectant or disinfectant towelettes
Paper towels or gauze pads
Material safety data sheet for cleaner/disinfectant
Gloves, mask, clothing, and eye protection

1. Put on utility gloves, mask, protective eyewear, and protective clothing.
   Rationale: Protective gear prevents contact with contaminants and chemicals through touching or splashing.

2. Choose a cleaner/disinfectant that is compatible with the surfaces to be cleaned and disinfected. Many manufacturers of dental equipment have determined which surface disinfectants are most appropriate for their products (e.g., dental chairs and unit accessories) from a material compatibility point of view.
   Rationale: One wants to cause the least damage possible to the surfaces being decontaminated.

3. Confirm that the precleaning/disinfecting product(s) have been prepared correctly (if diluted) and are fresh (if necessary). Read and follow the product label directions.
   Rationale: Using the product as directed helps ensure that the product works effectively.

4. For spray-wipe-spray: Spray the surface with the cleaning/disinfecting agent and vigorously wipe with paper towels. Holding paper towels behind appropriate surfaces during the procedure will reduce over-spray. Alternatively, saturate a paper towel or gauze pad with the cleaning/disinfecting agent and vigorously wipe the surface. Use a brush for surfaces that do not become visibly clean from wiping and consider covering them with a plastic barrier in the future. If cleaning large areas or multiple surfaces or large spills, use several towels or pads for cleaning so as not to transfer contamination to other surfaces. Disinfect the precleaned surface by respraying the disinfecting agent over the entire surface using towels to reduce overspray (or apply with a saturated pad). Let the surface remain moist for the longest contact time indicated on the product label (usually 10 minutes). Vertical surfaces may dry more quickly.

5. For wipe-discard-wipe: Obtain a disinfectant towelette from its container, close the container lid, and vigorously wipe (clean) the surface. Discard the towelette, obtain a fresh towelette, and wipe the surface again for disinfection. Discard the towelette and let the surface dry.
   Rationale: Proper precleaning (predisinfection) is essential to reduce the level of bioburden so the disinfecting step will have the best chance to kill remaining microbes. Using a disinfectant/cleaner begins to kill microbes on the surface during the cleaning step and helps protect the person doing the cleaning. Although the precleaning step removes/kills some microbes, the subsequent disinfection step helps ensure removal/death of the contaminants.

6. If the surface is still wet when ready for patient care, wipe dry. If the surface will come into direct contact with the patient's skin or mouth, rinse/wipe off residual disinfectant with water.
   Rationale: This prevents the cleaning/disinfecting chemicals from contacting the patient and staining clothing or irritating the skin.

- Sterilants (for killing all microorganisms on inanimate objects)

The Centers for Disease Control and Prevention has categorized disinfectants based on their microbial spectrum of activity. This categorization follows and is described further in Table 13-2:

- Sterilant/ high-level disinfectant (for killing all microorganisms on submerged, inanimate, heat sensitive objects)
- Intermediate-level disinfectant (for killing vegetative bacteria, most fungi, viruses, and *M. tuberculosis* var. *bovis*)

- Low-level disinfectant (for killing most vegetative bacteria, some fungi, and some viruses)

Labels on antimicrobial products can be confusing, but reading these labels carefully before using the product is very important. These labels commonly include the type of antimicrobial agent (active ingredients) and general properties such as the following:

- Virucidal (kills at least some viruses)
- Bactericidal (kills at least some bacteria)
- Fungicidal (kills at least some fungi)
- Tuberculocidal (kills the *M. tuberculosis* var. *bovis* bacterium)

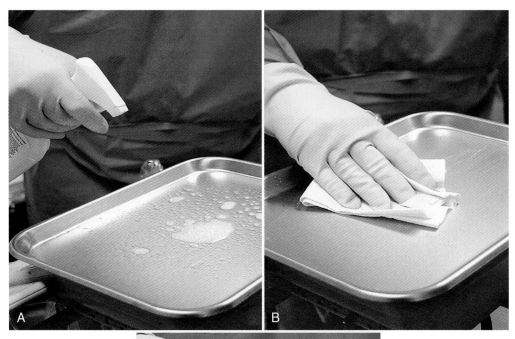

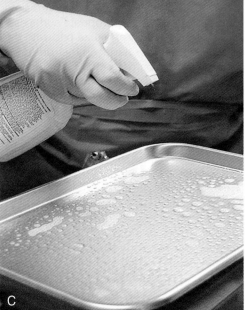

FIGURE 13-6 Surface precleaning and disinfecting by the spray-wipe-spray technique. Precleaning consists of **(A)** spraying with a surface disinfectant and **(B)** wiping the surface to clean it. Disinfection is **(C)** reapplying the disinfectant followed by the appropriate contact time. The surface may then be dried if needed.

- **Sporicidal** (kills bacterial spores, which means it is a sterilant)
- **Hospital disinfectant** (shown to kill the three representative bacteria: *Staphylococcus aureus*, *Salmonella choleraesuis*, and *Pseudomonas aeruginosa*)

The labels also commonly include the following:

- Specific microorganisms (genus and species) shown to be killed in laboratory testing (along with the necessary contact time)
- Directions for use of the product, including the need for precleaning

- Precautionary statements on handling the product
- Warnings such as toxic, poisonous, or flammable
- Treatment for accidental contact
- Storage and disposal information
- Shelf-life and use-life
- How to activate or dilute the product
- Name and address of the manufacturer/distributor, volume of the container, and Environmental Protection Agency (EPA) registration number

No perfect disinfectant exists that will kill all types of disease-producing microorganisms rapidly, have no toxic

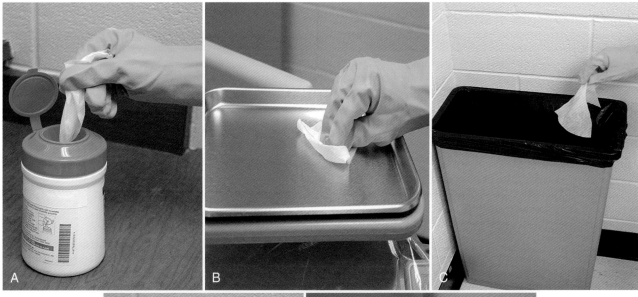

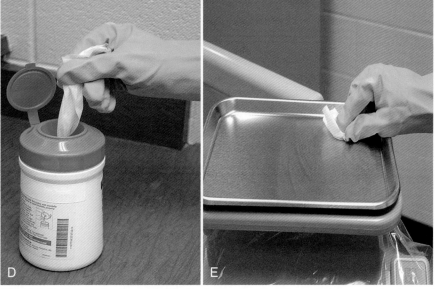

FIGURE 13-7 Surface precleaning and disinfecting by the wipe-discard-wipe technique. Precleaning consists of **(A)** obtaining a fresh surface wipe, **(B)** wiping the surface to clean it, and **(C)** discarding the wipe. Disinfection is **(D)** obtaining a fresh surface wipe and **(E)** wiping the surface again, followed by the appropriate contact time.

properties, be unaffected by organic materials, be odorless, not cause any damage to any surface, and be economical. Nevertheless, several classes of disinfecting chemicals have gained wide use in dentistry and medicine. These classes are identified by the type of antimicrobial agents present in the product, which are listed on the product label as active ingredients (Table 13-3). Because *M. tuberculosis* var. *bovis* is more difficult to kill than most other microorganisms, disinfectants with tuberculocidal activity are considered as strong disinfectants (see Chapter 12, Figure 12-1, *Mycobacterium* species). Stronger disinfectants are active against nonenveloped hydrophilic viruses also, as described in Table 13-4. Use of a water-based disinfectant is reported to provide better cleaning of biological material, such as blood, than use of

an alcohol-based disinfectant. For dental infection control, a water-based surface disinfectant that is Environmental Protection Agency (EPA)-registered and tuberculocidal (such as iodophors, phenolics, or chlorines) is appropriate if used as directed by the manufacturer and careful precleaning is performed.

Manufacturers of disinfectants must submit testing data on the antimicrobial activity and safety of their products to the EPA. If the data are consistent with claims stated on the product labeling and other requirements are met, the EPA registers the product. The U.S. Food and Drug Administration also must grant marketing clearance to liquid chemical sterilants/high-level disinfectants labeled for use on medical devices, such as heat-sensitive dental items.

TABLE 13-2 **Categories of Disinfecting/Sterilizing Chemicals**

Category	Definition	Examples	Use
Sterilant*	Destroys all microorganisms, including high numbers of bacterial spores	Glutaraldehyde, glutaraldehyde phenate, hydrogen peroxide, hydrogen peroxide with peracetic acid, peracetic acid	Heat-sensitive reusable items: immersion only
High-level disinfectant*	Destroys all microorganisms, but not necessarily high numbers of bacterial spores	Glutaraldehyde, glutaraldehyde phenate, hydrogen peroxide, hydrogen peroxide with per-acetic acid, peracetic acid, orthophthalaldehyde	Heat-sensitive reusable items: immersion only
Intermediate-level disinfectant	Destroys vegetative bacteria, most fungi, and most viruses; inactivates *Mycobacterium tuberculosis* var. *bovis* (is tuberculocidal)	EPA-registered hospital disinfectant† with label claim of tuberculocidal activity (e.g., chlorine-based products, phenolics, iodophors, quaternary ammonium compounds with alcohol, bromides)	Clinical contact surfaces; noncritical surfaces with visible blood
Low-level disinfectant	Destroys vegetative bacteria, some fungi, and some viruses; does not inactivate *M. tuberculosis* var. *bovis* (is not tuberculocidal)	EPA-registered hospital disinfectant with no label claim of tuberculocidal activity (e.g., quaternary ammonium compounds)	Housekeeping surfaces (e.g., floors, walls); noncritical surfaces without visible blood; clinical contact surfaces‡

Adapted from Kohn WG, Collins AS, Cleveland JL, et al; Centers for Disease Control and Prevention: Guideline for infection control in dental health-care settings-2003, *MMWR Recomm Rep* 52 (No. RR-17):66, 2003.
EPA, Environmental Protection Agency.
*Some, but not all, of these products can serve as high-level disinfectants and sterilants depending on the immersion time used.
†A hospital disinfectant is one that has been shown to kill *Staphylococcus aureus*, *Pseudomonas aeruginosa*, and *Salmonella choleraesuis*.
‡The Centers for Disease Control and Prevention indicates that low-level disinfectants can be used on clinical contact surfaces if the product has a label claim of killing human immunodeficiency virus and hepatitis B virus in addition to being an EPA-registered hospital disinfectant.

TABLE 13-3 **Active Ingredients in Surface Disinfectants**

Type of Disinfectant	Example of Active Ingredient(s) Listed on Product Label
Chlorines*	Sodium hypochlorite
	Chlorine dioxide
Iodophors*	Butoxypolypropoxypolyethoxyethanol-iodine complex
Water-based phenolics*	
Triphenolics	*o*-Phenylphenol, *o*-benzyl-*p*-chlorophenol, and tertiary amylphenol
Dual phenolics	*o*-Phenylphenol and *o*-benzyl-*p*-chlorophenol
PCMX	*p*-Chloro-*m*-xylenol
Alcohol-based phenolics*	Ethyl or isopropyl alcohol plus
	o-Phenylphenol or *o*-phenylphenol and tertiary amylphenol
Alcohols*	Ethyl alcohol, isopropyl alcohol
Quaternary ammonium compounds†	
First generation	Benzalkonium chloride
Second generation	Alkyldimethylethylbenzyl ammonium chloride or alkyl-dimethyl-3,4-dichloro-benzyl ammonium chloride
Third generation	Combination of first and second generation
Fourth generation	Dioctyldimethyl ammonium bromide or didecyldimethyl ammonium bromide
Fifth generation	Combination of first and fourth generation
Alcohol–quaternary ammonium compound*	A dimethyl-benzyl ammonium chloride plus isopropyl alcohol

*Tuberculocidal.
†Not tuberculocidal.

TABLE 13-4 **Types of Viruses Used in Testing Disinfectant**

Class	Virus	Solubility
Nonenveloped viruses	Poliovirus type 1	Hydrophilic*
	Coxsackievirus B1, B2	Hydrophilic
	ECHO type 6	Hydrophilic
	Rhinovirus type 17	Hydrophilic
	Adenovirus type 2 or 7	Intermediate†
	Reovirus	Intermediate
	Rotavirus	Intermediate
	V-40 virus	Intermediate
Enveloped viruses	Herpes simplex 1	Lipophilic‡
	Influenza A2	Lipophilic
	Vaccinia	Lipophilic
	Human immunodeficiency virus	Lipophilic

*Hydrophilic viruses do not have an envelope, and this makes them more difficult to kill with disinfecting chemicals and makes them more soluble in water.

†Intermediate viruses do not have an envelope, but their susceptibility to killing by disinfecting chemicals is intermediate between lipophilic and hydrophilic viruses, and they are more soluble in lipid materials than other nonenveloped viruses.

‡Lipophilic viruses have a lipid envelope that makes them easier to inactivate with disinfecting chemicals and makes them more soluble in lipid materials than in water.

Chlorine Compounds

Chlorine compounds have been used for many years to disinfect drinking water, swimming pool water, and various inanimate surfaces. These agents are intermediate-level disinfectants, kill a wide variety of microorganisms, and are tuberculocidal. Sodium hypochlorite (which is the main chemical in bleach) is an example of a chlorine compound used to disinfect surfaces. One should note that commercial bleach (which contains approximately 5.25% sodium hypochlorite) is a good surface disinfectant at a 1:10 to 1:100 dilution with water, even though the bleach product is not an EPA-registered disinfectant. However, EPA-registered disinfectants containing sodium hypochlorite or other chlorine compounds are available. Sodium hypochlorite can damage fabrics and metal surfaces (particularly aluminum), and its activity is reduced in the presence of organic material. If one uses diluted commercial bleach as a disinfectant, one should prepare the solution fresh daily. One should wear gloves, protective eyewear, a mask, and protective clothing when using any disinfectant.

Iodophors

Iodine and iodine-alcohol mixtures (known as tinctures of iodine) are well-known killing agents but have some undesirable properties of corrosiveness, staining, irritation of tissues, and allergenicity. When iodine is complexed with certain organic materials, the compound is referred to as an iodophor (see Table 13-3). Most iodophors are intermediate-level disinfectants and retain the broad-spectrum antimicrobial activity (including tuberculocidal activity) of iodine, but they are less corrosive, are less irritating to tissues, and have

reduced staining activity. Detergents are added to iodophor preparations used as surface disinfectants to enhance the cleaning ability of the solution. One may purchase iodophor disinfectants as concentrated solutions that must be diluted correctly before use. The diluted solution that is used should be prepared fresh daily, unless the manufacturer's label indicates otherwise. Because hard water may reduce antimicrobial activity, iodophor disinfectants should be diluted with distilled or deionized water. Iodophors still may be slightly corrosive to some metals and may cause slight staining with repeated use on light-colored surfaces. However, one usually can remove this stain by wiping with alcohol. One should wear gloves, protective eyewear, a mask, and protective clothing when using any disinfectant.

Alcohols

Isopropyl alcohol (isopropanol, sometimes referred to as rubbing alcohol) and ethyl alcohol (ethanol) have been used as antiseptics and disinfectants for many years because they are relatively nonirritating to the skin, although alcohol does "sting" when placed on mucosa (e.g., eye, mouth, and nostrils). Although alcohols at 50% to 70% concentration rapidly kill many microorganisms and are tuberculocidal, they evaporate rapidly when sprayed or wiped on surfaces. To counteract this drawback, extenders that retard evaporation of the alcohol after it is placed on a surface have been added to some isopropanol preparations sold as surface disinfectants. Nevertheless, alcohol has other properties that make it less desirable than other agents as a disinfectant. These properties include a reduction in activity by organic material, corrosiveness, and destruction of some plastic surfaces.

Alcohols also do not solubilize protein material in blood or saliva well and have been reported to be poor cleaners. Alcohols dry out the skin because they tend to dissolve fat and oil that serve as natural skin moisteners. The "waterless" alcohol-containing hand rubs also contain special skin moisteners to reduce these drying effects. Although other agents are more appropriate than alcohol as surface cleaners/disinfectants, alcohol is an important component of some disinfectant preparations (see Table 13-3).

Synthetic Phenolics

Phenol (also known as carbolic acid) has the distinction of being the first widely recognized disinfectant used in hospitals. Lord Joseph Lister suggested the use of phenol as an antiseptic during surgical procedures and as an environmental surface disinfectant more than 100 years ago. Although phenol clearly reduced postoperative infections, it was toxic to tissues, and its use on human beings was stopped. Several phenol-related (phenolic) compounds have been synthesized since and used for microbial killing. Thus, these compounds are referred to as synthetic phenolics, with some use today as active ingredients in surface disinfectants (see Table 13-3) and in mouth rinses and handwashing agents.

Most of the synthetic phenolic disinfectants are intermediate-level tuberculocidal agents and may contain one, two (dual phenolics), or three phenolics (triphenolics), as well as detergents to facilitate cleaning. Some of these disinfectants also contain alcohol. Some preparations must be diluted before use and should be prepared fresh daily unless otherwise stated on the product label. Some preparations are packaged in aerosol cans, and others are contained in pump-spray bottles. Some preparations may leave a film on the disinfected surface, degrade plastic surfaces with prolonged contact, or etch glass surfaces. One should wear gloves, protective eyewear, a mask, and protective clothing when using any disinfectant.

Quaternary Ammonium Compounds

Alcohol-free quaternary ammonium compounds

Quaternary ammonium compounds are also called "quats." These compounds are cationic detergents categorized as low-level disinfectants. A wide variety of quats has been developed over the years, and each time a new type of quat is developed, it is referred to as the next generation (see Table 13-3). All of the alcohol-free quat disinfectants have a low level of antimicrobial activity, and none are tuberculocidal. These disinfectants also may be inactivated by organic materials and soaps. Although they may be appropriate for disinfection of floors and walls, they are less desirable for items more directly involved in patient treatment that may be contaminated with body fluids. Because of these drawbacks, the American Dental Association recommended in 1978 that quaternary ammonium compounds (free of alcohol) not be used in dentistry. However, the Centers for Disease Control and Prevention has indicated that low-level disinfectants such as alcohol-free quats may be used on clinical contact

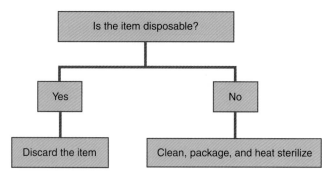

FIGURE 13-8 Management of equipment that will penetrate soft tissue or tooth structure.

surfaces if the product also has claims for killing human immunodeficiency virus and hepatitis B virus.

Quaternary ammonium compounds with alcohol

The addition of alcohol to quaternary ammonium compounds by manufacturers enhances their antimicrobial activity. These intermediate-level disinfectants are tuberculocidal and are appropriate for use in dentistry.

EQUIPMENT DECONTAMINATION

General Considerations

Some basic considerations for equipment decontamination exist. In general, one should try to prevent the equipment from becoming contaminated in the first place. If this is not possible, one should select heat sterilization first. If the equipment cannot be heat sterilized, then one should use a liquid sterilant or an appropriate disinfectant for decontamination. Following the manufacturer's directions for preventing contamination or for cleaning, sterilization, or disinfection of dental equipment is important.

One should use the following principles to reduce the spread of microbes from dental equipment used in the mouth that will penetrate soft tissue or tooth structure (Figure 13-8):
- If the item is disposable, one should dispose of it properly after use on one patient.
- If the item is not disposable, one should clean it, package it, and heat sterilize it.

One should use the following approach to decontamination if the item will be used in the patient's mouth but will not penetrate soft tissue or tooth structure (Figure 13-9):
- If the item is disposable, one should dispose of it properly after use on one patient.
- If the item is reusable, one should cover the parts that may become contaminated with an impervious barrier to prevent contamination.
- If the item is not disposable, cannot be covered completely, and becomes contaminated, one should clean it, package it, and heat sterilize it.
- If the item cannot be heat sterilized, one should clean and submerge it in a liquid sterilant/high-level disinfectant.

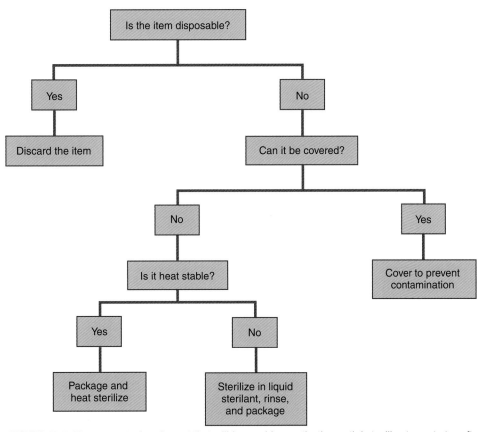

FIGURE 13-9 Management of equipment that will be used in a patient's mouth but will not penetrate soft tissue or tooth structure.

- If the item is not disposable and cannot be covered, heat sterilized, or submerged in a liquid agent, do not use the item.

One should use the following approach for items that are not used in the patient's mouth (Figure 13-10):

- If an item will not become contaminated with patient materials, one should just keep it clean.
- If an item will become contaminated with patient materials, one should clean it and, when possible, heat sterilize it.
- If the item cannot be heat sterilized because of its size or composition, one should clean and disinfect it.

Management of High-tech Equipment

New technologies are developed continually that aid the dental profession in treating patients. These technologies must be compatible with infection control or their use will be limited, but some technologies may present special infection control challenges, such as computers, cameras, and digital x-ray sensors.

For computers, one should avoid their contamination by performing hand hygiene before use. If this does not occur, recent studies have shown that the keyboards can be successfully decontaminated by using disinfectant wipes such as those containing quaternary ammonium compounds. Also,

the same study showed that no damage occurred to the keyboards after 300 disinfecting procedures. Care should be taken that disinfectant wipes used should not contain excess fluid that might that might enter the base of the keyboard. Also, protective covers for the keyboard are available as well antimicrobial keyboards.

For 35 mm, video, and digital cameras, one should try to avoid their contamination. They are not designed to be disinfected. One should cover them with plastic sheeting or operate them only with clean hands.

Computer-aided design/computer-aided manufacturing devices (CAD/CAMs) use close-up intraoral pictures to design and manufacture restorations. These devices use a small camera lens on the end of a wire that transmits pictures from the patient's mouth to a TV-type monitor. One should check with the manufacturer for proper decontamination of the camera and wire. One model has an outer removable prismatic device that slides over the camera lens, so the prism rather than the camera lens becomes contaminated. The prism can be sterilized in a dry heat sterilizer but not in a steam sterilizer, for the moist heat can damage the prism.

Digital radiography equipment needs special attention. This equipment uses intraoral sensors to provide a digital image that can be manipulated, viewed on a monitor, printed, or stored electronically. Because the sensors are

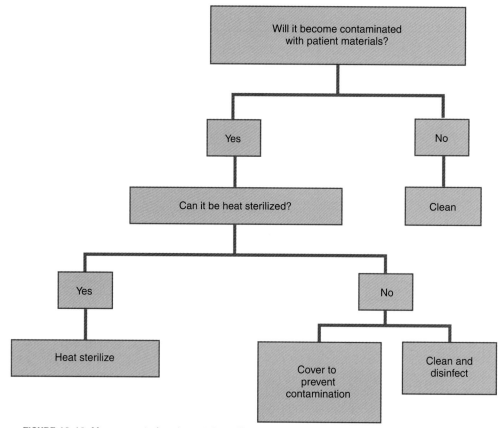

FIGURE 13-10 Management of equipment that will not be used in a patient's mouth but that may become contaminated by touching or by spatter.

reusable, one must handle them properly to prevent cross-contamination during subsequent use. One type of sensor, the charge-coupled device (CCD), is attached to a wire and should not be heat sterilized. Instead, one should cover the CCD with a plastic barrier that extends down the cable to prevent any contact with patient materials or contaminated hands. If the CCD does become contaminated, one may disinfect it by the spray-wipe-spray technique according to the manufacturer's directions. Another type of digital x-ray sensor is the complementary metal-oxide semiconductor with active pixel sensors. This device is wired and should be treated with plastic barriers just like the CCD sensor. A third type of sensor, the photostimulable phosphor plate sensor, is wireless and is placed in the patient's mouth much like a regular film packet. One must cover the device with a plastic barrier; it cannot become contaminated because it cannot be heat sterilized or chemically disinfected.

ASEPTIC DISTRIBUTION OF DENTAL SUPPLIES

Numerous supplies are used for patient care, and their storage and distribution present a major challenge to infection control. Examples of such items include cotton balls and rolls, gauze pads, floss, articulating paper, retraction cord, orthodontic wire, and tubes or bottles of dental materials,

to mention only a few. The major problems relate to surface asepsis and how these supplies are obtained for use at chairside without cross-contamination.

Aseptic Retrieval

If one stores supply items in bulk, such as a container of cotton rolls, one must use an aseptic retrieval system (rather than saliva-coated gloved fingers) to avoid contamination of unused items in the container. Providing sterile forceps (to retrieve the supply item) with the instruments needed for each patient is one approach to this problem (Figure 13-11). Storing supplies (or instruments) in drawers at chairside lends itself to cross-contamination of the drawer handle (if not covered or precleaned and disinfected) or of bulk items inside (if aseptic retrieval is not used).

Unit Dosing

The dental professional may protect supply containers, bottles, and tubes of materials used at chairside on more than one patient (multidose containers) with a surface cover for each patient or in some instances may preclean and disinfect these between patients. Many types of disposable supplies can be unit dosed, which means that the supplies are distributed or packaged in small numbers sufficient for care

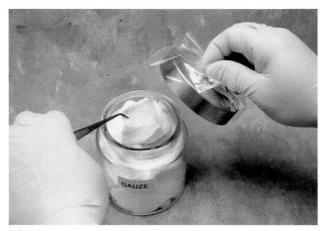

FIGURE 13-11 Aseptic retrieval using sterilized cotton pliers issued for each patient.

of just one patient and are placed at chairside before care begins. For example, a package may contain four cotton rolls, three cotton balls, two gauze pads, articulating paper, or whatever one anticipates for a single patient. Whatever is not used with a patient is discarded. Some supply items are unit dosed by the manufacturers, saving office staff time. Although unit dosing can solve some cross-contamination problems, unfortunately it can be expensive and wasteful if not organized properly.

SELECTED READINGS

Berendt AE, Turnbull L, Spady D, et al: Three swipes and you're out: how many swipes are needed to decontaminate plastic with disposable wipes? *Am J Infect Control* 39:442–443, 2011.

Kohn WG, Collins AS, Cleveland JL, et al: Centers for Disease Control and Prevention: Guidelines for infection control in dental health-care settings–2003, *MMWR Recomm Rep* 52(RR-17):1–61, 2003.

Miller CH: High-tech equipment: keeping it germ-free, *Dent Prod Rpt* 37:68–71, 2003.

Miller CH: Labels, a must read, *Dent Prod Rpt* 40:82–86, 2006.

Miller CH: Strategies for infection control in dentistry. In Ciancio SG, editor: *ADA guide to dental therapeutics*, ed 3, Chicago, 2003, ADA Publishing, pp 551–566.

Miller CH, Palenik CJ: Sterilization, disinfection and asepsis in dentistry. In Block SS, editor: *Sterilization, disinfection and preservation*, ed 5, Philadelphia, 2001, Lea & Febiger, pp 1049–1068.

Molinari JA, Gleason MJ, Cottone JA, Barrett ED: Cleaning and disinfectant properties of dental surface disinfectants, *J Am Dent Assoc* 117:179–182, 1988.

Rutala WA, Weber DJ: Sterilization, high-level disinfection and environmental cleaning, *Infect Dis Clin North Am* 25:45–76, 2011.

Rutala WA, White MS, Gergen MF, Weber DJ: Bacterial contamination of keyboards: efficacy and functional impact of disinfectants, *Infect Control Hosp Epidemiol* 27:372–377, 2006.

Westergard EJ, Romito LM, Kowolik MJ, Palenik CJ: Controlling bacterial contamination of dental impression guns, *J Am Dent Assoc* 142:1269–1274, 2011.

Williams HN, Singh R, Romberg E: Surface contamination in the dental operatory, *J Am Dent Assoc* 134:325–330, 2003.

REVIEW QUESTIONS

Multiple Choice

1. Which of the following microbes are not killed by inter-mediate-level disinfectants?
   a. Bacterial spores
   b. Tuberculosis agent
   c. Both a and b
   d. Neither a nor b

2. Which of the following types of antimicrobial agents should be used on floors?
   a. Sterilant/high-level disinfectant
   b. Intermediate-level disinfectant
   c. Low-level disinfectant

3. Which of the following antimicrobial agents should not be used for surface disinfection in dentistry?
   a. Sterilant/high-level disinfectant
   b. Intermediate-level disinfectant
   c. Low-level disinfectant

4. Which of the following agents is not tuberculocidal?
   a. Iodophor
   b. Quaternary ammonium compound
   c. Phenolic
   d. Glutaraldehyde

5. What types of surfaces should be covered rather than disinfected?
   a. Electric switches
   b. Surfaces that are difficult to clean
   c. Smooth surfaces
   d. Both a and b
   e. Both a and c

6. Why should disinfectants used on clinical contact surfaces in dentistry contaminated with blood or saliva have tuberculocidal activity?
   a. Tuberculosis is a common occupational disease of dental personnel, so a tuberculocidal agent is needed to prevent this type of spread in the office.

   b. The tuberculosis agent is spread most commonly by touching contaminated surfaces.
   c. Because the tuberculosis agent is one of the more resistant microbes to kill, tuberculocidal activity indicates sufficient potency to kill most other vegetative microbes.

7. Liquid sterilants such as a glutaraldehyde should be used only on reusable items that can be submerged and are:
   a. contaminated with blood
   b. made of metal
   c. heat sensitive
   d. classified as critical (penetrate tissue)

8. One should not use _____ as a surface cover.
   a. paper
   b. plastic-backed patient napkin
   c. plastic sheet
   d. formed plastic bags

9. Use of a disinfectant-type cleaner to preclean a contaminated operatory surface:
   a. should not be done
   b. starts the microbial killing process and helps protect the person doing the cleaning
   c. eliminates the need to follow up with a disinfectant wipe
   d. is necessary every time a surface cover is removed

10. When can a liquid sterilant/high-level disinfectant achieve sterilization?
    a. Sterilization will occur only when the solution is used at temperatures above 121° C (250° F).
    b. Sterilization will occur when the solution is used only for the longer exposure times.

Please visit http://evolve.elsevier.com/Miller/infectioncontrol/ for additional practice and study support tools.

Dental Unit Water Asepsis and Air Quality

OUTLINE

LEARNING OBJECTIVES

After completing this chapter, the student should be able to do the following:

1. Discuss the presence of microorganisms in dental unit water, and list the types and importance of these microbes.
2. Define biofilm and describe how it forms inside dental unit water lines.
3. Describe the concerns of having microbes present in dental unit water, the current infection control recommendations, and different approaches for reducing the microbial quantity in dental unit water.
4. Describe the procedures for monitoring the quality of dental unit water, what a "boil-water" notice means, backflow prevention measures, and contamination of dental air concerns.

KEY TERMS

Biofilm
Boil-Water Notice
CFU/mL

Endotoxins
Independent Water Reservoir
Planktonic

Potable Water
Surgical Procedures

The goal of infection control in dentistry is to reduce or eliminate exposures of patients and the dental team to microorganisms. Other chapters have discussed examples of how to accomplish infection control; this chapter describes contamination of the patient and the dental team with microorganisms present in dental unit water and what may be done to control the quality of dental unit water.

DENTAL UNIT WATER

Water enters the dental office from municipal supplies or from wells. As in homes, water then is routed to various sites, including sink faucets, toilets, water heaters, air conditioners, humidifiers, washers, and, in dental offices, dental units. At the dental unit, water enters plastic water lines that pass through a multichannel control box that allows the water to be distributed to the hoses that feed various attachments, such as high-speed handpieces, air/water syringes, and sometimes an ultrasonic scaler. The water lines in dental units have a small bore (about ¹⁄₁₆-inch inside diameter), and, in the standard four-hole handpiece hose, the water line is one of the two smaller lines (Figure 14-1). Thus the water that enters the dental unit is the same water that supplies the entire office.

PRESENCE OF MICROORGANISMS IN DENTAL UNIT WATER

The Environmental Protection Agency standard for the microbial quality of drinking water (called potable water) is no more than a total of 500 colony-forming units per milliliter (CFU/mL) of noncoliform bacteria. A colony-forming unit is considered to be one bacterial cell or a small number of bacterial cells, and a milliliter is approximately one-fourth of a teaspoon. Municipal water that enters the dental unit is not sterile and does have a low number of waterborne microbes present,

so the water that enters the dental unit usually contains just a few microorganisms (e.g., 0 to 500 CFU/mL). However, water exiting the dental handpiece, air/water syringe, and ultrasonic scalers may contain more than 100,000 CFU/mL. Table 14-1 lists the results of some studies conducted in the United States that have measured the concentration of bacteria in dental unit water. Maximum reported recoveries from dental unit water in the United States have been 1.2 million and 10 million CFU/mL. Dental unit water contamination occurs worldwide, with more than 35 articles in the scientific literature describing various levels of bacteria from Austria, Canada, Denmark, England, Germany, New Zealand, and the United States.

TYPES AND IMPORTANCE OF MICROORGANISMS IN DENTAL UNIT WATER

Although human oral microorganisms have been found in dental unit water, the vast majority of those present are waterborne microorganisms (Table 14-2). Most of the waterborne microorganisms are of low pathogenicity or are opportunistic pathogens causing harmful infections only under special conditions or in immunocompromised persons. Microorganisms of main concern are species of *Pseudomonas*, *Legionella*, and *Mycobacterium*.

Pseudomonas

Pseudomonas aeruginosa and *Pseudomonas cepacia* are common inhabitants of the environment, existing in soil and natural waters. Many strains can survive and even multiply in water of low nutrient content such as distilled water. Thus, to find *Pseudomonas* species in almost any type of domestic water supply, storage tanks, and drain lines is not unusual. *P. cepacia* is an important respiratory pathogen in patients with cystic fibrosis. *P. aeruginosa* is usually opportunistic in causing urinary tract infections, wound infections, pneumonia, and septicemia in burn patients, and, along with *P. cepacia*, usually has a higher degree of resistance than many bacteria to killing by disinfecting chemicals and by antibiotics. The only scientific report that directly implicates any microorganism from dental unit water as a health risk has involved *Pseudomonas*. The report from England implicated *P. aeruginosa* from dental unit water as the cause of oral infections in two medically compromised dental patients.

Legionella

Legionella pneumophila and other *Legionella* species are gram-negative bacteria that naturally occur in water and may gain some protection against the chlorine present in domestic water because they can exist inside certain free-living amebae also present in the water.

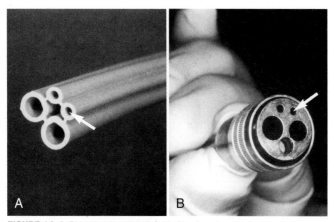

FIGURE 14-1 Dental unit water line. **A,** The four-hole high-speed handpiece hose. **B,** The connector at the end of the hose to which a high-speed handpiece is attached. (*Arrows* indicate the water lines.)

L. pneumophila is the causative agent of a type of pneumonia called legionnaires' disease, which was first recognized in 1976 when 182 attendees at an American Legion convention in Philadelphia became infected with this bacterium, which was present in water in the convention hotel. The bacterium usually is transmitted by inhalation of aerosolized contaminated water or by aspiration of organisms that have colonized the oropharynx. Specific examples of how *L. pneumophila* may have been transmitted to human beings from various sources of water involve cooling towers, heat exchange apparatuses, a mist machine spraying produce in a grocery store, humidifiers, shower heads, hot-water faucets, decorative fountains, tap water used to clean medical equipment, and whirlpools in hospitals. However, the route of spread has not been identified for all cases detected. *L. pneumophila* also may cause a nonpulmonary infection called Pontiac fever, and, rarely, wound infections following irrigation with *Legionella*-contaminated water. Although *L. pneumophila* is the principal pathogen in this genus, 30 other species of *Legionella* exist and may cause up to 20% to 30% of all *Legionella* infections.

L. pneumophila and other *Legionella* species have been detected in dental unit water. *L. pneumophila* was found in the water from approximately 10% of 42 units in 35 practices in Austria, from 3 of 5 units in a hospital dental clinic in London, from 4% of 194 dental units at levels greater than 100 CFU/mL in a London teaching hospital, and from several dental units at the University of Dresden in Germany. In the United States, *L. pneumophila* has been detected in dental unit water in an Ohio dental school clinic and in 8% of the water samples taken from 28 dental facilities in California, Massachusetts, Michigan, Minnesota, Oregon, and Washington. In the latter study, *L. pneumophila* was never detected at concentrations greater than 1000 CFU/mL, but other species of *Legionella* were found in 68% of the water samples tested and at levels of at least 10,000 CFU/mL in 19% of the samples.

As mentioned in Chapter 7, an 82-year-old woman died in Rome, Italy, in 2011, from legionnaires' disease that was contracted from a dental office. During the incubation period for this disease (2 to 10 days), the woman only left her home to attend two dental appointments and apparently had no other risks of exposure to this bacterium. Testing of water in her home was negative for *Legionella*. However, three different methods of testing showed the same genetic form of *L. pneumophila* serogroup 1 in the patient's bronchial aspirate and the dental office's tap water, dental unit waterline, and high-speed handpiece turbine. Although no other cases of legionnaires' disease or Pontiac fever were discovered among the patients of this dental practice, this incident shows that this disease can be acquired from dental unit water during routine dental treatment.

As of this writing, no scientific documentation exists for spread of legionnaires' disease from dental offices in the United States, but some dental offices have *Legionella* in untreated dental unit water used for patient care. Thus, some dental patients may be exposed to this bacterium, and if such patients are compromised somehow, may acquire the disease.

TABLE 14-1 **Presence of Bacteria in Dental Unit Water**

Location	Source	CFU/mL (Mean)
San Francisco*	10 dental units from 3 offices	180,000
	Tap water from same offices	15
Washington[†]	54 air/water syringe hoses	165,000
California[†]	22 high-speed handpiece hoses	739,000
Oregon[†]	10 faucets	<30
	4 water coolers	<30
	11 rivers and streams	28,200
Indianapolis[‡]	5 dental units	148,000
New Orleans[§]	6 dental units	188,333
Baltimore[¶]	8 dental units	110,000

*Abel LC, Miller RL, Micik RE, Ryge G: Studies on dental aerobiology: IV. Bacterial contamination of water delivered by dental units, *J Dent Res* 50:1567-1569, 1971.

[†]Santiago JI, Huntington MK, Johnston AM, et al: Microbial contamination of dental unit waterlines: short- and long-term effects of flushing, *Gen Dent* 42:528-544, 1994.

[‡]Unpublished data from the author, 1996.

[§]Mayo JA, Oertling KM, Abdrieu SC: Bacterial biofilm: a source of contamination in dental air-water syringes, *Clin Prev Dent* 12:13-20, 1990.

[¶]Williams HN, Brockington AM: Quantitation of bacteria in water delivered by dental units as determined by plate-count and direct-count methods, *Quintessence Int* 26:31-36, 1995.

TABLE 14-2   Microbes Isolated from Dental Unit Water

Microorganism	Probable Source	Pathogenicity
BACTERIA		
Achromobacter xylosoxidans	Water	Opportunistic
Acinetobacter sp.	Mouth	Low
Actinomyces sp.	Water	Opportunistic
Alcaligenes denitrificans	Water	Low
Bacillus sp.	Water	Low
Bacillus subtilis	Mouth	Low
Bacteroides sp.	Water	Low
Flavobacterium sp.	Mouth	Low
Fusobacterium sp.	Water	Low
Helicobacter pylori	Water	Low
Klebsiella pneumoniae	Mouth	Low
Lactobacillus sp.	Water	Opportunistic
Legionella pneumophila	Water	Opportunistic
Legionella sp.	Water	Low
Methylobacterium mesophilicum	Water	Low
Micrococcus luteus	Water	Low
Moraxella sp.	Water	Low
Mycobacterium gordonae	Water	Low
Nocardia sp.	Water	Low
Ochrobactrum sp.	Water	Low
Pasteurella haemolytica	Water	Low
Pasteurella sp.	Water	Low
Peptostreptococcus sp.	Mouth	Low
Pseudomonas aeruginosa	Water	Opportunistic
Pseudomonas cepacia	Water	Opportunistic
Pseudomonas paucimobilis	Water	Opportunistic
Pseudomonas sp.	Water	Opportunistic
Serratia marcescens	Water	Opportunistic
Staphylococcus aureus	Mouth	Intermediate
Staphylococcus sp.	Mouth	Low
Streptococcus sp.	Mouth	Low
Veillonella alcalescens	Mouth	Low
Xanthomonas sp.	Water	Low
FUNGI		
Alternaria sp.	Water	Low
Cephalosporium sp.	Water	Low

Continued

TABLE 14-2 **Microbes Isolated from Dental Unit Water—cont'd**

Microorganism	Probable Source	Pathogenicity
Cladosporium sp.	Water	Low
Exophiala mesophila	Water	Low
Penicillium sp.	Water	Low
Scopulariopsis sp.	Water	Low
PROTOZOA		
Acanthamoeba sp.	Water	Low
Naegleria sp.	Water	Low

Adapted from Miller CH: Dental unit waterline contamination, *Operatory Infect Cont Updates* 2:1-8, 1994.

Indirect evidence that dental team members may have occupational exposure to legionellae comes from two studies that showed higher rates of seroconversion with antibodies to legionellae in dental personnel than in nondental personnel. One of the studies also showed that seroconversion rates increased as the years of experience in dentistry increased. This information suggests that dental workers at least are exposed to *Legionella* through contact with aerosols from dental unit water coming out of high-speed handpieces, ultrasonic scalers, and air/water syringes.

Although no documentation indicates that dental unit water has ever caused legionnaires' disease in dental team members as well as in patients in the United States, a comment about unpublished data in a report about *Legionella* in dental unit water infers that a dentist in California who died of legionellosis may have contacted the causative agent from his dental unit water.

Mycobacterium

Nontuberculous mycobacteria (e.g., *Mycobacterium chelonae*) have been detected in some domestic water supplies. These bacteria are somewhat resistant to chemical killing, have caused infections in dialysis patients, and have been detected in the water used to process dialyzers. A case report describes an intraoral infection with *M. chelonae*, but the source of this bacterium was not known.

Other Bacteria

Acinetobacter, *Alcaligenes*, *Klebsiella*, and *Serratia* (see Table 14-2) are gram-negative opportunistic pathogens that may cause harmful infections in compromised hosts. No specific documentation exists that these bacteria from dental unit water have caused any infections in patients or in dental team members. The oral bacteria of *Bacteroides*, *Fusobacterium*, *Lactobacillus*, *Peptostreptococcus*, and *Streptococcus* are involved in causing dental caries or periodontal diseases and have opportunistic pathogenicity if allowed to accumulate on tooth surfaces in plaque. The majority of microbes present in dental unit water are bacteria, but fungi, such as *Cladosporium* and *Exophiala mesophila*, and protozoa, such as *Acanthamoeba* and *Naegleria*, also have been detected.

Endotoxins

Endotoxin is a component of the cell walls of gram-negative bacteria and also is known as lipopolysaccharide (see Chapter 2). One study showed that the dental unit water tested contained 1000 units of endotoxin per milliliter. Endotoxin can cause inflammation and shock and has been implicated in a variety of harmful infections involving gram-negative bacteria, including periodontal diseases. Although no endotoxin standard for drinking water exists, United States Pharmacopeia sterile water cannot have more than 0.25 units of endotoxin per milliliter.

BIOFILM IN DENTAL UNIT WATER LINES

General Nature of Biofilm

Water entering dental units usually has a low number of microorganisms present, but the water that passes out of the dental unit through handpieces, scalers, and air/water syringes is highly contaminated. Thus the incoming water becomes highly contaminated when inside the dental unit. This contamination comes from biofilm that forms on the inside of the dental unit water lines.

Microorganisms exist in dental unit water lines in two types of communities. One bacterial community exists in the water itself and is referred to as the planktonic (free-floating) microorganisms. The other exists in a sessile form attached to the inside walls of the water lines called biofilm.

Biofilm is defined as a mass of microorganisms attached to a surface exposed to moisture. Biofilms are common; they form just about anywhere one finds a moist, nonsterile environment, including the surfaces of rocks, plants, and fish associated with natural water environments in streams, lakes, and oceans, and those associated with "domestic/industrial" water environments, such as water lines, sewer systems, drain lines, wells, septic tanks, sewage treatment facilities, water storage containers, humidifiers, and spray heads. Biofilms also form on biomedical materials implanted in or associated with the human body, including many types of catheters, sutures, wound drainage tubes, endotracheal tubes, mechanical heart valves, and intrauterine contraceptive devices.

The best example of biofilm in dentistry is dental plaque, also referred to as oral biofilm. Thus a type of plaque develops inside of dental unit water lines that causes a permanent infection of the water delivery system.

Mechanisms of Biofilm Formation

Biofilm forms when bacterial cells adhere to a surface using cell surface polymers. Many of these polymers are highly hydrated exopolysaccharides, referred to as glycocalyx polymers that give the biofilm a "slimy" nature. As the attached cells multiply within the glycocalyx, the new cells remain embedded and form microcolonies on the surface. Continued multiplication results in the joining of microcolonies, and this with the continual recruitment of additional bacteria from the planktonic phase can result in a covering of the surface.

Biofilm forms on the inside of the dental unit water lines as the water is flowing through the unit. Several factors allow this to occur (Box 14-1). The water in the dental unit water lines moves at normal line pressures, which is slower than one might imagine. The water is not pressurized into the form of the handpiece spray until the water and air mix inside the handpiece. Intermittent stagnation of the water inside the units commonly occurs between patients, overnight, and over the weekend. This facilitates attachment of bacteria from the planktonic community. The dynamics of fluid flowing through a line are such that the maximum flow rate occurs in the center of the stream of fluid and the minimum flow rate occurs near the surfaces of the wall of the tubing. Thus the water is moving more slowly near the surface of the walls, facilitating attachment of bacteria. Another key factor in water line biofilm formation is that most waterborne bacteria have developed the ability to attach to surfaces more efficiently than most nonwaterborne bacteria. This feature allows these bacteria to become stabilized on a surface and let the nutrients in the water come to them. The small diameter of dental unit water lines causes a large amount of biofilm to form. As the diameter of pipes or tubings decreases, the surface-to-volume ratio increases. So the smaller the diameter, the more surface relative to volume there is for biofilm to form. In smaller lines, more bacteria have a chance to contact and attach to a surface than they have to remain in the fluid. Thus water coming out of a water line in a home that has a ½- to ¾-inch diameter will have less biofilm than the 1/16-inch diameter line in a dental unit.

BOX 14-1

Factors that Influence the Formation of Dental Unit Water Line Biofilm

1. Water stagnates. (Water in the tubing is not under high pressure, and the water flow rate in the lines is low near the walls of the tubing.)
2. Small-diameter tubing creates a large surface-to-volume ratio, giving bacteria a greater chance to contact and attach to the wall surfaces.
3. Even though bacteria are usually at low levels in the incoming water, they are continually present, providing the pioneer bacteria for biofilm formation.
4. Some bacteria in air or in patient materials may enter the dental unit water line system through contamination of water line openings or retraction through the handpiece or air/water syringe.
5. Waterborne bacteria entering the system have special abilities to attach to surfaces, facilitating biofilm formation.
6. Incoming water brings a continuous source of nutrients to the bacteria in the developing biofilm.
7. Bacteria that attach to tubing walls or to other attached bacteria multiply to increase the mass of the biofilm.
8. As water flows by the biofilm, it picks up bacteria from the biofilm and carries it through handpieces, air/water syringes, scalers, and cup fillers.

Rate of Biofilm Formation

The rate at which biofilm forms depends on the aforementioned factors. As we all know, the biofilm on our teeth (dental plaque) begins to reform immediately after we brush them. By the end of the day, most persons can even see this plaque. Dental unit water line biofilm forms more slowly but begins in a new dental unit within hours. One study showed that microbial levels in dental unit water reached 200,000 CFU/mL within 5 days after installation of new dental unit water lines.

Figure 14-2 compares the inside of a dental unit handpiece waterline (left side of the photo) with its adjacent airline (center of the photo). The whitish material in the waterline is biofilm. The inside of the airline appears clean. The right side of the photo shows a cross section of the handpiece hose.

Figure 14-3 shows what mature biofilm in dental handpiece water lines looks like under the scanning electron microscope. This particular water line was used in a dental unit for at least 5 years. Figure 14-4 shows scanning electron microscope photomicrographs of biofilm that formed in an air/water syringe water line of a new dental unit that was in operation for just 5.3 months.

Biofilm can serve as a continuous source of contamination of the flowing water as cells or chunks dislodge naturally or from physical stress placed on the line. The fact that biofilm serves as a source of microorganisms in the exiting water has been demonstrated. When water lines containing biofilm were flushed to remove planktonic bacteria and the lines were filled with sterile water, the sterile water became heavily contaminated after a few hours.

Although human beings cannot live without water, we commonly think of water as having little nutritional value. However, tap water contains low concentrations of inorganic and organic material that can serve as a source of nutrients for microorganisms. In fact, biofilm in water lines serves as a great mechanism by which bacteria can gain continuous access to the low levels of nutrients in a never-ending flow of water. The waterborne bacteria also are conditioned to an existence in a low-nutrient environment. For example, strains of *P. aeruginosa* and *P. cepacia* have been shown to multiply to high levels in water taken from distilled water reservoirs and commercially prepared distilled water.

NEED TO IMPROVE DENTAL UNIT WATER QUALITY

No evidence indicates the occurrence of any widespread public health problem from exposure to dental unit water. However, the sources of the microorganisms causing low levels of infectious diseases in the community are not always identified, and the presence of potential pathogens in dental unit water is of concern. Also, the goal of infection control is to eliminate or reduce exposure to microorganisms. Because infectious diseases may occur when human beings and microorganisms come into contact with each other, all health care providers have a responsibility to reduce this possible contact, particularly when it may occur between patients and microorganisms in a health care facility. Using dental unit water that is contaminated heavily with microorganisms of any kind for dental treatment is contrary to the goals of infection control.

Thus, improving the quality of dental unit water as means become available is a natural part of maintaining the high quality of patient care and staff protection for which dentistry is well noted.

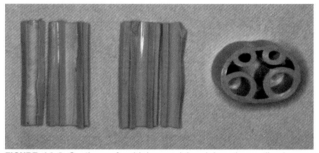

FIGURE 14-2 Sections of a high-speed handpiece hose sliced open. *Left*, waterline showing whitish biofilm inside. *Center*, airline showing a clean inner surface. *Right*, cross-section of the hose.

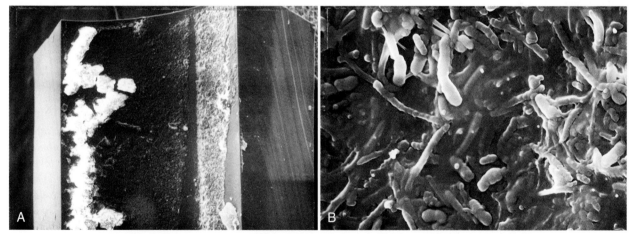

FIGURE 14-3 Scanning electron micrographs of the inside of a small section of high-speed dental handpiece water line. A ½-inch long section of handpiece hose attached to a dental unit was removed, and the water line was separated from the other three lines. The water line section was cut longitudinally with a clean sterile scalpel to expose the inner lumen. The water line section then was fixed in 5% glutaraldehyde in cacodylate buffer containing 0.15% ruthenium red. After rinsing with buffer, the section was treated with 4% osmium tetraoxide for 2 hours at room temperature, rinsed again, dehydrated in increasing concentrations of ethanol, incubated for 2 hours in hemamethyldisilazane, dried for 3 days, exposed to colloidal graphite, and sputter-coated with gold-palladium. **A**, Low-power magnification (80×) with cut edges of the water line on the right and left sides and the lumen with biofilm in the middle. **B**, High-power magnification (×6000) of the same sample showing biofilm in the lumen. (From Miller CH: Infection control, *Dent Clin North Am* 40:437-456, 1996. With permission.)

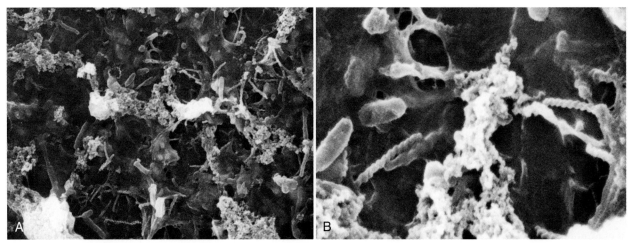

FIGURE 14-4 Scanning electron micrograph of biofilm on the inside of an air/water syringe water line. The samples were prepared as described in the legend of Figure 14-3. **A**, Original magnification, ×1500. **B**, Original magnification, ×6000.

CURRENT INFECTION CONTROL RECOMMENDATIONS

Centers for Disease Control and Prevention

Current (2003) recommendations from the Centers for Disease Control and Prevention (CDC) related to microorganisms in dental unit water are as follows:

- Dental offices use water that meets regulatory standards set by the Environmental Protection Agency for drinking water (fewer than 500 CFU/mL of heterotrophic water bacteria) for routine dental treatment output water.
- Consult with the dental unit manufacturer for appropriate methods and equipment to maintain the recommended quality of dental water.
- Follow recommendations for monitoring water quality provided by the manufacturer of the unit or water line treatment product.
- Discharge water and air for a minimum of 20 seconds after each patient from any dental device connected to the dental water system that enters the patient's mouth (e.g., handpieces, ultrasonic scalers, and air/water syringe).
- Consult with the dental unit manufacturer on the need for periodic maintenance of antiretraction mechanisms.

One should flush high-speed handpieces to discharge water and air for a minimum of 20 seconds after use on each patient. This procedure is intended to aid in physically flushing out patient material that may have entered the turbine and air or water lines. One should consider use of an enclosed container or high-velocity evacuation to minimize the spread of spray, spatter, and aerosols generated during discharge procedures. Additionally, evidence indicates that overnight or weekend microbial accumulation in water lines can be reduced substantially by removing the handpiece and

allowing water lines to run and discharge water for several minutes at the beginning of each clinic day. However, flushing of the water lines will not remove the biofilm in the lines. One should use sterile saline or sterile water rather than dental unit water as a coolant/irrigator when performing surgical procedures involving the cutting of bone.

American Dental Association

In 1995, the American Dental Association (ADA) board of trustees approved the following statement prepared by the ADA Council on Scientific Affairs:

The Council recommends an ambitious and aggressive course to encourage industry and the research community to improve the design of dental equipment so that by the year 2000, water delivered to patients during nonsurgical dental procedures consistently contains no more than 200 colony forming units per milliliter (CFU/mL) of aerobic mesophilic heterotrophic bacteria at any point in time in the unfiltered output of the dental unit; this is equivalent to an existing quality assurance standard for dialysate fluid that ensures that the fluid delivery systems in hemodialysis units have not been colonized by indigenous waterborne organisms. Manufacturers of dental equipment are encouraged to develop accessory components that can be retrofitted to dental units currently in use, whatever the water source (public or independent), to aid in achieving this goal. Further, the ADA should urge industry to ensure that all dental units manufactured and marketed in the USA in the future have the capability of being equipped with a separate water reservoir independent of the public water supply. In this way, dentists will not only have better control over the quality of the source water used in patient care, but also will be able to avoid interruptions in dental care when "boil-water" notices are issued by local health authorities. At the present time, commercially available options for improving dental unit water quality are limited and will involve some additional expense. They include the use of independent water reservoirs, chemical treatment regimens, daily draining and air purging regimens, and point of use filters.

The ADA reaffirmed this statement in 1999, and later indicated support of the 2003 CDC recommendations as described in Appendix G.

DENTAL UNIT WATER AND INFECTION CONTROL

Oral Surgical Procedures

The dental professional should follow CDC guidelines of not using dental unit water as an irrigant for oral surgery. The CDC defines oral surgical procedures as involving the "incision, excision, or reflection of tissue that exposes the normally sterile areas of the oral cavity. Examples include biopsy, periodontal surgery, apical surgery, implant surgery, and surgical extractions of teeth (e.g., removal of erupted or non-erupted tooth, requiring elevation of the mucoperiosteal flap, removal of bone and/or section of tooth, and suturing if needed)." Such surgeries may involve the use of sterile water delivery systems as mentioned in the next section or hand irrigation using sterile water in a sterile disposable syringe. Specialties, including oral surgery, endodontics, and periodontics, may have other recommendations concerning the use of irrigants.

Flushing of the Water Lines

One should flush water lines and handpieces between patients as recommended by the CDC (see the foregoing discussion). Although flushing will not remove biofilm from the lines (biofilm forms while water is moving through the lines), it may reduce the planktonic microbial count in the water temporarily and help clean the handpiece water lines of materials that may have entered from the patient's mouth. Flushing also brings into the dental unit a fresh supply of chlorinated water from the main water lines.

Minimizing Sprays and Spatter

The routine use of high-volume evacuation with the high-speed handpiece, ultrasonic scaler, and air/water syringe reduces exposure of the dental team to aerosol and spatter from the patient's oral fluids and from contamination with the water spray from handpieces, scalers, and syringes. This evacuation also may reduce exposure of the patient to these waterborne microorganisms.

Barriers for the Patient and Dental Team

The rubber dam serves as a protective barrier for the patient from dental unit water. The dam does not eliminate exposure totally but greatly reduces direct contact. The dam also greatly reduces the aerosolizing and spattering of patient microorganisms onto the dental team but does not reduce exposure of the dental team to dental unit water. However, protective barriers of eyewear, masks, and face shields do serve as barriers for the dental team against microorganisms coming from the patients' mouths and from the aerosols and sprays of dental unit water.

APPROACHES TO IMPROVE DENTAL UNIT WATER QUALITY

Developing approaches to improve the quality of water used for patient treatment is a rapidly advancing field, and additional breakthroughs could occur at any time. Box 14-2 gives basic considerations for designing approaches to improve dental water quality. Current approaches include independent water reservoirs, antimicrobial agents, filters, and sterile water delivery systems. In some instances, more than one of these approaches are combined. A listing of the specific products representing these approaches with links to the manufacturers can be found at the Organization for Safety, Asepsis and Prevention (OSAP) Web site (http://www.osap.org). Check with dental unit manufacturers for their recommendations to maintain the water quality in their units.

Independent Water Reservoirs

Although drinking water is not supposed to contain any more than 500 CFU/mL, contamination may be greater by the time the water passes through all of the distribution lines leading from the city water treatment facility to the dental office. Because accurately predicting the quality of municipal water when it enters dental units is not possible, one approach has been to disconnect from city water and supply another source of water. This process can involve installation of a water reservoir (e.g., a bottle) filled with good-quality water (e.g., distilled water) for patient treatment. This system also allows for the use of decontaminating or cleared antimicrobial agents (see below) for cleaning of the water lines. Some independent reservoir systems have dual bottles, one for treatment water and one for a cleaner. These independent water reservoirs (also known as self-contained water systems or clean water systems) provide a means for delivering treatment water and water-line cleaning agents.

Attacking the biofilm is important just before one starts using an independent reservoir system or any system designed to improve the quality of the incoming water. One also must periodically decontaminate the lines after installing the new water delivery systems, depending on

BOX 14-2

Considerations for Designing Improvements in Dental Water Quality

1. The quality of municipal water as it enters the dental unit cannot be guaranteed.
2. Biofilm will develop in any reusable water delivery system that is not maintained.
3. Any water that passes through lines containing biofilm will become heavily contaminated.
4. Development of approaches should include early testing in a dental unit to help ensure later success.
5. Several different approaches may be needed simultaneously.
6. Water or biofilm treatment chemicals must be compatible with the dental unit and be removed easily from the system by flushing or be nontoxic at the residual levels in the water lines.
7. Use of chemicals to treat water or biofilm must be consistent with the uses indicated by the manufacturer of the chemical.
8. Manufacturers of devices or antimicrobial chemicals for the control of microbes in dental unit water lines must be cleared by the Food and Drug Administration (device) or registered by the Environmental Protection Agency (chemical) before the products can be marketed for that use.
9. Products should not interfere with dental procedures or affect dental materials used for patient care.

the product/system used. One must remember that it is not enough to use good-quality incoming water. If one does not treat the biofilm in the water lines, even sterile water placed in the bottles will come out highly contaminated. Thus, the water lines need to be treated with an agent that will control the biofilm so as to maintain the quality of the water placed into the bottles as it passes through the lines. One also should not touch the pickup tube in the bottle with contaminated fingers when changing the bottle, and one needs to clean the bottles with soap and water every day.

Procedure 14-1 is an example of how one can use an independent water reservoir. Although this approach is labor intensive, it can yield high-quality water if one follows the steps faithfully.

Decontaminating and Antimicrobial Agents

Decontaminating and antimicrobial agents are available to use in independent water reservoirs to attack the biofilm. Some agents are placed in the bottles periodically (e.g., once a week) and flushed into the water lines, held there for various periods of time, and flushed out. Other chemical agents are added directly to the treatment water to provide

continuous antimicrobial activity in the lines. Other antimicrobial systems such as ultraviolet light, high heat, or antimicrobial chemicals (e.g., iodine, silver ions, and ozone) are used to treat municipal water before it enters the dental units. Chemical agents with antimicrobial claims are to be registered by the Environmental Protection Agency. Devices attached to the dental unit to deliver decontaminating agents should be cleared by the FDA as an accessory to a medical device.

Filters

Microbial filters are designed to remove free-floating microbes, and in one instance endotoxin, from the water. Placing a microbial filter in the water line just before the water enters the handpiece or air/water syringe can improve the quality of the treatment water greatly. Some of the concerns for this approach include knowing when to change the filter, positioning the filter in the line to avoid cross-contamination from any retraction of patient materials through the handpiece or air/water syringe, and the need to disinfect any part of the water line downstream from the filter. Even though filtering the output water does not address the biofilm problem, a filter at the end of the line may be an important safety measure to use along with other water quality improvement approaches. Some filters are used in combination with antimicrobial agents.

Sterile Water Delivery Systems

Oral surgical procedures (see the foregoing discussion) present an opportunity for microorganisms to enter the vascular systems and other normally sterile areas of the mouth, increasing the potential for a localized or systemic infection. Because dental units cannot reliably deliver sterile water, systems have been developed and cleared by the FDA that completely bypass the dental unit and deliver sterile solutions (e.g., water or saline) through sterile disposable or autoclavable lines to the patient. A sterile solution for irrigation also can be delivered through a hand syringe.

WATER QUALITY MONITORING

It is well known that untreated dental units produce water that is below the standard for drinking water. Thus, it is not necessary to actually test the water to see if it is contaminated. It will be! However, if equipment is being installed or products are being used to improve the microbial quality of water, baseline and periodic testing of the microbial levels in the exiting water may provide useful information as to whether the changes are working. Monitoring can detect not only how the system is functioning but also how the products/equipment are being used. The tests should determine total bacterial counts in the water after inoculation of diluted chlorine-neutralized water samples onto R2A agar plates and incubation of the plates at room temperature for

PROCEDURE 14-1

Using an Independent Water Reservoir

GOAL: To provide good-quality water for patient treatment in a previously unmodified dental unit

Materials Needed
Independent water reservoir
Detergent for bottle cleaning
Water-line cleaner/disinfectant
Material safety data sheet for chemicals used
Squirt bottle to rinse off pickup tube

1. Disconnect from municipal water and install an independent water reservoir (bottle) to deliver treatment water.
   Rationale: The quality of municipal water as it enters the dental unit is not known.

2. Place the appropriate amount of cleaner/disinfectant into the bottle, reconnect, and pressurize the bottle to flush through the cleaner/disinfectant. Leave all the lines full for the prescribed time (e.g., overnight). The next morning, remove the bottle, rinse off the pickup tube, connect a bottle filled with water, pressurize the bottle, and flush all the cleaner/disinfectant from the lines. Repeat this entire step 2 on three consecutive nights.
   Rationale: All unmodified dental units have biofilm in their water lines, and these procedures reduce the level of biofilm in the lines so that subsequent use of the self-contained reservoir system can maintain low levels of microbes in the water.

3. Fill a clean bottle with treatment water known to be of high microbial quality (e.g., distilled water), connect to the unit, and pressurize. Do not touch the pickup tube.
   Rationale: The water coming out of the unit cannot be any better than the water going into the unit. Contaminating the pickup tube will contaminate the treatment water.

4. After the last patient of the day, empty the bottle contents, place the bottle back on the unit, pressurize, and blow out the residual water in the lines.
   Rationale: Keeping the lines dry overnight aids in controlling the microbial levels.

5. At the beginning of the next day, place a clean bottle containing treatment water on the unit and pressurize.
   Rationale: If the bottles are not kept clean, they can host biofilm formation and contaminate the treatment water.

6. Once a week at the end of the day, remove the bottle and empty the contents. Repeat step 2 for one night only.
   Rationale: This process helps keep the biofilm to a minimum level and maintains the desired quality of the water.

(These steps may not apply to all independent water reservoir systems. Follow the manufacturer's directions.)

at least 1 week. One should keep water samples cold during transport if they are to be shipped to a laboratory for analysis. One should recognize that these counts may not always specifically reflect the degree of biofilm present in the lines, for this relationship has not been determined scientifically. Nevertheless, if one obtains high counts (above 500 CFU/mL), then the intended improvements are not working or are not being performed properly. If one obtains low counts, the improvements are working or the water analyzed did not reflect the true state of the system. Thus one may need multiple samples to confirm low counts. Commercial microbiology laboratories, hospital laboratories, some dental companies, and some dental schools can perform these water quality tests.

BOIL-WATER NOTICES

Water treatment facilities in our cities and towns are charged with providing safe drinking water to the public. Occasionally problems occur in the water treatment plant or with the water distribution system that brings the treated water to our homes and offices. One of the most common problems is a break in a water main that allows groundwater (contaminated with various microorganisms) to leak into the water distribution system and expose all sites downstream of the leak. Other problems are power failures or mechanical failures at the treatment plant that interrupt purification systems. When this occurs, the water company or health authorities issue a **boil-water notice** indicating that the water should not be consumed or should be boiled before use. Such water also should not be used for patient treatment of any type or for handwashing. This means that one must use syringe irrigation with nonmunicipal water when water is needed for treatment, or, if a dental unit has a self-contained water system and does not use municipal water, then no problem exists except with the office tap water. Otherwise, the dentist should see no patients until the water problem is solved. One can use alcohol hand rubs during a boil-water notice if the hands have no visible soil, or one can use an antimicrobial handwashing agent and bottled water if visible soil is present.

A dental office involved in a boil-water notice needs to contact the manufacturer of their dental units and determine exactly how to disinfect and flush the inside of the unit water lines after the "all clear" notice is given. If such directions are not available, a guideline is to flush the lines and faucets for 5 minutes.

BACKFLOW PREVENTION

In some locations, water regulators have required dental offices to install backflow prevention devices at the service connection or on individual dental operative units. These devices can be used to prevent back-siphonage of contaminated fluids into the public water supply. As indicated by the ADA, many of these requirements appear to be based on two assumptions. First, if a sudden drop in water pressure occurs, oral fluids may be aspirated from a patient's mouth into cross-connected water systems. Second, if aspiration does occur, it may result in a significant risk of transmission of bloodborne viruses from an infected patient to other patients or to persons who are using the same water system. Regulatory interventions requiring the installation of complex backflow prevention devices in certain dental offices are based on the conclusion that a high degree of hazard of contamination exists. Available science suggests, however, that there is an extremely low risk of such contamination of public water supplies from cross-connections in dental operative units. In the unlikely event that a sudden drop in water pressure caused backflow to occur, the volume of aspirated fluid would be minuscule. Also, information strongly suggests that the risk of transmission of a bloodborne disease through contaminated water supplies is very low.

DENTAL UNIT AIR

Very little is known about the microbial quality of dental unit air compared to dental unit water. However, this air contains much fewer microbes than the water, but it is not sterile. As shown in Figure 14-2, the handpiece air line appears clean compared to the biofilm present in the adjacent water line. The air taken into the compressor may contain some bacteria, and these bacteria may be able to multiply in the moisture that can accumulate in the bottom of the air tanks. As air is compressed moisture is "squeezed out" and settles to the bottom of the tank. Although air from the dental compressors is filtered, the filters may not be able to remove all the bacteria present.

SELECTED READINGS

American Dental Association: Council on Scientific Affairs: Dental unit waterlines: approaching the year 2000, *J Am Dent Assoc* 130:1653–1664, 1999.

Atlas RM, Williams JF, Huntington MK: *Legionella* contamination of dental-unit waters, *Appl Environ Microbiol* 61:1208–1213, 1995.

Centers for Disease Control and Prevention: *Backflow prevention and the dental operative unit.* http://www.cdc.gov/oralhealth/infectioncontrol/factsheets/backflow.htm. Accessed January 2012.

Challacombe SJ, Fernandes LL: Detecting *Legionella pneumophila* in water systems: a comparison of various dental units, *J Am Dent Assoc* 126:603–608, 1995.

Coan L, Hughes EA, Hudson JC, Palenik CJ: Sampling water from chemically treated dental units with detachable power scalers, *J Dent Hyg* 80:80, 2007.

Cochran MA, Miller CH, Sheldrake MA: The efficacy of the dental dam as a barrier to the spread of microorganisms during dental treatment, *J Am Dent Assoc* 119:141–144, 1989.

Fotos PG, Westfall HN, Snyder IS, et al: Prevalence of *Legionella*-specific IgG and IgM antibody in a dental clinic population, *J Dent Res* 64:1382–1385, 1985.

Kohn WG, Collins AS, Cleveland JL, et al: Centers for Disease Control and Prevention: Guidelines for infection control in dental health care settings–2003, *MMWR Recomm Rep* 52(RR-17):1–61, 2003.

Martin MV: The significance of the bacterial contamination of the dental unit water systems, *Br Dent J* 163:152–154, 1987.

Miller CH: Microorganisms in dental unit water, *Calif Dent Assoc J* 24:47–52, 1996.

Mills SE: The dental unit waterline controversy: defusing the myths, defining the solutions, *J Am Dent Assoc* 131:1427–1441, 2000.

O'Donnell MJ, Shore AC, Russell RJ, Coleman DC: Optimization of the long-term efficacy of dental chair waterline disinfection by the identification and rectification of factors associated with waterline disinfection failure, *J Dent* 35:438–451, 2007.

Palenik CJ, Burgess K, Miller CH: *Methods for microbial analysis of dental unit water.* Annual conference proceedings: Organization for Safety and Asepsis Procedures, Tucson, AZ, June 19–22, (abstract 0308), 2003.

Palenik CJ, Burgess KH, Miller CH: Effects of delayed microbial analysis of dental unit water line specimens, *Am J Dent* 18:87–90, 2005.

Pankhurst CL, Coulter WA: Do contaminated dental unit waterlines pose a risk of infection? *J Dent* 35:712–720, 2007.

Ricci ML, Fontana S, Pinci F, et al: Pneumonia associated with a dental unit waterline, *Lancet* 379:684, 2012.

Porteous NB, Redding SW, Thompson EH, et al: Isolation of an unusual fungus in treated dental unit waterlines, *J Am Dent Assoc* 134:853–858, 2003.

Reinthaler FF, Mascher F, Stunzer D: Serological examination for antibodies against *Legionella* species in dental personnel, *J Dent Res* 67:942–943, 1988.

Sajadi A, Noles DA, Galli D: *Prevalence of Helicobacter pylori in dental unit waterlines,* San Diego, 2011, IADR General Session (abstract 1369).

Tullner JB, Miller CH, Sheldrake MA, Gonzalez-Cabezas C: Accumulation of biofilm inside of dental unit waterlines, annual conference proceedings, Organization for Safety and Asepsis Procedures, Dallas, June 13–16, (abstract 9602), 1996.

Walker JT, Marsh PD: Microbial biofilm formation in DUWS and their control using disinfectants, *J Dent* 35:721–730, 2007.

REVIEW QUESTIONS

Multiple Choice

1. *Legionella* bacteria can cause what type of disease in susceptible persons?
   a. Damage to the liver
   b. Pneumonia
   c. Intestinal damage
   d. Skin disease

2. Besides *Legionella*, what other two bacteria that may be present in dental unit water are of the most concern in causing infections in compromised persons?
   a. *Streptococcus* and *Pseudomonas*
   b. *Fusobacterium* and *Micrococcus*
   c. *Micrococcus* and *Mycobacterium*
   d. *Pseudomonas* and *Mycobacterium*

3. What is the maximum acceptable level of bacteria in dental unit water as recommended by the Centers for Disease Control and Prevention?
   a. 200,000 CFU/mL
   b. 1000 CFU/mL
   c. 500 CFU/mL
   d. 200 CFU/mL

4. What role does dental unit water line biofilm play in the microbial contamination of dental unit water?
   a. Biofilm has no role.
   b. Biofilm traps all the bacteria in the incoming water and keeps the levels of bacteria in the outgoing water low.
   c. Biofilm sheds bacteria into the water, causing increased levels of bacteria in the outgoing water.

5. The level of microbes in water coming out of an unmodified dental unit is almost always:
   a. the same as drinking water
   b. higher than drinking water
   c. lower than drinking water

6. When does the Centers for Disease Control and Prevention recommend that dental unit water lines with the attached handpiece should be flushed?
   a. Between every patient
   b. Once a day
   c. Once a week
   d. Every 10 minutes during an appointment

7. What type of water should be used to irrigate during oral surgical procedures?
   a. Water that has passed through a dental unit
   b. Drinking water
   c. Distilled water
   d. Sterile water

8. All of the following are reasonable approaches to improve dental unit water quality except one. The exception is:
   a. replacing the water lines once a week
   b. using an independent water reservoir
   c. using antimicrobial chemicals in the water
   d. using filters to remove the microbes from the water

9. Potable water is the same as:
   a. dental unit water
   b. sterile water
   c. drinking water
   d. river water

10. Which of the following attacks dental unit water line biofilm?
    a. A filter inserted into the water line just before the handpiece
    b. Use of distilled water in an independent water reservoir
    c. Addition of an antimicrobial agent to the water

Please visit http://evolve.elsevier.com/Miller/infectioncontrol/ for additional practice and study support tools.

OUTLINE

Touching of As Few Surfaces As Possible

Minimization of Dental Aerosols and Spatter

High-volume Evacuation

Saliva Ejector

Use of The Rubber Dam

Preprocedure Mouth Rinse

Use of Disposables

Housekeeping and Cleaning

   Cleaning

   Flooring, Carpeting, and Upholstery

Other Aseptic Techniques

LEARNING OBJECTIVES

After completing this chapter, the student should be able to do the following:

1. Describe how to limit the spread of disease agents from the hands to environmental surfaces, and from dental aerosols and spatter.
2. Describe the importance of the high-volume evacuator in infection control and how to change a high-volume evacuator trap safely.

3. Describe the proper use of the saliva ejector and rubber dam.
4. Describe the use of preprocedure mouth rinses.
5. Describe the proper use of disposable items.
6. Describe proper housekeeping and cleaning considerations, as well as other aseptic techniques.

KEY TERMS

Aseptic Techniques

Dental Aerosols

Disposable Item

High-volume Evacuation (HVE)

Preprocedure Mouth Rinsing

Rubber Dam

Saliva Ejector

Single-use Device

Spatter

Some infection control techniques do not fall under the major infection control categories discussed in previous chapters. Collectively, they are referred to as aseptic techniques because they prevent or reduce the spread of microorganisms from one site to another, such as from patient to dental team, from patient to operatory surfaces, or from one operatory surface to another.

TOUCHING OF AS FEW SURFACES AS POSSIBLE

Gloves used for patient care are contaminated, and that contamination will be transferred to any surface touched. Thus, one should touch as few surfaces as possible with saliva- or blood-coated fingers. Any surfaces that may be touched should be protected with surface covers or pre-cleaned and disinfected (see Chapter 13). One should make every effort to dispense all items needed at chairside before patient care begins. This task reduces the need for leaving chairside with contaminated gloves, mask, and protective clothing, which may spread contamination to other parts of the office. As mentioned in Chapter 11, removal of contaminated gloves or use of an overglove before leaving chairside during patient care is the best practice. One should put on gloves or carefully remove and discard overgloves when returning to chairside. Another alternative is to have an uninvolved person retrieve items needed unexpectedly during patient care, which is particularly important during some types of surgery (e.g., implant surgery).

One should not rub the eyes, skin, or nose or touch hair with contaminated, gloved hands.

MINIMIZATION OF DENTAL AEROSOLS AND SPATTER

Dental aerosols and spatter are generated during use of high- and low-speed handpieces, ultrasonic scalers, and the air/water syringe. Dental aerosols are small, invisible particles of saliva that may contain a few microorganisms and may be inhaled or remain airborne for extended periods. Aerosol particles are less than 50 μm in diameter, and the smallest particles of 5 μm in diameter can be inhaled to the depths of the lungs (air sacs or alveoli). One should remember that the average diameter of a bacterial cell is only 1 μm, and viruses are much smaller than that. Spatter consists of particles larger than 50 μm. When these particles are propelled from the patient's mouth, they settle rapidly or land on nearby operatory surfaces or the face, neck, chest, and arms of the dental team member providing care to the patient. Minimizing the generation of dental aerosols and spatter by use of high-volume evacuation and the rubber dam and by proper positioning of the patient's head reduces the spread of microbes from the patient's mouth.

HIGH-VOLUME EVACUATION

High-volume evacuation (HVE) during use of rotary equipment and the air/water syringe greatly reduces the escape of salivary aerosols and spatter from the patient's mouth, which reduces contamination of the dental team and nearby surfaces. One should clean the HVE system at the end of the day by evacuating a detergent or water-based detergent-disinfectant through the system. One should not use bleach (sodium hypochlorite) because this chemical can destroy metal parts in the system. One should remove and clean the trap in the system periodically. A safer approach, however, is to use a disposable trap. These traps may contain scrap amalgam that should be disposed of properly. The dental team member must wear gloves, masks, protective eyewear, and protective clothing when cleaning or replacing these traps to avoid contact with patient materials in the lines from splashing and direct contact. Disinfection of the trap by evacuating some disinfectant-detergent down the line followed by water is best before one cleans or changes the trap.

SALIVA EJECTOR

Research has shown that in one in five cases, previously suctioned fluids might be retracted into the patient's mouth when a seal around the saliva ejector is created (i.e., when the patient closes his or her lips around the saliva ejector tip). The seal can cause a type of "suck back" or reverse flow in the vacuum line that might allow the contents of the line to reach the patient's mouth. Although disease spread, if this occurs, has not been demonstrated, reverse flow should

not be allowed to happen. Thus one should not tell patients to close their lips around the ejector and "spit" into the tip. Alternatively, some disposable saliva ejector tips now have a small hole in the side that relieves the pressure when the tip is closed off preventing reverse flow. Others have a closable valve that prevents backflow.

USE OF THE RUBBER DAM

Reduction in microorganisms escaping a patient's mouth in aerosols or spatter can approach 100% with proper use of the rubber dam, depending on the type and site of the intraoral procedure. Simultaneous use of HVE and the rubber dam provides the best approach to minimize dental aerosols and spatter. A sealant is also available for placement at the rubber dam–tooth interface to reduce further the leakage of saliva into the operative site.

Because the rubber dam reduces the amount of saliva present at the operative site, less saliva is available for retraction into water spray handpieces or air/water syringes if antiretraction valves in the dental unit fail.

Even though the rubber dam and HVE greatly reduce the salivary aerosols and spatter, one still must use gloves, mask, protective eyewear, and protective clothing when using these aseptic techniques. The rubber dam may not give a perfect seal, and microorganisms that may be present in biofilm on the inside of the dental unit water lines may be released into the flowing water and aerosolized and sprayed into the face, neck, chest, and arms of the care provider.

PREPROCEDURE MOUTH RINSE

The application of antiseptics to skin or mucous membranes before surgery or injections has been practiced for many years. The goal of such application is to reduce the number of microorganisms on the surface to prevent their entry to underlying tissues, which could cause bacteremia, septicemia, or local harmful infections.

The use of an antimicrobial mouth rinse by the patient before dental procedures is based on a similar principle of reducing the number of oral microorganisms. This reduction also lowers the number of microorganisms that may escape a patient's mouth during dental care through aerosols, spatter, or direct contact. Thus fewer microorganisms contaminate the dental team and operatory surfaces. Although studies have not yet shown that the aseptic technique of preprocedure mouth rinsing actually prevents diseases in dental team members, studies do show that a mouth rinse with a long-lasting antimicrobial agent (e.g., chlorhexidine gluconate, essential oils, and iodophor) can reduce the level of oral microorganisms for up to 5 hours. Use of non–antimicrobial mouth rinses allows the oral microorganisms to return to their original levels before most dental procedures are completed, thus having little infection control value.

Although a preprocedure mouth rinse can be used before any dental procedure, it may be most beneficial before a prophylaxis using a prophylaxis cup or ultrasonic scaler. During these procedures, one cannot use a rubber dam to minimize aerosol and spatter generation, and unless a hygienist has an assistant, HVE is not commonly used. The mouth rinsing may be the only approach to minimizing contamination from aerosols and spatter during such procedures.

USE OF DISPOSABLES

A disposable item is manufactured for a single use or for use on only one patient. Such items are manufactured from plastics or less-expensive metals that are usually not heat tolerant or are not designed to be cleaned adequately. Thus an item that is labeled as disposable must be disposed of properly after use, and one should not attempt to preclean and sterilize or disinfect it for reuse on another patient. A single-use device (SUD) is a device originally cleared by the Food and Drug Administration (FDA) for a single use on one patient. If one wishes to reprocess an SUD, the FDA now requires one to meet the same good manufacturing standards used by the original manufacturer. In other words, they will have to ensure that the reprocessed SUD is as safe and as effective as it was when originally manufactured. This includes:

- Submitting documents for premarket notification or approval
- Registering reprocessing firms and listing all products
- Submitting adverse event reports
- Tracking devices whose failure could have serious outcomes
- Correcting or removing from the market unsafe devices
- Meeting manufacturing and labeling requirements

From an infection control point of view, a single-use (disposable) item has major advantages over a reusable item. The disposable item absolutely prevents the transfer of microorganisms from one patient to another because the contaminated item is discarded and not reused on another patient. Another advantage is that the reusable counterpart may be difficult to clean and sterilize adequately (e.g., the lumen of a needle or the inside of the air/water syringe tip), thus increasing the risk of patient-to-patient cross-contamination. The disposable item eliminates this risk.

Disadvantages of disposables depend on the nature of the individual items, but may include less-efficient operation than the reusable counterpart, increased expense, and addition of nonbiodegradable materials to the environment on disposal. Determination of cost-effectiveness of disposables or reusables must include the cost of the items and also the labor dollars required to decontaminate the reusable items.

More and more disposable items are becoming available to dentistry and include injection needles, anesthetic carpules, air/water syringe tips, HVE tips, saliva ejector tips, curing light probes, certain hand instruments, prophylaxis angles, prophylaxis cups, high-speed handpieces, light handle attachments, impression trays, scalpel blades, and some burs. Other disposable items include patient care gloves, masks, gowns, some face shields, surface covers, patient bibs, sharps containers, biohazard bags, specimen containers, and vacuum line traps (Figures 15-1, 15-2, and 15-3).

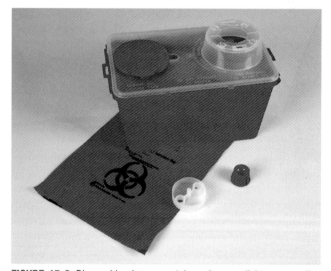

FIGURE 15-2 Disposable sharps container, dappen dish, vacuum line trap, and red bag for nonsharp waste.

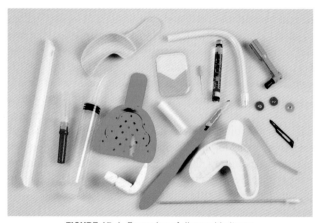

FIGURE 15-1 Examples of disposable items.

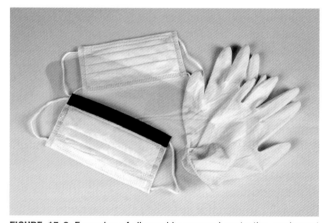

FIGURE 15-3 Examples of disposable personal protective equipment (mask, exam gloves, and combination mask-eye shield).

HOUSEKEEPING AND CLEANING

Cleaning

Dusting of surfaces or sweeping of floors in patient care areas can distribute microorganism-laden dust particles to other surfaces unless performed with a wet cloth or wet mop. One might consider dust covers for operatory and sterilizing room surfaces over the weekend or during vacation periods. One should clean mops and cloths after use and allow them to dry before reuse, or use single-use, disposable mop heads or cloths. Mop water should contain a low-level disinfectant to keep microorganisms from building up in the water and being painted onto the floor. One should prepare the mop water fresh at least daily. The filters in air vents and furnaces require frequent changing to avoid dust buildup.

See Chapter 20 for further information about general cleanliness of the entire office.

Flooring, Carpeting, and Upholstery

A smooth-surface floor rather than carpeting is more appropriate for patient care areas because of its cleanability and lesser likelihood of accumulating dust and dirt. Thus one should avoid using carpeting and cloth-upholstered furnishings in the dental operatory, laboratory, or instrument-processing areas.

OTHER ASEPTIC TECHNIQUES

During high-speed handpiece processing, one sprays a cleaner/lubricant into the drive air line and flushes excess lubricant out by connecting the dental unit air system on an air line installed in the sterilizing room. One must flush the air system so that the aerosol is not released into the air environment by flushing directly into the vacuum system or into a sink with water or a container with absorbent material that will catch the spray. Handpiece cleaning systems may become available that will minimize aerosolization.

Several aseptic techniques relate to instrument processing, as mentioned in Chapter 12. The sterilizing room should be separated into "clean" and "dirty" areas to avoid mingling of sterile and nonsterile instruments. Chemical indicators on instrument packaging also help differentiate between items that have or have not been heat processed. One should also handle and store sterile packages away from sinks in a dry area.

Unit dosing and use of a sterile retrieval system to prevent contamination of supply items were discussed in Chapter 13. A key point to remember is that gloves used for patient care are contaminated and that anything touched with those gloves will also be contaminated. Only items needed for the care of a single patient should be on the bracket table, portable unit, or countertops in the operatory. All other items should be stored elsewhere until dispensed for patient care to prevent their contamination.

SELECTED READINGS

Barbeau J, tenBokem L, Guathier C, Prevost AP: Cross-contamination potential of saliva ejectors used in dentistry, *J Hosp Infect* 40:303–311, 1998.

Cochran MA, Miller CH, Sheldrake MA: The efficacy of the dental dam as a barrier to the spread of microorganisms during dental treatment, *J Am Dent Assoc* 119:141–144, 1989.

Council on Dental Materials: Instruments and Equipment, American Dental Association: Dental units and water retraction, *J Am Dent Assoc* 116:417–420, 1988.

Food and Drug Administration: *Reprocessing of single use devices*, http://www.fda.gov/Medical Devices/DeviceRegulationandGuidance/ReprocessingofSingle-UseDevices/default.htm. Accessed January 2012.

Klyn SL, Cummings DE, Richardson BW, Davis RD: Reduction of bacteria-containing spray during ultrasonic scaling, *Gen Dent* 49:648–652, 2001.

Miller CH: Dealing with disposables, *Dent Prod Rpt* 39:58, 2006.

Miller CH: Swishful thinking: Can preprocedural mouthrinsing help prevent cross-contamination? *Dent Prod Rpt* 39:154, 2006.

Miller RL, Micik RE, Abel C, Ryge G: Studies on dental aerobiology. II. Microbial splatter discharged from the oral cavity of dental patients, *J Dent Res* 50:621–625, 1971.

Watson CM, Whitehouse RL: Possibility of cross-contamination between dental patients by means of the saliva ejector, *J Am Dent Assoc* 124:77–80, 1993.

REVIEW QUESTIONS

Multiple Choice

1. Particles of oral fluids that can be inhaled into the lung air sacs are called:
   a. spatter
   b. droplets
   c. aerosols

2. What is the key ingredient in a mouth rinse used for preprocedure mouth rinsing?
   a. Artificial sweetener
   b. Red coloring
   c. Antimicrobial agent
   d. Fluoride

3. A disposable air/water syringe tip can be used on how many patients?
   a. 1
   b. 2
   c. 3
   d. 4

4. Use of the rubber dam will not reduce spattering of what kinds of microbes?
   a. Plaque bacteria
   b. Salivary bacteria
   c. Dental unit water bacteria
   d. Periodontal bacteria

5. If a patient closes her lips around the _____ , patient-to-patient cross-contamination may occur.
   a. prophylactic angle
   b. high-volume evacuator tip
   c. air/water syringe tip
   d. saliva ejector tip

6. Which of the following may generate dental aerosols or spatter?
   a. High-speed handpiece
   b. Air/water syringe
   c. Ultrasonic scaler
   d. Prophylaxis angle
   e. All of the above
   f. Both a and c

7. What should be done before changing or cleaning a vacuum line trap?
   a. Heat sterilize the vacuum line.
   b. Flush concentrated bleach through the line.
   c. Evacuate a disinfectant-detergent into the line and flush with water.
   d. Do nothing.

Please visit http://evolve.elsevier.com/Miller/infectioncontrol/ for additional practice and study support tools.

Laboratory and Radiographic Asepsis

OUTLINE

LEARNING OBJECTIVES

After completing this chapter, the student should be able to do the following:

1. Describe how to properly disinfect microbially soiled prostheses and impressions.
2. Describe an acceptable laboratory receiving area.
3. List how to properly sterilize laboratory items used intraorally and correct disinfection procedures for laboratory items that are not used intraorally.
4. Design a system of proper environmental barriers and disinfection used during radiographic processes and the aseptic processing of radiographic films.

KEY TERMS

Daylight Loaders
Digital Radiographic Sensors

EPA-registered Disinfectant

FDA-cleared Barrier

LABORATORY ASEPSIS

Any instrument or piece of equipment used in the oral cavity or on orally soiled prosthetic devices or impressions is a potential source of cross-infection. It is impossible to identify all infectious patients from medical histories or patient conversations. Therefore, the only valid posture is to assume (and act as if) all patients are capable of transmitting highly infectious diseases. The dental team must use the same sets of criteria and techniques in all cases.

If contaminated items were to enter the laboratory environment, infectious materials could be spread to prostheses and appliances of other patients. Unsuspecting laboratory personnel also could be placed at increased risk for cross-infection.

Protective Barriers

All items coming from the oral cavity must be sterilized or disinfected before being worked on in the laboratory and before being returned to the patients. Asepsis procedures vary for each type of dental material. General recommendations for procedures and materials can be made. Laboratory infection control also involves, depending on need, the wearing of personal protective barriers such as gloves, safety eyewear, gowns, and masks. One must wear barriers when handling contaminated items until they have been decontaminated.

A successful laboratory infection control program requires meeting two major criteria: (1) the use of proper methods and materials for handling and decontaminating soiled items and (2) the establishment of a coordinated infection control program between dental offices and laboratories. This program will help dental practitioners and dental technologists create and maintain mutually effective infection control programs.

Receiving Areas

The dental team should create a receiving area to handle all items sent to the laboratory or handled in the laboratory areas within the dental practice. The area needs running water and handwashing facilities. To cover the area and the counter surfaces with impervious paper and to clean and disinfect the area regularly is the best practice. The amount of cleaning and disinfection depends on the rate of use of the area. No item (impression or prosthesis) should enter the receiving area until it has been disinfected properly.

One should use personal protective equipment when handling items received in the laboratory unit until they have been disinfected. Such equipment includes gloves and some type of gown. Protective eyewear may be needed to prevent contact with splashes.

Microbially Soiled Prostheses and Impressions

Any prosthesis coming from the oral cavity is a potential source of infection (see Chapters 6 and 7). Most prostheses and appliances cannot withstand standard heat sterilization procedures. An alternative technique for most prostheses is disinfection by immersion after a thorough cleaning. One should clean, disinfect, and rinse all dental prostheses and prosthodontic materials (e.g., impressions, bite registrations, and occlusal rims) using an Environmental Protection Agency-registered disinfectant (EPA-registered disinfectant) having at least an intermediate level of activity (tuberculocidal claim) before handling the items in the laboratory. One should consult with manufacturers regarding the stability of specific materials (e.g., impression materials) relative to disinfection procedures.

One also must wear gloves and protective outerwear when handling orally soiled prostheses until they have been disinfected properly. One also must wear masks and protective eyewear when handling hazardous chemicals such as disinfectants. Therefore one must always use personal protective barriers and adequate ventilation. Eye/face protection is mandatory whenever one uses rotary or air blasting cleaning equipment.

Some heavily soiled (e.g., with calculus or adhesive) prostheses require cleaning or scrubbing before disinfection. The most efficient (and safest) procedure is to place the prostheses into zippered plastic bags containing ultrasonic detergent and then to place the assembly into an ultrasonic cleaner (Figure 16-1). One also can use glass or plastic beakers or containers. Suspend the bags by pinning them in place at the lid of the ultrasonic cleaner. The goal is to position the

bag near the middle of the cleaning solution. Poorer cleaning occurs near the top and bottom of the solution pool. If further hand scrubbing or cleaning is required, keep personal barriers in place. Use air-powered blasters, such as shell blasters, only on cleaned and disinfected prostheses.

The team members must follow the same procedures when they receive prostheses from the dental laboratory. Prostheses that have been disinfected properly (treated and rinsed) can be returned to the patient office in a deodorizing solution such as a mouth rinse. Because of the increased risk for adverse tissue response (to the patient and the office staff), prostheses should never be sent out or returned in disinfectant solutions.

One should rinse impressions with tap water after removal and then shake them to remove residual water. Studies indicate that rinsing thoroughly serves an important function in the preliminary removal of adhering microorganisms. One then places rinsed impressions into glass beakers or zippered plastic bags containing an appropriate disinfectant (Figure 16-2). Limiting exposure to any disinfectant solution is best. One must keep all chemicals in well-sealed containers and avoid any contact, especially with skin and mucous membranes (see Chapter 13 for acceptable products). After 15 minutes, one removes the impressions, rinses them well with tap water, and gently shakes them. The impressions are now ready for pouring.

Some types of impressions are sensitive to immersion. Careful selection of disinfectant is required. As an alternative, one can spray these impressions thoroughly and wrap them with paper towels moistened well with the same disinfectant solution. The fibers from paper towels may stick to some impression materials. Check with the manufacturer. After 15 minutes, one removes the impressions, rinses them well, and shakes them gently, and they are ready to be poured.

Spraying has several advantages. Spraying is the treatment of choice for some types of dental materials, for it uses less solution and often one can use the same disinfectant for general disinfection of environmental surfaces. Spraying is probably not as effective as immersion, however, because

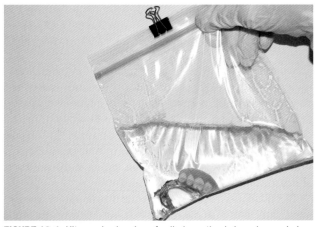

FIGURE 16-1 Ultrasonic cleaning of soiled prosthesis in a zippered plastic bag containing a detergent.

one cannot ensure constant contact of disinfectant with all surfaces of the impression. When given a choice, one always should select immersion. Spraying also releases disinfectant into the air, thus increasing the chances of personnel exposure. Most disinfectants can be used for spraying.

Disinfection of impression materials is an area of continuing research. Disinfection in certain types of chemical solutions harms some impression types. Other types of disinfectants, however, are safe for use on the same impression materials. Variation in response within a type of impression material (e.g., alginate) by manufacturing source has been noted. A small amount of in-house experimentation is highly recommended.

One should clean and heat sterilize heat-tolerant items used orally, including items such as metal impression trays and face-bow forks.

Grinding, Polishing, and Blasting

As stated before, perform laboratory work on previously disinfected impressions, appliances, and prostheses. Bringing untreated materials into the laboratory establishes the potential for cross-contamination.

Operation of a dental lathe provides an opportunity for the spread of infection and for injury. The rotary action of the wheels, stones, and bands generates aerosols, spatter, and projectiles. Whenever one is using the lathe, one should wear protective eyewear, properly place the front Plexiglas shield, and ensure that the ventilation system is operating properly. The use of a mask is highly recommended. The air-suction motor should be capable of producing an air velocity of at least 200 ft/min. Maximum containment of aerosols and spatter can be achieved when a metal enclosure with hand holes is fixed to the front of the hood of the lathe. One can sterilize or disinfect all attachments, such as stones, rag wheels, and bands, between uses or throw them away. The lathe unit must be disinfected twice a day.

One should use fresh pumice and pan liners for each case (Figure 16-3). The modest cost of the materials and the proven significant microbial contamination in reused pumice prohibits repeated use.

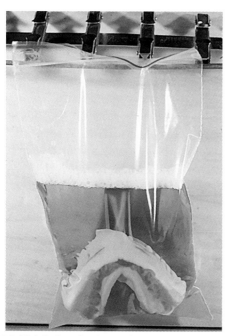

FIGURE 16-2 Disinfection of an impression within a zippered plastic bag.

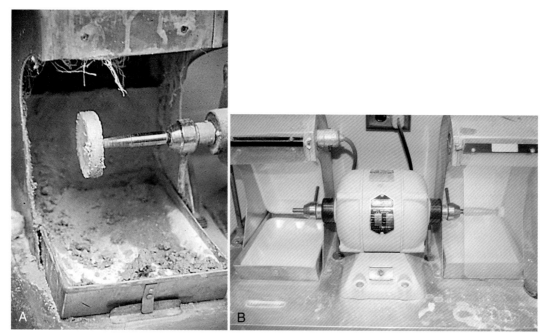

FIGURE 16-3 A, Improperly maintained lathe, pumice reused. **B,** Clean lathe setup, removable pan, single use of pumice.

Polishing of appliances and prostheses before delivery is a necessary activity. Polishing exposes the operator to potential cross-contamination and physical injury. However, if the item being polished has been prepared aseptically, the risks of infection are reduced to a minimum. To avoid the potential spread of microorganisms, one should obtain all polishing agents (e.g., rouge) in small quantities from larger reservoirs. One should never return unused material to the central stock but should throw it away. Most polishing attachments (e.g., brushes, wheels, and cups) are single-use, disposable items. One should sterilize reusable items between uses, if possible, or at least disinfect the items.

One should follow the manufacturer's instructions for cleaning and sterilizing or disinfecting items that become contaminated but that normally do not contact the patient (e.g., burs, stones, polishing points, rag wheels, articulators, case pans, and lathes). If manufacturer instructions are not available, one should clean and heat sterilize heat-tolerant items or clean and disinfect, depending on the degree of contamination.

Intermediate Cases

Complete and partial dentures often undergo an intermediate wax try-in stage. Crowns, splinted bridges, and partial denture frameworks often are "test seated" before cementation or soldering. These devices, like wax try-in step dentures, can become soiled with oral fluids. Before returning the items to the laboratory for further processing, one must disinfect them. The procedures in most cases are the same as those described for completed projects. Practices should include specific information regarding the disinfection technique used (e.g., solutions used and length of disinfection) when laboratory cases are sent off-site and on their return.

Return of Completed Cases

Appliances and prostheses being returned to the patient are not free of microbial contamination. These organisms could come from other cases and from the operator's body, if aseptic procedures are not followed rigorously. Many patients have open oral lesions or are traumatized sufficiently during treatment so as to facilitate easier microbial penetration. A growing number of patients also have impaired immune defense systems or are on chemotherapy programs that render them more susceptible to infectious diseases. The best location for disinfection procedures is chairside.

Other Thoughts

All laboratory infection control activities are designed to accomplish a single goal: breaking the chain of disease transmission. If the person-to-person flow of infection can be interrupted, the safety of the work environment is improved. The chances of patient acquisition of disease during treatment also are greatly reduced.

Infection control processes can be effective only when performed well consistently. For dental laboratory asepsis to be successful, offices and laboratories must perform essential tasks. Redundancies in the system should be identified and minimized. An overall increase in efficiency could be realized when offices and laboratories formally and properly coordinate their efforts.

RADIOGRAPHIC ASEPSIS

Proper infection control methods and materials for dental radiology differ little from those used for procedures more likely to result in blood exposure, such as periodontal therapy, surgical procedures, and many restorative treatments.

Consistent use of the most effective and efficient types of personal protective equipment—such as gloves, masks, gowns, and eyeglasses—decreases the chances of exposure to infectious agents. The team also must use appropriate environmental covers and perform cleaning and disinfection. For dental radiology, only a limited number of items require sterilization. In fact, the team should use heat-tolerant or disposable intraoral devices whenever possible (e.g., film-holding and positioning devices) and should clean and heat sterilize heat-tolerant devices between patients.

The dental team must use the correct materials along with a well-written office infection control procedures manual and regularly scheduled training sessions. A consistently appropriate level of personal and environmental protection must be extended.

The radiographic process also involves the handling of hazardous materials (see Chapter 26). It is imperative that all personnel involved with the development of radiographs be aware of the chemical hazards inherent to the process. Proper hazardous materials management is based on continuous employee training and active participation to minimize the chances of exposure and possible injury. Employees must know which chemical components are hazardous, the location of the hazardous materials list in the office, the labeling system used to identify and describe hazardous chemicals, the warning signs present, and the location and proper use of material safety data sheets.

Unit, Film, and Patient Preparation

The radiographic process offers the possibility that body fluids will contaminate disposable and reusable items. One must wear gloves of some type when taking radiographs and when handling orally soiled radiographic films. Because taking radiographs is a clinical activity, one also must consider the protective gowns and masks worn for restorative procedures. Protective eyewear is a barrier against contact with patient fluids but also prevents exposure to hazardous chemicals.

Plan ahead. Acquire all necessary disposables and heat sterilize materials and accessories. Many of the items used to take radiographs are used once and thrown away. Few reusable items touch unintact skin or mucous membranes or enter normally sterile body tissues. These items, however, still require sterilization. After cleaning, one sterilizes such materials by heat and reuses them. Because most of these reusable items can withstand sterilization temperatures, to process them in a steam autoclave or an unsaturated chemical vapor sterilizer is best. Heat-sensitive materials (e.g., some types of plastic) can be treated by immersion in a high-level disinfectant according to the manufacturer's instructions (see Chapters 12 and 13).

Environmental infection control requires surface cleaning and disinfection and the use of covers. In private practice, disinfection is preferred because such an item would be impossible to properly disinfect. However, the placement of plastic drapes, bags, or tubing over the x-ray unit (tube head, arm, and cone), chair head rest, and control panel probably is better than disinfection because of the numerous and large surfaces touched during the process (Figure 16-4).

Taking of Radiographs

Use films held within FDA-cleared barrier pouches (Figure 16-5).

Exposed films have to be oriented so as to differentiate them easily from unused films. A possible solution is to place exposed films into a disposable plastic cup or onto a labeled paper towel. This procedure helps to minimize contamination and also facilitates transport.

Environmental surfaces can be protected from contamination (see Figure 16-4) by use of covers, disinfection, or a combination of these. One must disinfect contaminated surfaces that are not covered. See Chapters 12 and 13 for proper disinfection agents, personal protective barriers, and procedures. Items such as control panel knobs and buttons, because of their shape and design, are best covered. Spraying of disinfectant into such areas may cause electric shortages. Because of time constraints, many offices elect to cover the majority of the involved surfaces, such as x-ray cones, rather than disinfect them.

Digital Radiographic Sensors

Digital radiographic sensors and associated computer hardware can be used in place of x-ray films. The digital system allows the image to be displayed on a computer monitor at chairside. The image can then be manipulated and stored for future retrieval. Unlike x-ray films, digital sensors are used repeatedly on multiple patients. Most, if not all, of these digital sensors cannot be heat sterilized or chemically disinfected. In these cases, the only alternative is to prevent the sensor from becoming contaminated. This is accomplished by using a disposable plastic surface cover over the sensor and part of the attached wire (unless the sensor is wireless) (Figure 16-6). When available, FDA-cleared barriers should always be used as covers. Consult with the sensor manufacturer for proper covering or decontamination of the particular type of sensor and computer hardware being used.

Darkroom Activities

One should transport exposed films to the darkroom in a plastic cup or within a folded paper towel but never in the pocket of a clinic gown or jacket. One should avoid touching any surfaces, such as doors, tabletops, or film processing equipment, with soiled gloves during transport.

One should open the films onto a new paper towel or sheet using disposable gloves and should drop the films out of the packets without touching them. One should accumulate the contaminated packets in a disposable towel or in a cup and, after opening all packets, should discard the packets and remove the gloves.

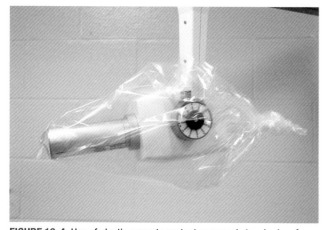

FIGURE 16-4 Use of plastic cover to protect commonly touched surfaces from contamination.

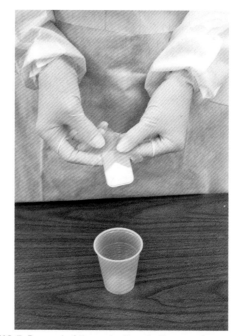

FIGURE16-5 Removal of the protective plastic cover from an exposed film packet.

One then washes one's hands and develops the films manually or uses an automatic processor. To prevent artifacts, one should avoid contact between gloves and uncovered film. One should note that developer and fixer, even when microbially contaminated, do not sustain bacterial or fungal growth.

For several years, x-ray films have been sold covered with protective plastic pouches. The pouches also can be purchased separately and placed onto x-ray films chairside (see Figure 16-5). Use of radiographic films in pouches has distinct infection control advantages. If one opens the pouches carefully in the operatory or the darkroom, one finds exposed but unsoiled film packets. Testing indicates that when properly placed, the covers do not allow penetration of fluids.

Daylight Loaders

Potential problems can arise with the use of **daylight loaders** attached to automatic processors (Figure 16-7) or with "portable darkrooms," which contain small beakers or cups of developing solutions. These units are equipped with portals that allow penetration of hands and arms with a maximum exclusion of light. This feat is accomplished using cloth or rubber sleeves, cuffs, or flaps. Because the units have limited operational space, chances of cross-infection are increased. The sleeves are difficult to impossible to disinfect properly after soiling.

The only aseptic way to use these units is to insert only disinfected or unsoiled film packets (those formerly in pouches) into the unit and to use powder-free gloves. One can group film packets into plastic cups and place them inside the daylight loader. One then can place unwrapped films into another clean cup or onto a paper towel. After one has opened all films, one can collect the waste packet wraps in a cup. Using a bare hand, one can pick up the films by the edges and feed them into the processor. Manual processing requires gloved hands and clips to dunk the films.

Waste Management

Orally soiled disposable items, such as gloves, paper towels, or x-ray film covers, are, in most locations, not considered to be infectious (and thus regulated) medical waste (see Chapter 17). This means that such items do not require special handling, storage, and neutralization procedures before disposal. However, every dental office and clinic has the responsibility to be aware of the current regulations for their location.

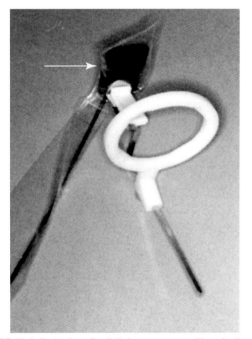

FIGURE 16-6 Protection of a digital x-ray sensor with a plastic cover.

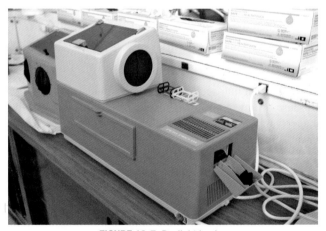

FIGURE 16-7 Daylight loader.

SELECTED READINGS

American Dental Association: Council on Scientific Affairs and Council on Dental Practice: Infection control recommendations for the dental office and the dental laboratory, *J Am Dent Assoc* 127:672–680, 1996.

Harte JA, Molinari JA: Infection control in dental radiology. In Molinari JA, Harte JA, editors: *Cottone's Practical Infection Control in Dentistry*, ed 3, Baltimore, 2010, Williams & Wilkins, pp 237–245.

Kohn WG, Collins AS, Cleveland JL, et al: Centers for Disease Control and Prevention: Guidelines for infection control in dental health-care settings–2003, *MMWR Recomm Rep* 52(RR-17):1–61, 2003.

Merchant VA: Infection control in the dental laboratory: concerns for the dentist, *Compendium* 14:382–390, 1993.

Merchant VA: Infection control in the dental laboratory. In Molinari JA, Harte JA, editors: *Cottone's Practical Infection Control in Dentistry*, ed 3, Baltimore, 2010, Williams & Wilkins, pp 246–260.

Miller CH, Palenik CJ: Sterilization, disinfection and asepsis in dentistry. In Block SS, editor: *Disinfection, sterilization and preservation*, ed 5, Philadelphia, 2001, Lea & Febiger, pp 1049–1068.

National Association of Dental Laboratories: *Health and Safety Committee: Infection control compliance manual for dental laboratories*, Alexandria, Va, 1992, National Association of Dental Laboratories.

Organization for Safety and Asepsis Procedures: OSAP position paper: laboratory asepsis, from http://www.osap.org/displaycommon.cfm?an=1&subarticlenbr=38, accessed May 2008.

Palenik CJ: Dental laboratory asepsis, *Dent Today* 24(52):54, 2005.

Palenik CJ, Miller CH: Infection control for dental radiology, *Dent Asepsis Rev* 17:1–2, 1996.

Puttaiah R, Langlais RP, Katz JO, Langland OE: Infection control in dental radiology, *J Calif Dent Assoc* 23:21–28, 1995.

White SC, Pharoah MJ: *Oral radiology: principles and interpretations*, ed 5, St Louis, 2004, Mosby.

REVIEW QUESTIONS

Multiple Choice

1. When given the choice, one should disinfect impressions by:
   a. immersion
   b. spraying

2. Air-suction motors on dental lathes should be capable of producing an air velocity of at least _____ ft/min.
   a. 15
   b. 80
   c. 135
   d. 200
   e. 650

3. If a denture is being sent to a dental laboratory for repairs, it should be disinfected:
   a. before being sent out
   b. after being received back
   c. before being sent out and after being received back

4. Today, dental radiographic films should be covered with protective plastic pouches before being used.
   a. True
   b. False

5. Disinfection of dental impressions should last _____ minutes.
   a. 5
   b. 15
   c. 30
   d. 60
   e. 180

Please visit http://evolve.elsevier.com/Miller/infectioncontrol/ for additional practice and study support tools.

Waste Management

OUTLINE

LEARNING OBJECTIVES

After completing this chapter, the student should be able to do the following:
1. Identify the federal agencies that regulate dental waste and design an acceptable action plan for the management of regulated dental waste.

2. Describe and differentiate the two basic types of waste generated in a dental office.
3. List the five types of regulated dental waste and discuss the proper handling of blood and pathogenic waste.
4. Describe the proper use of sharps containers

KEY TERMS

Hospital Waste
Infectious Waste
Medical Waste

Nonregulated Medical Waste
Pathology Waste
Regulated Medical Waste

Sharps
Sharps Containers

COMPREHENSIVE WASTE MANAGEMENT PLAN

Dental practices are subject to a variety of federal, state, and local regulations concerning infection control, hazardous materials handling, employee safety, and waste management issues. To be in compliance, all parties must make special efforts to be aware of an ever-increasing number of governmental mandates.

Because office and clinic personnel must have a working understanding of what actually is required, didactic and in-service training is needed. To meet a perceived need, many organizations and proprietary corporations now offer several consulting services, formal training sessions, and audiovisual materials. Because of the competitive nature of such businesses, the scope and value of some programs tend to be inflated. The question arises, "What kinds of programs do we really need and how can we choose the best ones for us?"

All employees must be knowledgeable of Occupational Safety and Health Administration (OSHA) regulations concerning bloodborne pathogens (see Chapter 6), hazardous materials (see Chapter 26), and safe use of chemicals in the laboratory (see Chapter 26). The Environmental Protection Agency (EPA) has standards, many of which are applicable to dentistry, for workplace exposure levels to chemicals, heat, and radiation and for discharge and final treatment of waste materials. Employees also must be aware of their state (and possibly local) requirements concerning sterilization, disinfection, and medical waste management. The Centers for Disease Control and Prevention (CDC) and the American Dental Association (ADA) guidelines/recommendations contain important and valuable information (see related topics in Chapters 8, 23, and 24).

Most offices elect to use external sources (including this book) to become more knowledgeable about the involved rules and regulations. After one understands the rules, the process of compliance is far less imposing. OSHA and the ADA indicate that personnel who are knowledgeable about the general rules and the specific discipline(s) of the audience must provide the training. OSHA also requires that training include opportunities for questions. Even though many audiovisual kits contain elements of programmed learning and sets of review questions, such training aids do not involve the presence of a knowledgeable, "live" facilitator.

A bare minimum for personnel training should be attendance at some type of annual program. Unless all required topics are covered, participation in several (more narrowcast) conferences is required. Currently, the trend in many states is to reinstate or increase the number of continuing education hours required to obtain or renew a dental license. Apparently, some of the required continuing education time should be devoted to infection control and employee safety issues.

The 2003 CDC guidelines for infection control make two recommendations for general medical waste. First, a medical waste management program for the practice needs to be developed. This written program must follow federal, state, and local regulations. Second, dental practices also need to ensure that all personnel who handle and dispose of potentially infective waste are trained in appropriate methods and that they are informed of the possible safety and health hazards. More specific CDC guidelines related to dental waste are discussed in this chapter.

TYPES OF WASTE

Two basic types of waste in dental offices are regulated medical waste and nonregulated medical waste. Many persons mistakenly consider the terms hospital waste, medical waste, and infectious waste as synonymous. Hospital waste, like dental office waste or household waste, refers to the total discarded solid waste generated by all sources within a given location, according to the EPA (Table 17-1). In a hospital, this waste includes biological waste materials such as medical, food services, or animal facility waste, in addition to nonbiological refuse such as clerical paper

and plastic items. Medical waste includes materials generated during patient diagnosis, treatment, or immunization in medical, dental, or other health care facilities. Infectious waste is a small subset (estimated at 3% of the total) of medical waste that has shown a capability of transmitting an infectious disease. This type of waste is also called regulated medical waste—waste that requires special care. One should note that factors such as the number and virulence of the microorganisms present, host resistance, and the presence and availability of portals of entry have important roles in whether an infection occurs (see Chapter 3).

INFECTIOUS WASTE MANAGEMENT

Over the last 20 years, differences among federal agencies concerning the definition of infectious medical waste have narrowed. These definitions may be superseded (additional soiled items included) by some states and local jurisdictions. However, no state or local agency can mandate a regulation that does not first encompass all federal rules.

The prevailing view is that no epidemiological evidence suggests that most medical waste is any more infective than residential waste. Also, no epidemiological evidence indicates that current medical/dental waste handling and disposal procedures have caused disease in the community. Therefore identifying wastes for which special precautions are necessary is largely a matter of judgment concerning the relative risk of disease transmission.

What now is commonly agreed upon is that only a limited amount of medical waste needs to be regulated (requiring special handling, storage, and disposal methods). Regulated waste as defined by OSHA and some dentistry-related examples are given in Table 17-2. The key factor in defining regulated medical waste rests upon the presence of blood or other potentially infectious material (OPIM). In dentistry, OPIM is mainly saliva. Most of the regulated waste in dental offices consists of contaminated sharps and extracted teeth. Some

TABLE 17-1   Definitions of Waste

Term	Definition
Contaminated waste	Items that have had contact with blood or other body secretions
Hazardous waste	Waste posing a risk or peril to human beings or the environment
Infectious waste	Waste capable of causing an infectious disease
Medical waste	Any solid waste* that is generated in the diagnosis, treatment, or immunization of human beings or animals in research pertaining thereto, or the production or testing of biologicals (the term does not include hazardous waste or household waste; only a small percentage of medical waste is infectious and needs to be regulated)
Regulated medical waste	Infectious medical waste that requires special handling, neutralization, and disposal
Toxic waste	Waste capable of having a poisonous effect

Adapted from Environmental Protection Agency: Standard for the tracking and management of medical waste (40 CFR parts 22 and 259), *Fed Regist* 54:326-395, 1989.
*Solid waste includes discarded solid, liquid, semiliquid, or contained gaseous materials.

offices involved with surgeries may also generate a small amount of nonsharp solid medical waste such as 2 × 2s or cotton rolls saturated/caked with blood or saliva.

BLOOD IN A LIQUID OR SEMILIQUID FORM

All federal agencies consider free-flowing/bulk blood to be infectious medical waste that needs to be regulated. In an overwhelming number of areas, blood (even mixed with other fluids, such as saliva) can be poured or evacuated into the office/clinic waste water system. One should rinse sink traps and evacuation lines thoroughly at least daily. Also helpful is the drawing of a nonbleach disinfectant solution through the lines and final rinsing with water.

Although generally allowed, several locales are attempting to restrict the volume of blood entering their sanitary sewers. These areas have had traditional waste disposal problems of all types, especially with the EPA water quality requirements. Personnel always should be aware of the regulations in their area and become actively involved in attempts to change the current situation.

The 2003 CDC infection control guideline has a recommendation for discharging blood or other body fluids to sanitary sewers or septic tanks. The CDC indicates that one should pour blood, suctioned fluids, or other liquid waste carefully into a drain connected to a sanitary sewer system, provided that local sewage discharge requirements are met and that the state has declared that this is to be an acceptable method of disposal. One must beware of splashing and wear gloves, mask, safety eyewear, and protective clothing while performing this task.

PATHOGENIC WASTE (TEETH AND OTHER TISSUES)

Teeth and other waste tissues are considered potentially infectious pathology waste, and thus their disposal is regulated. One always should use a color-coded and labeled container that prevents leakage (e.g., biohazard bag) to contain nonsharp regulated medical waste. Extracted teeth can be placed in sharps containers.

Many areas allow in-house neutralization of such items. The easiest and most effective procedure is sterilization by heat. Steam autoclaving is the method of choice. However, published information indicates that an unsaturated chemical vapor sterilizer is effective in neutralizing pathological waste. Because the operation parameters (time, pressure, and temperature) of the unsaturated chemical vapor sterilizer are similar to those of the steam autoclave, it seems logical that such a sterilizer also would be capable of pathological waste sterilization. One should never use dry heat ovens for this purpose.

The dental team must monitor the operation of the sterilizer routinely (see Chapter 12). Monitoring includes mechanical (physical) examination, chemical indicators, and biological (spore test) monitors.

Offices and clinics should be discreet about the final disposal of treated infectious medical waste. Reports indicate that waste haulers have refused to empty dumpster boxes or garbage cans if blood and blood soiled items were visible. The best option probably is to place treated items into some type of sealed container, such as a cardboard box, before disposal.

One common problem involves the treatment of teeth containing amalgam restorations. The heat of sterilization could create dangerous mercury vapors. Amalgam-restored teeth can be disinfected before disposal. Ideally, one should use a sterilizing chemical (e.g., full-strength glutaraldehyde). A tooth could be added to a small volume of fresh glutaraldehyde held within a sealed container. Exposure should be for at least 30 minutes. One should then rinse treated teeth well.

One stimulus for the return of teeth involves younger children and the "tooth fairy." Jurisdictions vary on the validity of such requests and on the procedures to follow to satisfy such an inquiry. However, the 2003 CDC guideline allows extracted teeth to be returned to the patient.

One must dispose of treated teeth and other tissues according to local regulations. Many areas allow these

TABLE 17-2   Regulated Waste According to OSHA

Waste*	Examples in Dentistry
Liquid or semiliquid blood or other potentially infectious material (OPIM)	Liquid blood or saliva
Contaminated items that would release blood or OPIM in a liquid or semiliquid state if compressed	2 × 2s or cotton rolls saturated with blood or saliva
Items that are caked with dried blood or OPIM that are capable of releasing these materials during handling	2 × 2s or cotton rolls saturated/caked with blood or saliva
Contaminated sharps	Used needles, scalpel blades, orthodontic wire, broken sharp instruments, burs
Pathological or microbiological wastes containing blood or OPIM	Biopsy specimens, excised tissue, extracted teeth not returned to the patient

*OSHA. *Blood-borne pathogens standard*, http://www.osha.gov/pls/oshaweb/owadisp.show_document?p_table=STANDARDS&p_id=10051, accessed April 2012.

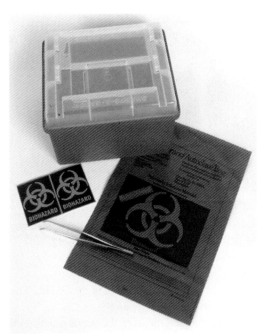

FIGURE 17-1 Examples of a sharps container and a red bag for non-sharp waste, biohazard symbols, and cotton pliers for safely picking up dropped sharps.

treated items to be added to the nonregulated waste stream. Pathological waste is best hidden from the view of the public. Final disposal should be in a secured receptacle.

Treated regulated medical waste is waste treated (usually by the application of heat or by incineration) to reduce or eliminate its pathogenicity substantially. This does not necessarily mean that the waste is destroyed or the volume is reduced significantly. For example, autoclaving does not appreciably affect the volume of treated waste materials.

SHARPS

Another form of regulated medical waste known to be capable of transmitting disease is contaminated **sharps**. Sharps are items that can penetrate intact skin or other tissues, and Chapter 18 describes how to prevent sharps injuries. All federal agencies consider contaminated sharps to be infectious waste. Don't throw loose sharps into the trash, flush sharps down the toilet, or put sharps in a recycling bin (they are not recyclable). The OSHA bloodborne pathogens standard indicates that immediately after use, disposable sharps are to be placed in closable, leakproof, puncture-resistant containers (**sharps containers**; Figure 17-1). These containers must be labeled with a biohazard symbol and color coded for easy identification. The CDC recommends that sharps containers be located as close as is practical to the work area. This means that each operatory should have at least one sharps container. Take the following precautions when using sharps containers:

- Use FDA-cleared containers.
- Pay attention to cautionary statements on sharps containers.

BOX 17-1

Recommended Procedures for In-house Sterilization of Sharps Containers in Moist Heat Sterilizers

1. Use only containers specified and labeled by their manufacturers for the collection of sharps (which must be autoclavable).
2. Regularly biologically spore test the sterilizer (steam or unsaturated chemical vapor) used.
3. Consider the following procedural recommendations:
   a. Fill containers no more than three quarters full.
   b. Leave container vents open.
   c. Place containers in an upright position within the sterilizer chamber (containers placed on their sides are sterilized more readily, but this increases the chances of needlestick accidents).
   d. Process the containers for 40 to 60 minutes (usually two cycles unless a longer single cycle can be used) to cover differences in container size, type and fill level, and model and operational status of the sterilizer used.
   e. Remove containers after processing and allow them to cool and then carefully close the vents.
   f. Label and dispose of containers according to local governmental regulations.

- Use containers with larger bottoms to avoid tipping them over.
- Don't exceed the recommended fill line.
- Avoid forcing sharps into containers.
- Drop syringes horizontally into containers.
- Use the containers for nothing other than sharps.
- Before handling filled containers, check carefully for protruding sharps.
- Close containers before moving them.
- Replace containers as soon as they're filled.

Education regarding needle safety and sharps containers should be available for all workers who are at risk for needlestick injury (see Chapter 18).

Because waste haulers charge a premium for the removal of medical waste, where legally permissible, dental offices should consider treating their sharps containers in-house if allowed by state regulations. Box 17-1 provides specific recommendations for in-house treatment of sharps containers. Figure 17-2 demonstrates placement of a sharps container and a red bag for nonsharp waste into a steam autoclave. Be sure the tops are open during sterilization so that the steam can enter the containers. The size and shape of the containers also can influence overall efficiency of sterilization. Be sure the container is labeled as "sterilizable" so it does not melt in the sterilizer.

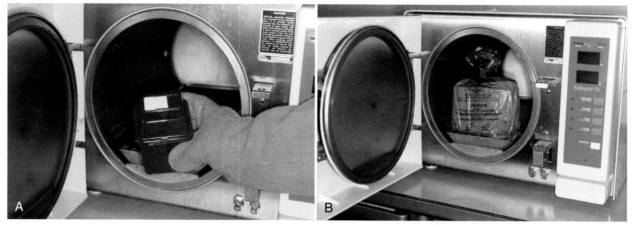

FIGURE 17-2 Sterilization of waste containers. **A,** Sharps container. **B,** Red bag for nonsharp waste. ***Do not*** sterilize with the tops closed as shown.

In some areas, regulated medical waste must be removed, neutralized, and disposed of by an approved waste hauler. In some cases, facilities elect to contract for such disposal even though not required to do so. These services are often expensive, especially if the office or clinic is not in the same building with other practices.

One should remember that although another party physically is removing and disposing of the medical waste, the generating facility has the responsibility to ensure use of acceptable and correct methods. One should ask the waste hauler to provide some training materials approved by the Department of Transportation. This material is in addition to the training required or recommended by OSHA. The CDC and local regulations also may apply.

If waste was dumped illegally, the dental practice involved would also be held responsible. Therefore, one should establish the credentials of any waste hauler. Speaking to other clients and to local health authorities is essential. The EPA usually approves haulers. They are awarded a unique identifying contractor number, which should appear on all paperwork. A receipt of shipment should be provided by the hauler on removal of the waste. Several weeks after removal, a manifest from the hauler should come through the mail indicating the exact manner in which the waste was treated and its final site of disposal.

SELECTED READINGS

American Dental Association: Council on Scientific Affairs and Council on Dental Practice: Infection control recommendations for the dental office and the dental laboratory, *J Am Dent Assoc* 127:672–680, 1996.

Blumstein S, Zeller J, Sharbaugh R: APIC commentary on "healthcare" waste management: a template for action, *Am J Infect Control* 28:E1, 2000.

Centers for Disease Control and Prevention. *Selecting, evaluating and using sharps disposal containers,* http://www.cdc.gov/niosh/docs/97-111/, accessed April 2012.

Gordon JG, Denys GA: Infectious wastes: efficient and effective management. In Block SS, editor: *Disinfection, sterilization and preservation,* ed 5, Philadelphia, 2001, Lippincott Williams & Wilkins, pp 1139–1160.

Kohn WG, Collins AS, Cleveland JL, et al: Centers for Disease Control and Prevention: Guidelines for infection control in dental health-care settings–2003, *MMWR Recomm Rep* 52(RR-17):1–61, 2003.

Miller CH: No wasted effort, *Dent Prod Rept* 41:130–134, 2007.

Miller CH, Palenik CJ: Sterilization, disinfection and asepsis in dentistry. In Block SS, editor: *Disinfection, sterilization and preservation,* ed 5, Philadelphia, 2001, Lippincott Williams & Wilkins, pp 1049–1068.

Palenik CJ: Managing regulated waste in dental environments, *Dent Today* 23:62–63, 2004.

US Department of Labor: Occupational Safety and Health Administration: Occupational exposure to blood-borne pathogens: final rule (29 CFR part 1910.1030), *Fed Regist* 56:64004–64182, 1991.

US Environmental Protection Agency: *EPA guide for infectious waste management (EPA/530–5W-86-014),* Washington, DC, 1986, Author.

REVIEW QUESTIONS

Multiple Choice

1. On average, what percent of all waste materials generated by a dental practice should be considered as being infectious?
   a. 0.1%
   b. 3%
   c. 11%
   d. Approximately 25%
   e. 39%

2. Which of the following should not be considered an example of regulated medical/dental waste according to OSHA?
   a. An extracted tooth
   b. A used latex examination glove
   c. Liquid blood
   d. A used anesthetic needle
   e. A used bur

3. You have just removed two small bags used to cover the light handles of your unit. In most cases, you should:
   a. place them into the nearest sharps container
   b. find a red biohazard bag and put them inside
   c. place them into the regular trash

4. Which type of waste can best be described as items that have had contact with blood or other body fluids and secretions, such as saliva?
   a. Contaminated waste
   b. Infectious waste
   c. Medical/dental waste
   d. Hospital waste

5. What should be done to a full sharps container before moving it?
   a. Empty it.
   b. Push down any protruding items.
   c. Label it as being sterile.
   d. Close the top.

Please visit http://evolve.elsevier.com/Miller/infectioncontrol/ for additional practice and study support tools.

LEARNING OBJECTIVES

After completing this chapter, the student should be able to do the following:
1. Describe some of the risks from sharps injuries.
2. List some examples of when sharps injuries may occur in a dental office. (p. 199, When Can Injuries Occur?)

3. Describe a culture of safety and list the three basic approaches to preventing sharps injuries.

KEY TERMS

Culture of Safety   Sharps   Sharps Containers
Percutaneous

RISKS FROM SHARPS INJURIES

"Sharps" is a term for devices with sharp points or edges that can puncture or cut skin or other tissue. Dental examples include injection needles, orthodontic bands and wire, scalpel blades, burs, suture needles, instruments, and broken glass (Figure 18-1). The most serious types of occupational exposure to bloodborne pathogens are accidental percutaneous (through the skin) injuries involving sharps. The Centers for Disease Control and Prevention (CDC) estimates that each year 385,000 needlesticks and other sharps-related injuries are sustained by just hospital-based health care personnel. Similar injuries occur in other health care settings, such as dental facilities, nursing homes, clinics, emergency care services, and private homes. Nonhospital health care workers experience approximately 205,000 such injuries per year for a total of almost 600,000 injuries annually. Such injuries involve a risk of infection, possible reactions to related prophylactic medications, and psychological stress related to the threat of infection. Thus, reducing contaminated sharps injuries is an important goal.

Sharps injuries are primarily associated with occupational transmission of hepatitis B virus (HBV), hepatitis C virus (HCV), and human immunodeficiency virus (HIV), but they have been implicated in the transmission of more than 20 other pathogens. Even though chances of acquiring an infectious disease from a sharps injury are relatively low, we can't say that the risk is zero. The United States Public Health Service (USPHS) has indicated that in health care personnel who had sustained injuries from needles contaminated with blood containing HBV, the risk of developing clinical hepatitis was 22% to 31% if the blood was both hepatitis B surface antigen (HBsAg)-positive and hepatitis B e antigen (HBeAg)-positive. The risk of developing serological evidence of HBV infection was 37% to 62%. HCV is not transmitted efficiently through occupational exposure to blood. The average incidence of anti-HCV seroconversion after occupational percutaneous exposure from an HCV-positive source is 1.8%, with a range of 0% to 7%. The average risk of HIV transmission after a percutaneous exposure to HIV-infected blood is estimated to be 0.3%. After a mucous membrane exposure, it is estimated

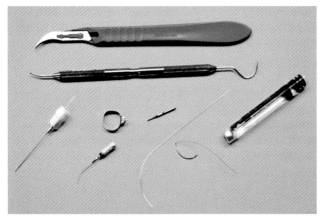

FIGURE 18-1 Examples of sharps (scalpel, anesthetic needle, suture needle, wire, file, band, broken instrument, bur, anesthetic carpule [if broken]).

at 0.09%. A vaccination against hepatitis B virtually eliminates the risk for contracting hepatitis B; to date, however, there are no such vaccinations that protect against hepatitis C or HIV.

WHEN CAN INJURIES OCCUR

Sharps injuries can occur anytime when handling a sharp item (Box 18-1). If the sharp has been used on a patient or has otherwise contacted a patient's blood or saliva, it is contaminated and has a potential to transmit microbes. Everyone is concerned about any type of injury that occurs in the office, but contaminated injuries offer the added grief of a potentially harmful infection (Figure 18-2).

PREVENTION OF SHARPS INJURIES

Culture of Safety

There are several prevention strategies, but establishing a "Culture of Safety" in the office is one overall strategy recommended by the CDC–National Institute for Occupational Safety and Health (NIOSH). Culture refers to factors that influence overall attitudes and behavior in the office. A safety culture reflects the shared commitment of the employer and employees toward ensuring the safety of the work environment. The employer should openly support a safety culture by:
- providing an adequate supply of resources;
- engaging worker participation in safety planning;
- making available appropriate safety devices and protective equipment;
- introducing workers to a safety culture when they are first hired.

Other components of a safety culture include:
- identifying and removing sharps injury hazards; (see below);
- developing feedback systems to communicate safety (e.g., newsletters, bulletin boards, brochures, meeting

---

BOX 18-1

Examples of When Sharps Injuries Can Occur

At chairside
  When preparing the anesthetic syringe
  When giving injections
  When sharps are passed
  When needles are recapped
  When needles are discarded
  When exposed sharps are picked up
  When using sharp hand instruments
  When sharps are laid down
  When manipulating scalpels and blades
  When making incisions
  When suturing
  When placing/removing burs from handpieces
  When contacting protruding burs on handpieces still in their holders
  When manipulating wires, orthodontic bands, and dental appliances
  When gathering items after patient appointments

During instrument processing
  When sharpening instruments
  When removing needles, scalpel blades, broken items left in tray setups
  When hand-scrubbing and rinsing sharps
  When placing/retrieving sharp instruments from cleaning solutions
  When packaging sharp items for sterilization
  When organizing tray setups
  When handling sterile packages of sharps

At other times
  When handling laundry with hidden sharps in pockets
  When handling and cleaning dental appliances with clasps
  When handling sharps in the dental laboratory

---

agendas, rewards for identifying dangerous situations, celebrations for success and improvements);
- promoting individual accountability (e.g., assess safety compliance, have staff sign a pledge to promote safety);
- measuring improvements in safety (e.g., before-and-after survey of staff perception of safety in the office, sharps injury reports).

Occupational Safety and Health Administration's Needlestick Prevention Act

The Occupational Safety and Health Administration (OSHA)'s approach to help protect health care and other workers from exposure to bloodborne pathogens is the bloodborne pathogens standard that became effective in

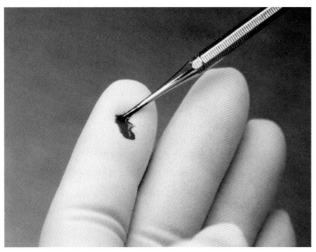

FIGURE 18-2 Simulated instrument puncture.

early 1992 (see Chapters 8, 23, and 24, and Appendix G). It requires employers to protect their employees from exposure to human body fluids. In 2001, OSHA revised the bloodborne pathogens standard to include requirements of the Needlestick Safety and Prevention Act. The revisions modified or added new terms in the definitions section of the standard; made additions to the Exposure Control Plan; required the employer to solicit input from employees in the identification, evaluation, and selection of engineering controls and work practices that prevent exposure; and required the maintenance of a sharps injury log for some employers.

Changes in Definitions

The revised standard added the following to the definitions section of the standard: (1) "Sharps with Engineered Sharps Injury Protections: a non-needle sharp or a needle device used for withdrawing body fluids, accessing a vein or artery, or administering medications or other fluids, with a built-in safety feature or mechanism that effectively reduces the risk of an exposure incident." (2) "Needleless Systems: a device that does not use needles for [A] the collection of bodily fluids or withdrawal of body fluids after initial venous or arterial access is established; [B] the administration of medication or fluids; and [C] any other procedures involving the potential for occupational exposure to bloodborne pathogens due to percutaneous injuries from contaminated sharps." The definition of "Engineering Controls" has been modified to include as examples "safer medical devices, such as sharps with engineered sharps injury protections and needleless systems."

Changes in the Exposure Control Plan

The review and update of the Exposure Control Plan is required to "[A] reflect changes in technology that eliminate or reduce exposure to bloodborne pathogens; and [B] document annually consideration and implementation of appropriate commercially available and effective safer medical devices designed to eliminate or minimize occupational

exposure." Thus, the written Exposure Control Plan is to include a description of (1) how newer medical devices that may reduce exposure will be identified and considered for adoption; (2) the methods used to evaluate the devices and the results of the evaluations; and (3) the justification as to why a device was or was not selected for use. An example of compliance with this change would be an annual review and evaluation of newly available devices designed to reduce percutaneous exposures to bloodborne pathogens. The information added to the Exposure Control Plan must be updated at least annually, like all other parts of the plan.

Input from Employees

The changes require that "An employer, who is required to establish an Exposure Control Plan, shall solicit input from non-managerial employees responsible for direct patient care who are potentially exposed to injuries from contaminated sharps in the identification, evaluation, and selection of effective engineering and work practice controls, and shall document such solicitation in the Exposure Control Plan." This may involve documented discussions with employees or more formal procedures, such as problem-solving groups, safety audits, inspections, pilot studies, or other types of investigations. Evidence of employee input can include meeting minutes, copies of written requests for employee participation, and signed reports.

Injury Log

This change in the standard relates only to employers who are required to maintain an OSHA log of occupational injuries and illnesses (those with 11 or more employees covered under the bloodborne pathogens standard). The change indicates that "The employer shall establish and maintain a sharps injury log for the recording of percutaneous injuries from contaminated sharps. The information in the sharps injury log shall be recorded and maintained in such manner as to protect the confidentiality of the injured employee. The sharps injury log shall contain at a minimum: [A] The type and brand of the device involved in the incident, [B] the department or work area where the exposure incident occurred, and [C] an explanation of how the incident occurred."

In 2005, OSHA determined that offices and clinics of dentists are of a low hazard and **do not** have to keep an OSHA injury and illness record unless the government asks for it. But all employers still have to report any workplace incident that results in a fatality or the hospitalization of three or more employees.

Specific Prevention Approaches

There are three basic approaches to preventing sharps injuries.

- Eliminate the use of the sharp when possible—this is seldom possible in dentistry.
- Apply engineering controls (a device that removes the potential hazard; for example, engineered medical

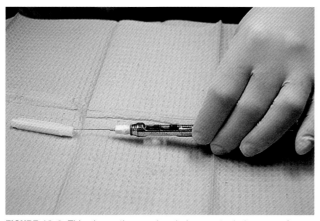

FIGURE 18-3 This shows the one-handed scoop technique, a safe way to recap a needle.

devices with sharps injury prevention features such as a protective needle sheath [sharps containers]).

- Apply work practice controls (actions that alter the manner in which a task is performed; for example, the one-handed scoop technique for recapping a used needle).

Proper handling of sharps is essential because common personal protective barriers such as exam gloves often do not prevent sharps punctures or cuts. Box 18-2 gives some examples of sharps safety. To minimize the potential for accidents with injection needles, use some type of protective cap-holding device or replace the cap sheath using the one-handed scoop technique (Figure 18-3). Chapter 17 describes the proper procedures for disposing of contaminated sharps.

BOX 18-2

Examples of Sharps Safety

1. Avoid bending, breaking, or manipulating needles before disposal.
2. Do not recap a needle by hand (Figure 18-4).
3. Safely recap used needles before removing from nondisposable syringes.
4. Recap needles using a cap holder or the one-handed scoop technique.
5. Avoid removing needles from disposable medical syringes before disposal.
6. Dispose of used needles as soon as possible after use (e.g., at chairside).
7. Evaluate needle safety devices for possible use when they become available.
8. Avoid putting others at risk for an injury.
9. Avoid hand-to-hand passing sharps to another person; use a neutral zone (Figure 18-5).
10. Be extra careful when giving a second aesthetic injection to the same patient.
11. Use round-tipped scalpel blades instead of pointed-tipped blades.
12. Consider using instruments rather than fingers to retract tissue when giving injections or suturing.
13. Use tongs or cotton pliers (rather than fingers) to pick up sharps from the floor (Figure 18-6).
14. Consider distributing your instrument in instrument cassettes; this greatly reduces direct handling of the instruments as they remain in the cassettes during cleaning, packaging, sterilizing, and distributing to chairside.
15. Organize sharp instruments in trays/cassettes so that their tips are not pointing up.
16. Make sure handpieces in their holders have the bur pointing away from the operator.
17. Use instrument cassettes thick enough to avoid sharps from protruding out of the cassette.
18. Place sharp instruments back in a stable fashion when returning them to trays, cassettes, or bracket table (Figure 18-7).
19. Look before reaching for a sharp instrument or instrument package.

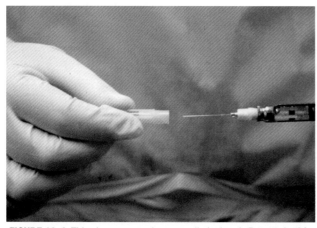

FIGURE 18-4 This shows recapping a needle by hand. ***Do not do this.***

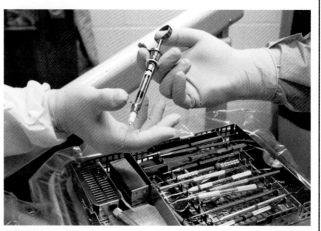

FIGURE 18-5 This shows the passing of an exposed needle. ***Do not do this.***

BOX 18-2

Examples of Sharps Safety—cont'd

20. Carefully check instrument packages for protruding instruments before handling.
21. Do not reach blindly into a container of sharp items.
22. Wear heavy duty gloves during operatory clean-up and instrument processing.
23. Do not sharpen contaminated instruments.
24. Reduce the need for chairside sharpening by providing multiples of an instrument in the setup.
25. If discarding a disposable medical needle syringe, discard the entire unit without removing the needle.
26. Use puncture-resistant, closable, labeled sharps containers for sharps disposal (Figure 18-8).
27. Close sharps containers before moving them to avoid spillage if dropped.
28. Fill sharps containers only three-fourths full to avoid sharps protruding from the top.
29. Use sharps containers with wide enough bases so they do not easily fall over.
30. Do not routinely hand scrub sharp instruments (use ultrasonic or automatic washer units) (Figure 18-9).
31. Use a basket or cassette rack to place instruments/cassettes into an ultrasonic cleaner.
32. If an instrument must be hand-scrubbed on occasion, use a long-handled brush.
33. Consider using tongs or cotton forceps rather than fingers to remove burs from the high-speed handpieces.

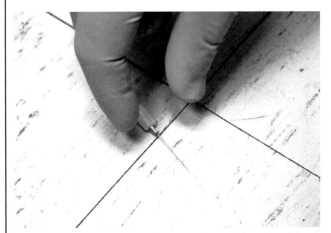

FIGURE 18-6 This shows picking up a sharp with a gloved hand. ***Do not do this***.

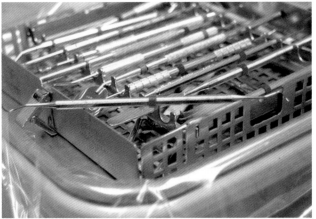

FIGURE 18-7 The sharp instrument was placed by on the cassette in an unstable position. ***Do not do this***.

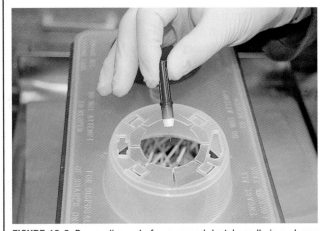

FIGURE 18-8 Proper disposal of a recapped dental needle in a sharps container.

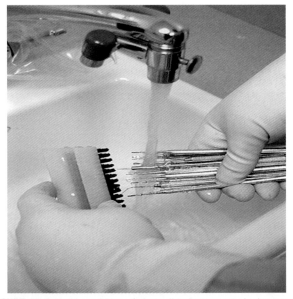

FIGURE 18-9 Hand scrubbing of sharp dirty instruments is dangerous. ***Do not do this***.

SELECTED READINGS

Bell DM: Occupational risk of human immunodeficiency virus infection in healthcare
workers: an overview, *Am J Med* 102(Suppl
5B):9–15, 1997.

Centers for Disease Control and Prevention, Workbook for designing, implementing and evaluating
a sharps injury prevention program, http://www.
cdc.gov/sharpssafety/pdf/sharpsworkbook_2008.
pdf, accessed January 2012.

Centers for Disease Control and Prevention:
Updated U.S. Public Health Service guidelines
for the management of occupational exposures
to HBV, HCV and HIV and recommendation
for postexposure prophylaxis, *MMWR Recomm
Rep* 50(RR-11):1–52, 2001.

Gooch BF, Cardo DM, Marcus R, et al: Percutaneous exposures to HIV-infected blood. Among
dental workers enrolled in the CDC Needlestick
Study, *J Am Dent Assoc* 126:1237–1242, 1995.

Ippolito G, Puro V, De Carli G: Italian Study
Group on Occupational Risk of HIV Infection: The risk of occupational human
immunodeficiency virus in health care workers, *Arch Intern Med* 153:1451–1458, 1993.

Miller CH: Beyond the sticking point, *Dent Prod
Rep* 42:112–116, 2008.

Occupational Safety and Health Administration:
Recordkeeping handbook, 2005, http://www.
osha.gov/recordkeeping/handbook/index.
html#1904.2. accessed January 2012.

REVIEW QUESTIONS

Multiple Choice

1. Which of the following is not an acceptable technique for the handling of sharps?
   a. Recapping a needle using a cap holder
   b. Recapping a needle using the "scoop technique"
   c. Disposing of a needle in a general trash bag
   d. Disposing of a needle in a puncture-resistant container

2. Where should sharps containers be placed in the office?
   a. In the sterilizing room and the storage room
   b. In the storage room and the clinic
   c. In the clinic and the dental laboratory
   d. Wherever disposable sharps are used or may be found

3. A plan referring to factors that influence overall attitudes and behavior in the office regarding sharps safety is:
   a. a culture of safety
   b. the bloodborne pathogens standard
   c. the needlestick prevention act
   d. universal precautions

4. Sharps safety procedures indicate what type of gloves should be worn during operatory clean-up and instrument processing?
   a. Latex exam gloves
   b. Nitrile exam gloves
   c. Utility gloves
   d. Sterile gloves

5. Sharps injuries are primarily associated with occupational transmission in which of the following diseases?
   a. Hepatitis B, hepatitis C, and human immunodeficiency virus disease
   b. Influenza, herpes, and tuberculosis
   c. Legionnaires' disease, hepatitis B, and the common cold
   d. Meningitis, chickenpox, and human immunodeficiency virus disease

Please visit http://evolve.elsevier.com/Miller/infectioncontrol/ for additional practice and study support tools.

CHAPTER 19

A Clinical Asepsis Protocol

OUTLINE

Before Seating the Patient
After Seating The Patient
During Patient Treatment
After Patient Treatment

Radiographic Asepsis
Unit/Patient Preparation
Darkroom Processing
Daylight Loader Processing

LEARNING OBJECTIVES

After completing this chapter, the student should be able to do the following:

1. Describe what type of infection control preparation is necessary for a patient appointment.
2. Describe infection control procedures used after the patient is seated but before beginning the actual treatment.

3. Describe the infection control procedures to be performed during patient treatment.
4. Describe infection control procedures to be performed after the patient appointment is completed.
5. Describe infection control procedures to be performed when taking radiographs.

KEY TERMS

Antimicrobial Mouth Rinse
Aseptic Retrieval
Gloves
Hand Hygiene

Handwashing
Mask
Protective Clothing
Protective Eyewear

Radiographic Asepsis
Surface Covers

O ther parts of this book describe a variety of separate infection control procedures. The information in this chapter is intended to organize these procedures into a usable protocol based on the sequence of patient treatment activities. Some steps in the protocol may change from one office to the next. The procedures are grouped into five sets of activities that are conducted as follows:

1. Before seating the patient
2. After seating the patient
3. During patient treatment
4. After patient treatment
5. **Radiographic asepsis**

BEFORE SEATING THE PATIENT

1. Put on **protective clothing**, **protective eyewear**, **mask**, and **gloves**, and clean and disinfect those surfaces that may be touched during patient treatment and which will not be protected by **surface covers**. These surfaces can include the following:
   a. Cuspidor rim and control knob
   b. Countertops
   c. Drawer pulls and top edges of drawers that may be used
   d. Sink faucet handles
   e. Handpiece connectors

2. Clean and disinfect items brought into the area to be used during patient procedures (e.g., articulators, casts, dies, custom impression trays, record bases, fixed and removable prostheses, and face-bows). Disinfection procedure is as follows:
   a. Spray the surface with the surface disinfectant that has been prepared properly.
   b. Clean the surface by vigorously wiping with paper towels or 4 × 4 gauze pads.
   c. Disinfect the precleaned surface by respraying it and letting it air dry or by wiping it dry if it is still wet after the prescribed contact time.
   d. Alternatively wipe with a disinfectant towelette, discard towelette, wipe with a second fresh towelette, and let dry.
3. Remove and discard mask and gloves and wash hands. Follow the procedure for removing gloves.
   a. Pinch one glove in the wrist area on one hand with the thumb and forefinger of the other hand.
   b. Stretch the glove out away from the wrist, slide it off toward the fingertips—but only halfway.
   c. Repeat that step on the other hand, except slide that glove completely off and drop it directly into the waste receptacle.
   d. Move back to the first hand and place the ungloved thumb under the edge of the glove, which now has the noncontaminated surface inside of the glove turned out. Stretch the glove out away from the hand, slide it completely off toward the fingertips, and drop it directly into the waste receptacle. Wash hands.
4. Obtain surface covers, supplies, and sterile instruments and other equipment from the supply area.
5. Cover the following surfaces with the appropriate cover:
   a. Headrest
   b. Control buttons on side of chair
   c. Light handles
   d. Unit light switch and view box switch
   e. Air/water syringe buttons/handle
   f. High-volume evacuator control
   g. Unit control switches and handpiece, air/water syringe, and high-volume evacuation holders
   h. Saliva ejector, handpiece, and air/water syringe hoses
   i. Bracket table
   j. Stool backs
6. Remove all items not used during patient treatment from countertops (e.g., datebooks, articulator boxes, and cardboard and plastic boxes).
7. Make sure a sharps container is available at chairside.

AFTER SEATING THE PATIENT

1. Adjust chair and headrest.
2. Place patient napkin.
3. Take or update medical history, discuss treatment, and do necessary paperwork.

4. Remove chart from the countertop.
5. Have patient rinse thoroughly with an **antimicrobial mouth rinse**.
6. Open instrument packages or tray without touching the instruments.
7. Put on mask and eyeglasses.
8. Perform **hand hygiene** (preferably in view of patient).
   a. **Handwashing** procedure
      • Remove jewelry and gently clean your fingernails.
      • Lather for 15 seconds with the liquid antimicrobial or non-antimicrobial detergent.
      • Rinse under cool water and towel dry.
   b. Or, use an alcohol-based hand rub.
   c. Perform surgical scrub for procedures so indicated.
9. Put on gloves (preferably in view of patient). Use sterile gloves for procedures so indicated; otherwise, use nonsterile examination gloves.
10. Use powder-free gloves. Alternatively, rinse nonsterile, powdered examination gloves with plain, cool water (no soap) to remove excess powder and towel dry before making impressions and bite registrations. If desired, remove excess powder by rinsing with water and drying before other types of procedures. Explain to the patient that these are new gloves being rinsed to remove the powder.
11. Connect sterile handpieces and sterile or disposable air/water syringe tip, high-volume evacuation tip, and saliva ejector tip.

DURING PATIENT TREATMENT

1. Restrict spread of microorganisms from patient's mouth.
   a. Use rubber dam.
   b. Use high-volume evacuation.
   c. Touch as few surfaces as possible with saliva-coated fingers.
   d. Keep gloved hands out of hair, and do not rub eyes or bare skin or adjust mask or glasses.
   e. If leaving chairside during treatment is necessary, remove and discard the gloves. Wash hands and reglove with fresh gloves on return. Do not wear protective clothing in lunchrooms, restrooms, or outside the building; change protective clothing if obviously soiled.
   f. Remove contaminated gloves and wash hands before handling cameras for intraoral photographs.
2. Do not use items dropped on the floor or on other nonsterile surfaces. Obtain sterile replacements. Remove and replace gloves, preferably in view of the patient.
3. If gloves are torn during treatment, remove, discard, wash hands, and reglove with fresh gloves.
4. Do not recap needles by hand. Insert the needle into the cap using the one-handed "scoop" technique or a cap holder that will not permit contact of the needle with any part of the body. Do not pass syringes with uncapped needles to someone else.

5. Look first before reaching for a sharp instrument.
6. When placing sharp instruments back on the instrument tray, make sure sharp tips are not pointed up and make sure they are placed in a stable position.
7. If equipment is brought to chairside (e.g., light curing apparatus), make sure it is protected with a surface cover or has been disinfected before use.
8. Use an **aseptic retrieval** technique to obtain supplies from bulk containers at chairside.
9. If one must obtain supplies (e.g., amalgam, varnish, or cavity liner) from a central storage area, do not take a container to the unit unless it is covered with plastic wrap or is cleaned and disinfected after use.
10. Disinfect contaminated items before taking them to the dental laboratory.
11. Do not handle charts with contaminated gloves. Use an overglove or remove gloves and wash hands.
12. If exposed to a patient's blood or saliva, immediately contact the appropriate person to institute a postexposure medical evaluation. An exposure is any sharps injury or contact with the eye, mouth, other mucous membrane, or nonintact skin involving blood or saliva.

AFTER PATIENT TREATMENT

Anyone who will be cleaning contaminated instruments must wear heavy utility gloves, protective clothing, a mask, and a face shield or protective eyewear. If instruments are hand scrubbed, they should be submerged in detergent while scrubbing with a long-handled brush to prevent splattering.

1. Remove gloves and then the mask by touching only the ties or elastic band and discard them in a plastic-lined waste container at the unit and then wash hands or use an alcohol-based hand rub.
2. Send the patient to the front desk for dismissal or reappointment.
3. Put on fresh gloves and mask.
4. Place all instruments back in the tray.
5. Place all disposable sharps, including capped or uncapped needles, directly into the sharps container at chairside. Do not place needles or other sharps into the regular trash receptacle. This would be a serious violation of procedures. Sharps include needles, scalpel blades, carpules, broken instruments and files, burs, orthodontic wire, and other disposable items that could penetrate the skin.
6. Place nonsharp disposable items in the plastic-lined waste container at the unit.
7. Flush the air/water syringe, high-speed handpiece, and ultrasonic scaler into the sink, cuspidor, or container for 20 to 30 seconds and disconnect from hoses.
8. Remove all surface covers (without touching the underlying surface) and discard in plastic-lined waste container at the unit.
9. Clean and disinfect patient care–related surfaces that were not covered and were contaminated during treatment. Cleaning and disinfection of surfaces that were

covered is unnecessary unless they become contaminated during removal of the covers (see the aforementioned disinfection procedures).
10. Take instruments and handpieces to the decontamination/sterilizing area.
11. Remove and wash contaminated eyeglasses, and rinse and dry them. Avoid contaminating hair.
12. Remove and dispose of the disposable gown (if used) in the plastic-lined waste container at the unit. Untie the gown and pull it off over gloved hands, and do not touch underlying clothing or skin.
13. Remove gloves and discard them in the plastic-lined waste container.
14. Wash, rinse, and dry hands or use an alcohol-based hand rub.

RADIOGRAPHIC ASEPSIS

Unit/Patient Preparation

1. Before seating the patient, prepare the unit by covering or disinfecting all surfaces that will be touched or exposed to potentially infectious fluids.
2. Review or update the medical history of the patient.
3. After washing hands, gowning, and gloving, determine the appropriate number and type of films to be taken.
4. Obtain the films from a central distribution area or film dispenser while wearing clean gloves or cover the digital x-ray sensor with the appropriate barrier.
5. Reglove and expose the films or sensor in the recommended manner.
6. Place exposed films on a paper towel or in a cup. If film packs are precovered with plastic protectors, carefully remove the contaminated covers after exposure and drop the film packs onto a clean surface. Do not touch the film packs with contaminated gloves.
7. Remove surface covers from the unit or disinfect contaminated surfaces.
8. Remove gloves and wash hands or use an alcohol-based hand rub.

Darkroom Processing

1. Place new gloves on hands.
2. Carry the films to the darkroom using caution not to touch doors, walls, work areas, or processors with contaminated gloves.
3. With gloved hands, carefully open the film packets and drop the films onto a clean paper towel. Place contaminated film wrappers into the designated refuse containers.
4. Remove contaminated gloves and place the films in the processor and perform hand hygiene.
5. After processing, place the films into the appropriate mounts using care not to contaminate the films, mounts, or charts with instruments that were used in the operatory.

Daylight Loader Processing

1. Because of the limited operating space inside the loader and because the hand insertion sleeves cannot be disinfected, place only films that are not contaminated in the loader. This can be accomplished in two ways:
   a. *Film disinfection:* After the films have been exposed, rinse them with water, soak them in an appropriate bleach or iodophor solution for 10 minutes, and while wearing clean gloves, rinse them with water and dry them with a clean paper towel. Place the films into the loader through the top. (Only plastic film packets may be disinfected.)
   b. *Preexposure wrapping:* Wrap the film in plastic before placing it in the patient's mouth. Film packs already protected with a removable plastic cover are available. After exposure, carefully open the outer wrapping or remove the cover and drop the film packet onto a clean surface. Use caution so that the clean packets do not touch the contaminated gloves or wrapping. Place the films in the loader through the top, and after donning new gloves, pass the hands through the insertion sleeves.

SELECTED READINGS

Miller CH: Handling negative issues: taking patient x-rays, *Dent Prod Rep* 39:72, 2006.

Miller CH: Infection control strategies for the dental office. In Ciancio S, editor: *ADA guide to dental therapeutics*, ed 3, Chicago, 2003, ADA Publishing, pp 551–566.

Miller CH: Prevent invisible problems: follow standard operating procedures, *Dent Prod Rep* 38:96, 2004.

Miller CH, Palenik CJ: Sterilization, disinfection and asepsis in dentistry. In Block SS, editor: *Sterilization, disinfection and preservation*, ed 5, Philadelphia, 2001, Lippincott Williams &Wilkins, pp 1049–1068.

Miller CH, Palenik CJ, Schaaf JE: *Infection control manual*, Indianapolis, 2003, Indiana University School of Dentistry.

REVIEW QUESTIONS

Multiple Choice

1. All of the following surfaces except one may need to be cleaned and disinfected before each patient appointment. Which one is the exception?
   a. Cuspidor rim and control knob
   b. Floors
   c. Drawer pulls and top edges of drawers that may be used
   d. High-volume evacuation connector
   e. Handpiece connectors

2. When should handpiece lines be flushed?
   a. Before attaching the sterile handpiece
   b. After attaching the sterile handpiece
   c. Before removing the contaminated handpiece
   d. After removing the contaminated handpiece

3. Operatory surfaces that were covered with plastic barriers during patient treatment are to:
   a. remain covered for the next patient
   b. be cleaned and disinfected for the next patient
   c. be recovered for the next patient

4. Gloves to be used in the patient's mouth are to be put on:
   a. before preparing the unit for the patient
   b. after preparing the unit and seating the patient
   c. just before seating the patient

5. When should an uncovered, contaminated operatory surface be cleaned and disinfected?
   a. Before the next patient is seated
   b. Just after treatment but before the patient leaves the chair
   c. Each time the operatory surface is contaminated during patient treatment

Please visit http://evolve.elsevier.com/Miller/infectioncontrol/ for additional practice and study support tools.

PART THREE

Office Safety

General Office Safety and Asepsis

OUTLINE

LEARNING OBJECTIVES

After completing this chapter, the student should be able to do the following:

1. Describe examples of potentially dangerous or injurious incidents that may occur in a dental office and how training is essential for safety management.
2. Describe how to maintain asepsis in the dental office reception room.
3. Describe the types of people that may bring their microbes into a dental facility.
4. Describe how air, water and dirt contribute to contamination of a dental facility.
5. Describe one way to evaluate the cleanliness of a dental office.

KEY TERMS

Cleanliness
Entry Floor Mats

Green Products
Plan Ahead

Potable
Walk Through

BE PREPARED

From a safety point of view, it's important to identify possible events that could be potentially dangerous or injurious to patients or office staff (Box 20-1). Thus plans need to be developed to manage such events. Some of these events may recur (e.g., sharps injuries) and plans can be developed based upon past experience. In other instances (e.g., a flood), plans must be developed in anticipation of the event.

Training

The more you know about a potential hazard, the better you can manage it or prevent its occurrence. Thus training becomes an essential to adequate preparation. As indicated by the Bloodborne Pathogens Standard from the Occupational Safety and Health Administration (OSHA) (see Chapter 8 and Appendix G), examples of training include:

- Recognizing tasks in the office that may involve exposure to patient's blood or saliva
- Knowing appropriate actions to take and persons to contact if a blood or saliva exposure incident occurs, including the method of reporting the incident and the postexposure evaluation and the medical follow-up that will be made available
- The warning signs and labels and/or color coding used to identify biohazards
- Various aspect of the transmission and prevention of bloodborne diseases

Training associated with OSHA's Hazard Communication Standard (see Chapter 26 and Appendix H) includes knowing:

- The tasks that include the use of hazardous chemicals
- The location and availability of the written hazard communication program
- The methods and observations that may be used to detect the presence or release of hazardous chemicals in the work area
- The physical and health hazards of the chemicals used
- The measures to take to protect yourself from those hazards, including the specific procedures the employer has implemented to protect employees from exposure to hazardous chemicals
- The details of the hazard communication program developed by the employer, including an explanation of the labeling system and the material safety data sheets, and how employees can obtain and use the information
- About any new physical or health hazard introduced into the workplace on which the employees have not been previously trained

Plan Ahead

Chapter 27 describes Emergency Action Plans for fires, bad weather, and other emergencies. Chapter 18 describes preventing sharps injuries. Chapter 14 describes what to do in case of a boil-water notice. Management of equipment failures includes knowing who to contact (names, addresses, and phone numbers) in case of a failure and knowing if your local supplier has back-up equipment available. For sterilizer failures, follow the recommendations from the Centers for Disease Control and Prevention (see Chapter 12 and Appendix B).

BOX 20-1

Examples of Possible Dangerous or Injurious Events

- Exposure to patient's body fluids (e.g., needle-sticks, cuts, abrasions, instrument punctures, spatter to the skin or eyes)
- Exposure to hazardous chemicals (e.g., splash of disinfectant in the eyes or mouth)
- Boil-water notices (e.g., break in a nearby water main)
- Equipment failures (e.g., sterilizer malfunction, air compressor failure, vacuum line clogging)
- Utility emergency (e.g., faulty electrical cord or outlet, natural gas leak, water heater failure)
- Bad weather (e.g., tornado, hurricane, lightning strikes, flooding)
- Medical emergencies (e.g., patient heart attack, chocking, allergic reaction)

THE RECEPTION AREA

Cleanliness and asepsis need to extend beyond the operatory and laboratory. Pay particular attention to the waiting room, which offers the first impression about cleanliness of the office. Patients can't see microbes, but they can see dust, fingerprints, smudges, cobwebs, and dirt, and they can feel sticky surfaces. Shiny surfaces imply cleanliness, but can show dirt if not kept up. Attention needs to be paid to every surface in the reception area.

Make sure the door knobs (Figure 20-1) and the arms of chairs (Figure 20-2) are not sticky. Check the magazines periodically for torn covers and smudges. The countertop at the reception window needs to be spotless, and the carpeting needs to be clean. Vacuum cleaners need to contain HEPA (high-efficiency particulate air) filters. Consider removing artificial plants from the office or keep them dusted. Damp-dust all horizontal surfaces regularly. Make sure appropriate caution signs are out if tile or wooden floors may be wet.

The Centers for Disease Control and Prevention (CDC) has published guidelines for environmental infection control in health care facilities, and these can apply to the dental office reception area (Box 20-2).

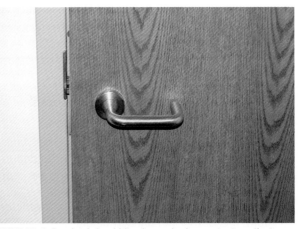

FIGURE 20-1 Doorknob (could involve main door, entry to patient care area, patient bathroom).

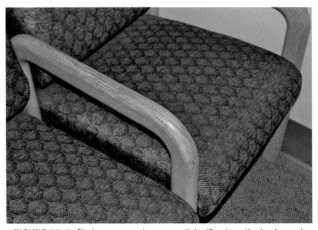

FIGURE 20-2 Chair arms can become sticky if not routinely cleaned.

To help prevent the spread of respiratory agents from patients in the waiting room, provide a box of facial tissue and a waste container. Also, CDC posters, such as "Cover Your Cough" (available at http://www.cdc.gov/flu/protect/covercough.htm) and "Germ Stoppers" (available at http://www.cdc.gov/germstopper/materials.htm), can be posted in the reception area.

Keep patient bathrooms clean. Use a liquid soap rather than bar soap and preferably use a hands-free soap dispenser and paper towels. Make sure it's free of staff personal items.

CONTAMINATION FROM THE OUTSIDE

People

When patients enter the office, they bring with them their associated microbes, which is one of the main reasons infection control is practiced. However, other people also enter the office including the doctor(s), regular and temporary staff, cleaning crew, student trainees, sale representatives, medical waste haulers, and repair persons. Because these folks work in, or at least pass through, the clinical areas, they need to be protected by, aware of, and adhere to proper infection prevention procedures. Other people, including mail persons, delivery persons, patients' family members, and other visitors, enter the office and usually remain in the waiting room.

BOX 20-2

Some CDC Guidelines for Environmental Infection Control

- Avoid placing decorative fountains and fish tanks in patient-care areas; ensure disinfection and fountain maintenance if decorative fountains are used in public areas of the health care facility.
- Flowers and potted plants need not be restricted from areas for immunocompetent patients but should not be allowed near immunosuppressed patients.
- Designate care and maintenance of flowers and potted plants to staff not directly involved with patient care.
- If plant or flower care by patient care staff is unavoidable, instruct the staff to wear gloves when handling plants and flowers and perform hand hygiene after glove removal.
- Advise families, visitors, and patients regarding the importance of hand hygiene to minimize the spread of body substance contamination (e.g., respiratory secretions or fecal matter) to surfaces.

Centers for Disease Control and Prevention: *Guidelines for environmental infection control in healthcare facilities,* http://www.cdc.gov/mmwr/preview/mmwrhtml/rr5210a1.htm, accessed January 2012.

However, some delivery persons may enter the back door or a parent or other caregiver may accompany a patient to the operatory. All of the people who enter the office may use the restroom facilities, so maintaining cleanliness there is essential for both image and infection prevention.

Temporary Staff

Temporary hygienists, assistants, dentists, and student trainees who may be in the office should already be familiar with infection prevention techniques. Some degree of training will be necessary to describe the location of personal protective equipment (PPE), safety data sheets, and eye wash stations. They'll need to know about the emergency action plan, where the exits and fire extinguishers are located, and who to report to in case of an exposure. A one-page summary containing some of this information might be helpful.

Housekeeping Staff

The outside housekeeping staff needs to be trained about infection control and bloodborne pathogens by their original employers, but this needs to be confirmed. Their training should include how to manage waste, recognize hazardous materials and situations, how to properly clean and disinfect appropriate surfaces, what PPE they need, plus whatever OSHA-required training is needed. It's important to know exactly what the housekeeping staff will clean and what products they will use. For example, if they use "green products" that are supposed to be more friendly to the environment, make sure these are not just diluted products that add lower amounts of chemicals to the environment. Diluted products are usually much less effective. The cleaning staff needs to know what areas or equipment that they should not touch (e.g., items in the sterilizing room, disinfected and covered dental units, x-ray equipment, certain countertops, sharps containers). The clinical staff needs to know that sharps are never to be disposed of in regular trash containers, for this can result in serious exposure of the cleaning staff when they collect the trash.

Observers

Observers—such as those interested in applying to dental, assisting, or hygiene schools; those in such school having their first exposure to the clinics; family members of patients; scouts working on merit badges—are usually lacking in their infection prevention knowledge. So they need to be instructed on what they can and cannot touch and appropriate PPE needs to be provided if there is a chance they may contact contaminated surfaces.

Repair and Delivery Persons

Repair personnel should know not to work on clinical equipment without wearing appropriate PPE or confirming that the equipment has been disinfected or, as required by OSHA, properly labeled as contaminated. Hazardous waste haulers coming to pick up regulated waste (e.g., sharps containers, red bags) should already know how to properly handle hazardous materials. Delivery persons need to be instructed where to enter the office to minimize disruption (e.g., the back door) and where to place their deliveries. They, along with sales representatives, should be instructed not to touch any clinical or laboratory surfaces.

Natural Resources

There are other things besides people that enter a dental office, including air, water, and dirt.

Air

All air carries microbes and these are also present in dental aerosols, droplet nuclei, and spatter, and on dust particles. Open windows in the office allow entry of dust and insects. Fans in the clinical area or sterilizing room should be avoided for they simply collect airborne microbes and redistribute them throughout the area. Also, warm air hand dryers (sometimes placed in restrooms) draw in air and any contaminants present and blow them directly on your previously washed hands. Hand drying after routine handwashing is best accomplished with disposable paper towels.

The compressed air used by air/water syringes and to drive high-speed handpieces is not sterile but usually is quite low in microbial counts. In some instances, small amounts of water that might accumulate on the inside bottom of compressed air tanks (as the water is "squeezed out" of the compressed air) may harbor microbes that could become aerosolized.

Water

As described in Chapter 14, the water that enters a dental office is supposed to be potable (drinkable) but is not sterile. Thus dental units are continually inoculated with the microbes in the incoming water and some attach to the inside of the dental unit waterlines to form a biofilm. This biofilm releases microbes into the flowing water, resulting in high counts of microbes being delivered to patient's mouths. The Environmental Protection Agency (EPA) standard for good quality drinking water is water having less than 500 colony-forming units per milliliter (CFU/mL) of noncoliform bacteria. This level is also that which the CDC recommends for dental unit water entering a patient's mouth. There are a variety of equipment and chemicals available to maintain good quality dental unit water.

Dirt

Soil on the bottom of shoes can contain many microbes that are mainly deposited on the waiting room carpet and elsewhere. The International Sanitary Supply Association reports that most of the dirt within a building is tracked in on people's shoes and that 85% of this can be eliminated if proper entry floor mats are used and maintained. To effectively remove most pollutants from shoes requires a combination of mat materials, textures, and lengths. The

combination may vary depending on your climate and location. For example, a snowy climate may require a greater amount of scraper mat; a rainy location more absorption mat; and a muddy location more of each of the mats. As described by the EPA, the scraper mat is located outside the entry doors and removes the bulk of dirt and snow with some form of knobby or squeegee-like projections. Generally, the higher the projection, the better the cleaning and holding capacity. Surface mats are typically made of nitrile rubber. The absorption mat is located just inside the entry doors. It's generally made from nylon or combinations of nylon and heavily textured piles of polypropylene that can perform both a scraping action and a moisture wicking action. The finishing mat follows immediately after the absorption mat. It's generally made from polypropylene with a course fiber surface that will both capture and hold any remaining particles or moisture. These mats should be cleaned, and daily vacuuming of the carpeting also helps maintain a good indoor air quality.

Food

All food needs to be protected from the environment and kept frozen or refrigerated until heated or served. Foods that are moved from the cold or heat into the ambient environment need to be covered unless served immediately. Be particularly careful of food that has never been through a heating process. Fruits should be washed. Hands used to prepare, serve, or eat food need to be clean, as should associated countertops, utensils, and dishes. Food and drink should not be kept in refrigerators, shelves, cabinets, countertops, or bench tops where blood, saliva, or hazardous materials are present.

Deliverables

Items received from a dental lab should be placed at a specific receiving area in the office that is kept clean and disinfected. The decontamination status of these items needs to be confirmed with the lab to determine if disinfection is needed before delivering to the patient. Supply and equipment items shipped to the office should be unpacked and bulk-stored in nonclinical areas. Items stored for use in a clinical area need to be covered and retrieved only with an aseptic, such as using cotton pliers or fresh gloves, as described in Chapter 13.

WALK THROUGHS

A good way to assess the cleanliness of the office is to pretend you are a patient and periodically walk through the office and observe the environment. Check out the entry door knob. Walk in and look for the lighted exit signs and other signage directing the patients to the proper areas. Sit in a reception chair and look at the carpet, reception window, corners on the floor and ceiling, magazine rack, plants, and toys if there are any. Check out the patient/staff restroom (floor, mirror, toilets, sink, soap, and paper towel dispensers) and move back to the clinical area, noting the floor, walls, and any hand rails. Sit in all the dental chairs and look for cobwebs on the ceiling. Are the air vents clean? Are there dead gnats or flies in the plastic fluorescent light diffusers? Are the nontouch surfaces (e.g., bracket table arm, countertop, front of the dental light) and around the chair clean and dust-free? Observe the checkout area, proceed out the reception room door, and check the cleanliness of that inside doorknob.

SELECTED READINGS

Environmental Protection Agency: *Controlling pollutants and sources*, http://www.epa.gov/iaq/schooldesign/controlling.html#EntryMatBarriers. accessed January 2012.

Hubar SI, Pelon W, Gardiner DM: Evaluation of compressed air used in the dental operatory, *J Am Dent Assoc* 133(7):837–841, 2002.

Miller CH: Bringing the outside in, *Infect Control Pract* 8(4):1–5, 2009.

Miller CH: When stuff happens, *Infect Control Pract* 7(2):1–5, 2009.

Miller CH: The reception room, *Infect Control Pract* 7(2):1–5, 2008.

Miller CH: Before you walk in the door, *Infect Control Pract* 7(1):1–5, 2008.

REVIEW QUESTIONS

Multiple Choice

1. What is potable water?
   a. Water that has not been sterilized
   b. Water that is carried in a metal pot
   c. Water that boils at 80° C (176° F)
   d. Water suitable for drinking

2. The International Sanitary Supply Association reports that most dirt within a building enters the building:
   a. in the air
   b. in the water
   c. on people's shoes
   d. on delivered packages and mail

3. The dental office outside housekeeping staff needs to be trained about infection control and bloodborne pathogens by:
   a. OSHA
   b. EPA
   c. their original employer
   d. the dental office where they are contracted to work

4. What type of patients may be particularly sensitive to the presence of plants or flowers in a dental office waiting room?
   a. All patients
   b. Patients older than age 20 years
   c. Immunosuppressed patients
   d. Female patients

5. Green products:
   a. are friendly to the environment
   b. are manufactured by Green, Inc. in Indianapolis, Indiana
   c. turn green when their expiration date occurs

Please visit http://evolve.elsevier.com/Miller/infectioncontrol/ for additional practice and study support tools.

Greener Infection Control

OUTLINE

LEARNING OBJECTIVES

After completing this chapter, the learner should be able to:
1. Describe what going green means.
2. Give examples of adverse environmental impacts.
3. Define recycling and biodegradation.
4. Describe some logos that indicate green products.
5. Give specific examples of how to develop a greener infection control program.

KEY TERMS

Biodegradation
Carbon Footprint
Environmental Impact

Going Green
Greenhouse Effect
Greenhouse Gases

Ozone-depleting Substances
Recycling
Volatile Organic Compounds

GOING GREEN

The concept of green infection control is based on reducing adverse health and environmental impacts. **Going green** means to use products and procedures that have lower adverse impacts on health and the environment than the regular products and procedures. Going green is a personal decision that takes many things into consideration such as:

- Your basic philosophy (e.g., making changes is difficult)
- Scientific evidence (e.g., does a product really benefit the environment?)
- Infection control efficacy (e.g., changes must not compromise infection control)
- Cost
- Ability or authority to take action
- Availability of quality products and equipment

The information in this chapter is not meant to convince anyone to go green. Rather, it provides information related to environmental impacts and infection control should one consider taking this approach to disease prevention.

It is difficult to imagine an infection control procedure that would improve the environment. Most have a negative effect—increased waste, spread of harmful chemicals, or deleterious effects on humans. Taking a green approach usually requires some changes and change is rarely easy. It requires organization and dedication. It not only involves research, experimentation, and new materials or procedures but also behavioral change, and changing behaviors may be the most difficult. Table 21-1 addresses the four steps or stages in the development an infection prevention program with a reduced **environmental impact**. Reviewing infection control procedures may help identify pathways for change. For example, using disinfectant wipes instead of spraying

TABLE 21-1   **The Four Steps in the Development of an Infection Prevention Program with Reduced Environmental Impact**

Step	Step Description	Outcomes
1	Inventory of infection control procedures	Will determine the nature and frequency of current practices and establish baselines (helps to measure improvement)
2	Develop a plan	All good plans have steps or goals that have measurable outcomes (always consider alternative methods and materials)
3	Implement the plan	Establish a timeline for implementation
4	Review and monitoring	Ensure that all issues have been addressed and monitored for change

disinfectants could reduce the amount of chemicals in the environment and exposure by patients and practitioners.

A successful plan not only addresses all possibilities for change, but also other issues. These include costs, including upfront expenses, such as new equipment. Proper training of workers is required for success; however, it also involves costs and lost work time. On the other hand, the time and resources spent on training will result in a smoother, quicker implementation.

Identify a reasonable amount of time and resources to establish the program. Having intermediate goals is often useful. Staying on task is necessary.

Once you think that the entire program is in place, review all points to establish completion. Monitoring will help determine if the desired effects are being accomplished. Reviewing and monitoring may indicate areas for further improvement. Any plan should always be open to change.

ADVERSE ENVIRONMENTAL IMPACTS

One type of environmental impact is measured as the carbon footprint left by the production or consumption of an item, and this footprint is defined as the amount of greenhouse gases directly or indirectly emitted. Carbon dioxide (CO_2), methane (CH_4), nitrous oxide (N_2O), and hydrofluorocarbons (HFCs) are greenhouse gases with CO_2 being the most prominent. These gases are generated in a variety of ways, including humans breathing, the burning of fossil fuels (coal, oil, natural gas), some manufacturing processes, and deforestation (trees use CO_2). The greenhouse effect is a natural occurrence that helps regulate the temperature of our planet. Heat (infrared radiation) from the sun warms the earth. Some of this heat escapes back into space, but the rest is trapped in the atmosphere by greenhouse gases and water vapor. So, the more greenhouse gases in the atmosphere, the more heat that is retained on earth, which is referred to as global warming. The carbon footprint of a single product is difficult to assess for it involves the collective impacts of gathering the raw materials, production, transport, distribution, use, and disposal.

Other environmental impacts occur when some chemicals are added to the environment that are nonbiodegradable, biotoxic, or enhance the production of respiratory irritants such as smog (the "bad" ozone at ground level) like volatile organic compounds (VOCs—some solvents, paints, benzene, gasoline vapors, and compounds in car exhaust).

$$\text{VOC} + \text{oxides of nitrogen} + \text{sunlight} \rightarrow \text{ozone}$$
$$(\text{ozone is the main component of smog})$$

Another impact comes from ozone-depleting substances (ODSs) that destroy the "good" atmospheric ozone such as some solvents, aerosol propellants, and coolants. Ozone is produced naturally in the upper atmosphere. This ozone layer filters out 95% to 99% of the sun's harmful ultraviolet radiation. The action of ODSs (see below) lets more ultraviolet (UV) light through to the earth's surface effecting cataracts, skin cancer, and damage to plants.

$$\text{ODS} + \text{sunlight} \rightarrow \text{chlorine and bromine that destroy ozone}$$

One molecule of chlorine can destroy 100,000 molecules of ozone and one molecule of bromine destroys six million molecules of ozone.

RECYCLING AND BIODEGRADATION

The three "Rs" of going green are:
- Reduce
- Reuse
- Recycle

Recycling is reported to reduce emission of greenhouse gases and water pollutants by minimizing the manufacturing process from virgin materials. This saves energy, supplies, and valuable raw materials and reduces the need for disposal facilities such as landfills. Recycling also may help sustain the environment for future generations.

The term "recycled" on a product label means that the product or its packaging is made of recycled material, but what percent is actually from recycled material? The term "recyclable" suggests that the product can be collected and used again or made into other products. The phrase "please recycle" assumes that there is a place that will accept the item for recycling. The SPI (Society of the Plastics Industry) symbol is the triangular symbol on many plastic items that identifies the chemical nature of seven different types of plastics. It consists of a triangle with a number 1 through 7 inside. Many communities will collect only numbers 1 and 2 plastics (1 is on water bottles and pop bottles; 2 is on milk cartons and some detergent bottles).

Biodegradation is the breakdown of materials by microbes in the environment. Not all biodegradation is beneficial. Uncontrolled biodegradation in a landfill can cause ground water pollution, methane gas emissions, and unstable subsoil conditions. As a result, modern landfills are kept as dry and airtight as possible to prevent biodegradation. Federal standards require landfills to have a membrane overlaying 2 feet of clay soil lining the bottom and sides of the landfill to protect groundwater and underlying soil from the liquid released from the waste. This liquid is drawn off for treatment and disposal. The waste in landfills is continually being covered with soil to help reduce odor, control insects and rodents, and reduce oxygen availability that reduces biodegradation. Biodegradable materials (e.g., food scraps, wet and soiled paper, leaves, grass, and certain plastics) are still being sent to some landfills where they will sit in an airless, dry environment to mummify rather than biodegrade.

GREEN INDICATORS

Environmental claims for products or procedures need to be as specific as possible. Beware of the following terms frequently used to advertise products, for their meanings are vague and confusing:

- Safe
- Nontoxic
- Biodegradable
- Eco-friendly
- Eco-safe
- Environmentally conscious

For example, water can be toxic under certain situations. An item may be biodegradable but in what time frame will it actually be broken down by environmental microbes. Aluminum cans are biodegradable, but it takes approximately 350 years. Food and paper may take decades. "Eco-friendly" and "environmentally conscious" sound warm and fuzzy, but what do they mean?

There are a few programs available that give manufacturers logos indicating a product has a reduced environmental impact. Examples include:

- **Green Seal:** organized in 1989 as a third-party certification program in the United States for products that meet specific standards; is accredited by the American National Standards Institute (see http://www.greenseal.org)
- **EcoLogo:** the Canadian green certification program (see http://www.ecologo.org/en/)
- **LEEDS**: Leadership in Energy and Environmental Design, a certification by a nongovernmental nonprofit group related to the efficient use of water and energy and good air quality
- **Energy Star:** an Environmental Protection Agency (EPA) and Department of Energy program that rates the energy efficiency of products and equipment (see http://www.energystar.gov)
- **DfE certified:** Design for the Environment, an EPA program that allows manufacturers to put the DfE label on household and commercial products such as cleaners and detergents that meet stringent criteria for human and environmental health (see http://www.epa.gov/dfe)

BOX 21-1

EPA's EPP Program of Properties for Quality Green Products

- Minimizes exposure to concentrates
- No ozone depleting substances
- Recyclable packaging
- Recycled content in packaging
- Reduced packaging
- Reduced bioconcentration factor
- Reduced flammability
- Reduced or no added dyes, except when added for safety purposes
- Reduced or no added fragrances
- Reduced or no skin irritants
- Reduced or no volatile organic compounds

- **EPP:** the EPA's Environmentally Preferable Purchasing program that helps governmental agencies purchase "green" products (see http://www.epa.gov/epp)

Box 21-1 shows the desired properties of green products as indicated by the EPA's EPP program. Governmental agencies are required to review these properties when purchasing products.

EVALUATING SPECIFIC INFECTION CONTROL PROCEDURES

Hand Hygiene

Although cloth towels for drying the hands after handwashing are reusable, they also perpetuate contamination. They contain microbes that may not have been washed off the hands. Using a cloth towel once and then washing it could be done, but this doesn't seem very practical. Warm air hand dryers also have problems, as discussed in Chapter 10. Even though paper towels are disposable and will add to the waste stream, they are more appropriate for infection prevention.

Instrument Processing

Proper reprocessing of oral contaminated instruments is an essential component of every dental office's infection control program. Sterilization is an eight-step process: holding/precleaning, cleaning, drying, corrosion and inspection, packaging, sterilization, storage and distribution, and monitoring. The steps involve considerable use of energy, water, chemicals, and packaging materials. Unfortunately, there are limited ways to reduce the impact of sterilization. One might use a reusable instrument packaging material, but do not use plain cloth as a sterilization wrap for it is not a microbial barrier. Also, do not reuse regular sterilization pouches wraps or bags, for these are FDA-cleared products for single use.

Make sure the sterilizer is fully loaded for each run, if possible, to reduce the number of runs and save energy.

Using mechanical methods for cleaning reduces water and chemical use. Some large instrument washers can handle as many as 25 instrument cassettes and are more efficient than ultrasonic cleaners. Because of their large capacity, they usually use less water and chemicals per instrument.

Radiology

Use of digital radiography instead of traditional film-based x-rays would help to reduce the impact on the environment. If using traditional x-rays, recycle fixer and developer solutions and lead foil from x-ray films.

Personal Protective Barriers

Many personal protective equipment (PPE) items are single use and disposable. Gloves and masks are not reusable. Protective eyewear can be cleaned and disinfected. Clinic gowns may be single use or reusable. Some single-use clinic gowns are recyclable. An alternative is to use washable gowns. This, of course, uses energy, chemicals, and water, and requires more labor. Energy Star washers and driers, which are more energy efficient, should be used.

Regulated Medical Waste

Only approximately 3% of waste generated in dental offices is regulated medical waste requiring special holding, neutralizing, and disposal methods (see Chapter 17). That means the remaining 97% can enter the normal waste stream. Some waste materials are biodegradable or can be recycled. Using less means less to throw away.

Environmental Asepsis

Use of physical barriers can protect clinical contact surfaces from contamination. Disinfection will kill and remove potential pathogens. Both have advantages and disadvantages as described in Chapter 13. Most dental offices use a combination of physical barriers and disinfection.

Applied and removed properly, physical barriers will not allow soiling. They are single-use, disposable items and thus increase the amount of waste generated. Do not use regular cloth as a surface barrier, for it is not impervious to moisture. Most physical barriers are plastic, and some that fit over medical devices are regulated by the FDA. Always limit the amount of physical barriers used.

Disinfection involves use of chemicals, PPE, and exposure of patients and practitioners to chemicals. As described previously, disinfectant wipes release less chemical into the environment, but they do add to the waste stream. An acceptable disinfectant should be able to kill *Mycobacterium tuberculosis* var. *bovis* in 10 minutes or less, not be deleterious to surfaces, and be as benign to humans as possible. There are no perfect disinfectants. Be careful that a disinfectant labeled as good for the environment is not just a diluted product. Dilution of the active ingredient usually results in less killing power and a compromise in infection prevention.

Use of Paper

A survey of dental offices reported that 12.8 pages of paper were included in a typical patient chart. By reducing this number to 6, an average office having 2000 patient charts would save 12,600 pages per year. All paper used should be made of chlorine-free pulp with a high recycled content. When possible, all paper should be recycled. Digital patient records could have a positive effect on the amount of paper used.

SUMMARY OF PROCEDURES FOR GREENER INFECTION PREVENTION

Improving the environmental impact of your infection control procedures includes elimination of some practices, using less, or employing a different product or procedure. Table 21-2 lists some ideas about greening the office.

FINAL COMMENTS AND FUTURISTIC THINKING

There are a limited number of changes that dental offices can make in order to reduce their impact on the environment and human safety and health. New materials and processes are developed every day. It is imperative for offices to stay current with emerging developments.

- Do not compromise infection control so you can go green.
- Check the Centers for Disease Control and Prevention (CDC) guidelines and Occupational Safety and Health Administration (OSHA) regulations before making changes in the infection control program.
- Continue to use only EPA-registered disinfectants and appropriate FDA-cleared products.
- Don't reuse items that should be discarded after a single use.

TABLE 21-2   Ideas for Greening the Office

Ideas	Comments
Compare reusables vs. disposables	Make sure the reusable does not compromise infection control and be sure to factor in the increased labor costs to decontaminate the reusables
Increase use of alcohol-based hand rubs vs. handwashing to save water and reduce chemicals in the waste stream	Occasionally wash and rinse hands to remove the build-up of glove materials, dead bacteria, sweat, and other debris that remain with use of hand rubs
Consider disinfectant pump sprays and wipes that may reduce adding chemicals in the waste stream	Disposable surface covers also will reduce chemical use but will increase the waste stream
Increase inventory control and proper mixing of chemicals to reduce discarding of expired/outdated products	Be mindful of the shelf-life (expiration) and in-use dates
Consider recycling plastic, paper, metal, and glass	Depends on what local recycler will accept
Always run full instrument loads through cleaning units and sterilizers to save energy, water, and detergents	Does not apply to emergency needs of a small number of instruments
Purchase supplies that are packaged in recycled materials and have a minimum amount of packaging	May not have a choice of alternative products
Consider digital radiography to reduce use of and exposure to chemicals	Relatively expensive but may pay off in the long run
Recycle foil from x-ray films	Or consider digital
Use refillable soap dispensers and other containers	Make sure to clean out these before refilling as just topping them off will perpetuate any contamination present
Using instrument cassettes may reduce sharps injuries during instrument processing	Make sure the thinner cassettes will not allow sharp or pointed tips of instruments to protrude
Consider using amalgam separators	These eliminate almost all of the mercury from the waste stream
Use energy efficient light bulbs and turn off lights and electrical equipment when not in use	The fluorescent types are approximately 70% more efficient. Incandescent lights lose approximately 90% of the energy they use as heat

SELECTED READINGS

Adams E: Eco-friendly dentistry: not a matter of choice, *J Can Dent Assoc (Tor)* 73:581–583, 2007.

Daschner DF: Environmental protection in hospital infection control, *Am J Infect Control* 28:386–387, 2000.

Eagle A: Clean + green. Instituting a "green" floor care program, *Health Facil Manage* 17:25–28, 2004.

Kelsch N: It IS easy going green (Part 2), *RDH* 30(No. 8):75–76, 2010.

Lee BK, Ellenbecker MJ, Moure-Eraso R: Analyses of the recycling potential of medical plastic wastes, *Waste Manage* 22:161–170, 2002.

Smith M: Waste not. Hospitals reduce, recycle and manage waste, *Healthtexas* 48:10–18, 1992.

Transcedentist: *A dentist for tree huggers.* http://www.springwise.com/eco_sustainability/a_dentist_for_treehuggers. accessed June 2008.

REVIEW QUESTIONS

Multiple Choice

1. What's the main reason one should not use and reuse regular cloth as a sterilization wrap?
   a. Its color will fade.
   b. It will fall apart.
   c. It is not a good microbial barrier.
   d. It will catch on fire.

2. What is the main component of smog?
   a. CO_2
   b. Ozone
   c. Ozone-depleting substances
   d. Chlorine

3. How many pages would the average dental office save in 1 year by reducing the number of pages in patient files by one-half?
   a. 1250
   b. 5500
   c. 12,600
   d. 38,000

4. What percent of waste generated in a dental office is regulated medical waste, thus requiring special handling, neutralization, and disposal?
   a. 3%
   b. 12.5%
   c. 37%
   d. Almost half

5. If you regularly use alcohol-based hand rubs, why should you periodically wash and rinse your hands?
   a. The hand rubs do not kill microbes.
   b. Glove materials and dead bacteria are not removed by the hand rubs.
   c. Handwashing does not dry out your hands.
   d. The hand rubs can dissolve latex gloves.

Please visit http://evolve.elsevier.com/Miller/infectioncontrol/ for additional practice and study support tools.

Cross-contamination Between Work and Home

CHAPTER 22

OUTLINE

Routes of Spread from the Office to Home
  Clothing
  Personal Items, Hands, and Hair
Routes of Spread from Home to the Office
  Work Restrictions

Clothing and Personal Items
Food Preparation and Storage
Taking Lunches or Other Foods to Work
General Home Hygiene

LEARNING OBJECTIVES

After completing this chapter, the student should be able to do the following:

1. Describe how microbes from work can be carried home.
2. List some diseases of health care workers that would preclude them from caring for patients at work.

3. Describe how microbes from home can be carried to work and how to keep food safe during preparation and storage.
4. List several ways to reduce cross-contamination in kitchens and bathrooms.

KEY TERMS

Common-touch Surfaces
Cross-contamination

Food Safety
Personal Protective Equipment

Work Restrictions

We all know that microbes are everywhere, and one aspect of infection prevention is to reduce their spread to other sites by trying to keep them in their place. The other chapters in this book concentrate on reducing the spread of microbes within the office, but here we look at the potential for cross-contamination between work and home. The overriding rule here is to reduce the number of microbes shared between work and home. Certainly we can't totally eliminate this cross-contamination, but if we become aware of the routes of spread, we can apply prevention techniques to keep this at a minimal level.

ROUTES OF SPREAD FROM THE OFFICE TO HOME

Clothing

Chapters 10 and 11 show how dental workers become contaminated while caring for patients at work. If that contamination

is not properly managed, we'll take it wherever we go. This is why one of the rules of the Occupational Safety and Health Administration (OSHA)'s Bloodborne Pathogens Standard states "all personal protective equipment shall be removed before leaving the workplace." Another rule addresses this concern by requiring the use of personal protective equipment at work to cover work clothes, street clothes, and undergarments, in addition to skin, eyes, mouth, and other mucous membranes. So, protective clothing (the other layer worn in the office when there is a chance for contamination with patient fluids) is not to be worn home or anywhere out of the office. Thus the outer layer, whatever it is (e.g., scrubs, gown, uniform, lab coat), needs to be removed before leaving the office.

Another OSHA rule requires employers to be responsible for cleaning and maintaining personal protective equipment. This means that contaminated personal protective clothing cannot be taken home and laundered. It needs to be laundered in the office or sent out to a medical laundry service.

Personal Items, Hands, and Hair

Although shoes are not considered as protective clothing, their soles do become grossly contaminated, which is why shoe covers are used in some hospital environments. Commonly, after a hard day at work, one relaxes a few minutes at home in an easy chair with the feet propped up. This places the shoes at eye level for toddlers who may play with them or even chew on them as we doze off. This can also happen when we take off our shoes and leave them on the floor. Although shoe covers could be used at work, the concept of having work shoes and leaving them at work is another option.

Anything carried home from the office may be contaminated if not properly stored or handled at the office. These items (e.g., purses, containers, packages, nonprotective outer clothing, boots, garment bags) need to be kept in nonclinical areas at work and not handled with contaminated hands. When these items are taken home, do not place them any place where food is prepared or eaten or where children may play with them.

Of course, hands need to be washed before leaving work. If alcohol-based hand rubs are commonly used throughout the day, it's a good idea to actually wash and rinse your hands at the end of the workday to remove accumulated materials. One's hair can become contaminated at work with aerosols and spatter material, but wearing a hair cover is more common during some surgical procedures than during routine dentistry. Routinely washing your hair at home is a good idea.

ROUTES OF SPREAD FROM HOME TO THE OFFICE

Work Restrictions

If you're sick, especially with a respiratory or skin disease, stay home from work. The Centers for Disease Control and Prevention (CDC) has suggested work restrictions for health care personnel infected with or exposed to certain microbes. These specific restrictions and their durations are detailed in Table 1 of "Guidelines for Infection Control in Dental Health-Care Facilities–2003," which can be found at http://www.cdc.gov/mmwr/preview/mmwrhtml/rr5217a1.htm. A summary of the CDC suggestions for restriction from patient contact include those health care workers with:

- Conjunctivitis
- Diarrheal disease
- Hepatitis A
- Herpes on the hands
- Measles
- Meningococcal infection
- Mumps
- Pediculosis
- Pertussis
- Rubella
- Active *Staphylococcus aureus* infections
- Group A streptococcal infection
- Active tuberculosis
- Chickenpox
- Shingles

Clothing and Personal Items

Wear clean clothes to work. Personal items taken in from home (e.g., purses, gifts, food, lunch containers, packages, nonprotective outer clothing, boots, and garment bags) should not be taken into the clinical areas at work.

Food Preparation and Storage

Food prepared at home is often taken to work for lunch or parties. Because foodborne illnesses can occur with improper preparation or storage, care must be taken for the safety of yourself, your work colleagues, and your family. A famous case of foodborne illness in the home was that involving "Typhoid Mary" (Mary Mallon) who was a private household cook and asymptomatic carrier of *Salmonella*. She gave typhoid fever to 51 people (3 of whom died) over the course of her career in the early twentieth century. More recently, in 2011, whole cantaloupes were implicated in one of the deadliest foodborne outbreaks in the United States. The cantaloupes were contaminated with *Listeria monocytogenes* during processing and packaging at a farm in Colorado. The outbreak involved 146 people with 30 deaths in 28 states.

Most raw foods are contaminated with varying levels of microbes, and foods that haven't been thoroughly cleaned or through some heat process are still contaminated when they reach our homes and kitchens. For example, if good quality ground beef is left wrapped and unused in the refrigerator, it will eventually spoil. This occurs because bacteria contaminating the outside of the meat used to prepare the product are ground into the meat and will slowly grow and break down (spoil) the meat. Unopened milk kept in the refrigerator will eventually spoil from growth of the naturally occurring bacteria present. Unopened packages of bread will eventually mold because of the contaminating fungi. The following are some general suggestions for food safety:

- Clean (removing microbes from the surfaces helps prevent their spread to other surfaces).
  - Wash hands frequently especially after handling fresh meats.
  - Wash countertops, utensils, dishes, and cutting boards after each use.
  - Use paper towels or a clean cloth to wipe surfaces and spills.
  - As an extra precaution, use a kitchen cleaning/disinfecting agent on surfaces.
  - If using a sanitizing wipe, use one wipe for one surface. Don't use one wipe for all surfaces as you may be transferring microbes from one surface to the next.
  - Rinse fresh fruits and vegetables with running water but don't use soap, bleach, or commercial produce

washes. A produce brush can be used on firm produce like cucumbers and melons.

- Don't wash meats as this can spread bacteria found on their surfaces and in their juices to nearby areas through splashing.
- Separate (separating foods from each other helps prevent cross-contamination)
  - Use separate cutting boards and plates for produce, meat, poultry, seafood, and eggs.
  - Keep meat, poultry, seafood and eggs and their juices away from ready-to-eat foods during preparation, in the grocery bags, and in the refrigerator.
- Cook (contaminated food is safe only after it has been heated to high enough temperatures to kill harmful bacteria).
  - Use a food thermometer and cook food to appropriate temperatures (Table 22-1).
  - Keep foods hot after cooking until eaten or properly stored.
  - Microwave food thoroughly to 74° C (165° F). Stir in the middle of the heating process. If the food label says to "let stand for x minutes after cooking," do it. This helps the food cook more completely. After microwaving, use a food thermometer to confirm a temperature of at least 74° C (165° F).
- Chill (at room temperature, some bacteria can double in numbers every 20 minutes; the higher the number of bacteria consumed, the greater the chances of becoming sick; cold temperatures prevent or slow down multiplication of most bacteria).

- Refrigerate perishable foods as soon as possible within a maximum of 2 hours—1 hour if the temperature is 32° C (90° F) or higher.
- Never thaw or marinate foods on the counter at room temperature. The safest way is to thaw in the refrigerator. Frozen items can be placed in a water-tight plastic bag and submerged in cold water changing the water every 30 minutes. For faster thawing, place in a microwave following manufacturer's instructions for thawing. Foods thawed in cold water or the microwave should be cooked immediately. Alternatively, frozen foods can be cooked without thawing, but this requires much longer cooking time.
- Chill foods using shallow containers to promote more rapid even cooling.
- Remember, refrigerated foods can still spoil, but frozen foods may remain safe indefinitely. Table 22-2 presents some safe time limits for refrigerated food.
- Smart serving (serving food improperly can contribute to unnecessary contamination).
  - When serving food for an office party or buffet, distribute the food in small platters, and when needed, set out fresh platters of food that have been stored hot or cold. Don't add fresh food to a platter that already had food in it, for that platter and remaining food may be contaminated from sitting out and possibly touched by several people.
  - When serving snacks (e.g., cubed cheese, uncooked broccoli or carrots, peanuts, mints, etc.), provide toothpicks or small spoons for self-serving to prevent people from using their fingers.
  - Covering food that has been set out for serving keeps airborne contamination at a minimum.

TABLE 22-1 Cooking Temperatures for Some Foods

Food	Minimum Internal Temperature*
Ground beef, pork, veal, or lamb	71° C (160° F)
Poultry	74° C (165° F)
Egg dishes	71° C (160° F)
Leftovers and casseroles	74° C (165° F)
Fresh pork/ham, stakes, roasts, chops	63° C (145° F) + let stand 3 minutes
Precooked ham (reheat)	60° C (140° F)
Fin fish	63° C (145° F)
Shrimp, lobster, crab	Cook until flesh is pearly and opaque
Clams, oysters, mussels	Cook until shells open during cooking
Scallops	Cook until flesh is milky white or opaque and firm

*As measured with a food thermometer.
From http://www.foodsafety.gov/keep/charts/mintemp/html.

Taking Lunches or Other Foods to Work

Because foods taken to the office usually won't be eaten for a while, take special precautions to keep them safe. Use the above guidelines for preparing foods and always keep everything involved in preparation clean—hands, utensils, containers, surfaces, fruits, vegetables, etc.

It's fine to prepare the food the night before and store the packed lunch in the refrigerator.

Prepare cooked food ahead of time to allow for thorough chilling in the refrigerator. Keep hot foods hot by using an insulated bottle. Keep cold foods cold by using an insulated lunch box or container along with a frozen gel pack or frozen juice box. Store the food in a refrigerator (if available) at work. When finished eating, throw away the perishable leftovers, and don't reuse the packaging. If using a microwave to reheat lunches, heat to 74° C (165° F), and carefully follow any heating instructions on prepackaged items.

General Home Hygiene

Reducing the spread of microbes in the home may help reduce their carryover to the workplace. Remember that as

TABLE 22-2   **Storage Times for Refrigerator and Freezer**

Category	Food	Refrigerator at 60° C (140° F) or above	Freezer at −18° C (0° F) or below
Salads	Egg, chicken, ham, tuna, macaroni	3 to 5 days	Does not freeze well
Hot dogs	Opened package	1 week	1 to 2 months
	Unopened package	2 weeks	1 to 2 months
Luncheon meats	Opened package or deli sliced	3 to 5 days	1 to 2 months
Bacon	Bacon	7 days	1 to 2 months
Sausage	Raw sausage—chicken, turkey, pork, beef	1 to 2 days	1 to 2months
Ground meats	Hamburger, ground beef, turkey, veal, pork, lamb, and mixtures of them	1 to 2 days	3 to 4 months
Fresh beef, veal, lamb, pork	Steaks	3 to 5 days	6 to 12 months
	Chops	3 to 5 days	4 to 6 months
	Roasts	3 to 5 days	4 to 12months
Fresh poultry	Chicken or turkey, whole	1 to 2 days	1 year
	Chicken or turkey, pieces	1 to 2 days	9 months
Soups and stews	Vegetable or meat added	3 to 4 days	2 to 3 months
Leftovers	Cooked meat and poultry	3 to 4 days	2 to 6 months
	Chicken nuggets or patties	3 to 4 days	1 to 3 months
	Pizza	3 to 4 days	1 to 2 months

From http://www.foodsafety.gov/keep/charts/mintemp/html.

in health care facilities, hands are very common microbe spreaders in the home.

Here are some suggestions:

- Wash or sanitize your hands after you come home from public places. Also, wash your hands before preparing foods or eating, before placing your hands in multiuse snack bags, after blowing your nose, after toilet use, and between handling uncooked fruits, vegetables, and raw meats.
- Keep all floors clean/vacuumed—more frequently if babies and toddlers in the home crawl, lie, and sit on the floors.
- Dust frequently.
- Keep common-touch surfaces (e.g., drawer/cabinet/door knobs and latches, refrigerator/freezer/toilet handles, dishes, utensils, dials, and switches) clean.
- If you're sick with a respiratory infection, such as the common cold or flu, let others help you in the kitchen, if possible, and reduce contacting those common-touch surfaces. If sneezing or coughing, cover your mouth and nose with a handkerchief or facial tissue.
- After sneezing, coughing, or blowing your nose, place the used tissues directly in a plastic bag or paper sack

for discarding rather than letting them lie around for someone else to pick up.

- Don't share drinking glasses or eating utensils.
- Don't share hand/bath towels, washcloths, back scrubbers, razors, toothbrushes, or other personal items.
- Don't use bar hand soaps.
- Don't just add liquid soap or lotion (i.e., top off) to partially empty dispensers. Wash them before refilling.
- Toilet bowls, sinks, showers and bathtubs need regular cleaning and disinfecting. Work from the "top down" moving from the cleanest to the dirtiest.
- When disinfecting kitchen and bathroom surfaces, clean the surface of visible soil then disinfect.
- Clean/disinfect kitchen countertops after contact with grocery bags and before preparing foods.
- The bottoms of purses are commonly contaminated, so keep them off kitchen countertops.
- Kitchen towels and sponges need to be replaced or washed using hot water and thoroughly dried weekly or sooner if visibly soiled.
- Don't let wet towels lay on the floor to promote mold growth.
- Use plastic liners in all waste containers.
- If injection needles are used (e.g., in diabetes), discard in plastic puncture-resistant containers.

SELECTED READINGS

Association for Professionals in Infection Control and Epidemiologists: *Infection prevention outside the hospital*, http://www.apic.org/For-Consumers/IP- Topics/Article?id=infection-prevention-outside-the-hospital, accessed April 2012.

Centers for Disease Control and Prevention: *Cover your cough*, http://www.cdc.gov/flu/protect/covercough.htm, accessed April 2012.

Centers for Disease Control and Prevention: *Foodborne illnesses*, http://www.cdc.gov/ nceh/vsp/training/videos/transcripts/foodborne .pdf, accessed April 2012.

Larson E, Duarte C: Home hygiene practices and infectious disease symptoms among household members, *Pub Health Nurs* 18(2):116–127, 2001.

U.S. Department of Labor: Occupational Safety and Health Administration: 29 CFR Part 1910.1030: Occupational exposure to blood-borne pathogens: final rule, *Fed Regist* 56:64004–64182, 1991. (actual regulatory text, pp 64175–64182). Available at http:// www.osha.gov/pls/oshaweb/owadisp.show _document?p_table=STANDARDS& p_id=10051, accessed April 2012.

U.S. Food and Drug Administration: *Information on the recalled Jensen farms whole cantaloupes*. updated January 1, 2012, http://www. fda.gov/Food/FoodSafety/CORENetwork/ ucm272372.htmcantelopes. accessed April 2012.

U.S. Department of Health and Human Services: *Food safety*, http://www.foodsafety.gov, accessed April 2012.

REVIEW QUESTIONS

Multiple Choice Questions

1. What minimum temperature should food reach when microwaving?
   a. 38° C (100° F)
   b. 52° C (125° F)
   c. 63° C (145° F)
   d. 74° C (165° F)

2. What does Occupational Safety and Health Administration's Bloodborne Pathogens Standard say about personal protective clothing?
   a. Place it in a garment bag before taking it home for cleaning or laundering.
   b. Remove it before leaving the workplace.
   c. Cover it up with work clothes before leaving the workplace.
   d. Identify one employee to home launder all of the protective clothing for the facility.

3. Which of the following foods should not be washed before eaten or prepared for eating?
   a. Broccoli
   b. Melons
   c. Cucumbers
   d. Raw meats

4. The Centers for Disease Control and Prevention recommends that health care workers with which of the following diseases be restricted from patient contact?
   a. Measles or periodontal disease
   b. Pertussis or dental caries
   c. Diarrheal disease or conjunctivitis
   d. Mumps or periapical infection

5. Which of the following is suggested for reducing cross-contamination in bathrooms?
   a. Clean a surface before disinfecting.
   b. Use bar soaps.
   c. Always "top off" liquid soap containers when they are about half full.
   d. Be sure to rinse out washcloths thoroughly before others use them.

Please visit http://evolve.elsevier.com/Miller/infectioncontrol/ for additional practice and study support tools.

About the Occupational Safety and Health Administration

OUTLINE

Mission of the Occupational Safety and Health Administration

Purposes of the Occupational Safety and Health Administration

Coverage of the OSHA Act

Standards

Standards Development

State Safety and Health Programs

Department of Labor 2011-2016 Strategic Plan

Strategic Challenges

LEARNING OBJECTIVES

After completing this chapter, the student should be able to do the following:

1. Describe the mission statement of the Occupational Safety and Health Administration (OSHA) and list the seven reasons (purposes) why OSHA was formed.
2. List what persons OSHA standards cover.

3. Define an OSHA standard and describe how standards are developed.
4. Discuss state OSHA plans.
5. List the five major points of the OSHA 2011-2016 Strategic Management Plan, and discuss the strategic challenges OSHA faces.

KEY TERMS

Federal Register

National Institute for Occupational Safety and Health (NIOSH)

Occupational Safety and Health Act of 1970

Occupational Safety and Health Administration (OSHA)

OSHA General Duty Clause

Almost 135 million Americans are employed in more than 8.9 million workplace environments. Thirty years ago, more than 14,000 workers died annually because of work-related accidents, almost 2.5 million workers had been disabled while working, and an estimated 300,000 new cases of occupational diseases and injuries occurred each year. Since then, the Occupational Safety and Health Administration (OSHA) has helped to cut workplace fatalities by more than 60% and occupational injury and illness rates by 40%.

The effect of worker injuries in terms of lost productivity and wages, medical expenses, and disability compensation was enormous. Also immense was the amount of human suffering.

In response, Congress passed the Occupational Safety and Health Act of 1970, which became effective in April, 1971. The purpose of the act was "to assure so far as possible every working man and woman in the Nation safe and

healthful working conditions and to preserve our human resources." Under the act, OSHA was created within the Department of Labor (DOL). March, 2013, marks the 100th anniversary of the founding of the DOL.

MISSION OF THE OCCUPATIONAL SAFETY AND HEALTH ADMINISTRATION

OSHA conducts a broad range of programs and activities to promote workplace safety and health and to protect the nation's workers. These programs and activities are based on three strategies.

1. Strong, fair, and effective enforcements
2. Outreach, education, and compliance assistance
3. Partnerships and other cooperative programs

PURPOSES OF THE OCCUPATIONAL SAFETY AND HEALTH ADMINISTRATION

OSHA was formed for several purposes, including the following:

1. Encourage employers and employees to reduce workplace hazards and to implement new or existing safety programs.
2. Provide research in occupational safety and health problems.
3. Establish "separate but dependent responsibilities and rights" for employees and employers to help achieve better working conditions.
4. Maintain a reporting and record keeping system to monitor injuries and illnesses.
5. Establish training programs to increase competence of occupational safety and health personnel.
6. Develop and enforce mandatory job safety and health standards.
7. Provide for the development, analysis, evaluation, and approval of state occupational safety and health programs.

COVERAGE OF THE OSHA ACT

The act covers almost all employers and employees in the United States. Coverage is applied directly by the federal OSHA or through an OSHA-approved state program (in 25 states plus Puerto Rico and the Virgin Islands). The act does not cover self-employed persons, farms worked by family members, and working environments controlled by other federal agencies. States and territories that have approved local plans for private sector occupational safety and health programs must also have a similar program for state and local government employees.

STANDARDS

In general, standards require the employers to do the following:

- Maintain conditions or adopt practices reasonably necessary and appropriate to protect workers on the job.
- Be familiar with and comply with standards applicable to their establishments.
- Ensure that employees have and use personal protective equipment when required for safety and health.

OSHA issues standards for a wide variety of workplace hazards, including the following:

- Toxic substances
- Harmful physical agents
- Electric hazards
- Fall hazards
- Trenching hazards
- Hazardous waste
- Infectious diseases
- Fire and explosion hazards
- Dangerous atmosphere
- Machine hazards

OSHA performs its duties by promulgating legally enforceable standards. Standards may describe conditions or the use of practices, means, methods, or processes that are reasonably necessary and appropriate to protect employees on the job. Standards often are "performance standards" or "performance achievements." For example, 8-hour occupational exposure limits for many chemicals have been identified. The employer is challenged to ensure that exposures are within the stated limits. This is the expected performance. The employer can use a combination of work practices, engineering controls, and personal protective equipment to achieve the goal. OSHA does not require specific equipment or processes; rather, it reviews the outcome of the preventive efforts by the employers and employees.

Employers must be aware of all standards applicable to their work environments; ensure that employees are informed, knowledgeable, and participating in health and safety programs; and provide materials that accomplish the desired protection.

OSHA has produced many standards. However, when a specific standard does not exist for a situation, the OSHA General Duty Clause applies. The clause states that employers "shall furnish…a place of employment which is free from recognized hazards that are causing or are likely to cause death or serious physical harm to their employers." State plans must set standards that are at least as demanding as the federal standards.

Copies of standards are available from several sources. The U.S. Government Printing Office in Washington, DC, sells print and electronic copies (telephone: 202-512-0000). All formative stages of standards, as well as amendments, corrections, insertions, or deletions, appear in the *Federal Register,* which is available in larger libraries. Materials published in the *Federal Register* since 1994 are available electronically (www.gpoaccess.gov/fr/index.html). The Office of the Federal Register annually publishes all current regulations and standards in the *Code of Federal Regulations*, which is available in many libraries.

OSHA regulations are collected in Title 29 of the *Code of Federal Regulations*, Parts 1900-1999. One can order information concerning OSHA regulations (various booklets and lists) from the U.S. Department of Labor, OSHA Publications, PO Box 37535, Washington, DC, 20013-7535; telephone: 800-312-6742. One can download many publications from the OSHA Web site (http://www.osha.gov/pls/publications/pubindex.list). To find contact information about state OSHA offices, go to http://www.osha.gov/dcsp/osp/index.html.

STANDARDS DEVELOPMENT

OSHA can begin the standard promulgation process on its own or in response to petitions from other parties, including other federal agencies, state and local organizations, industry self-regulating groups, employers, labor representatives, or any interested person.

If OSHA determines that a specific standard is needed, it establishes advisory committees. Some are ad hoc; others are standing federal committees. All such committees are composed of governmental workers and members from management, labor, and local agencies. Recommendations also may come from the National Institute for Occupational Safety and Health (NIOSH), a division of the Centers for Disease Control and Prevention, which conducts research on safety and health issues and provides technical assistance to OSHA.

If OSHA wants to propose, amend, or revoke a standard, it publishes its intention in the *Federal Register* as an "Advanced Notice of Proposed Rulemaking" or as a "Notice of Proposed Rulemaking." Advanced notices usually involve solicitation of information that can be used in drafting the proposal. Usually some time period (e.g., 30 to 60 days) is allowed for public response. Interested parties who submit written arguments and pertinent evidence may request a formal public hearing. OSHA always announces the times, dates, and locations of its hearings in the *Federal Register*. A full report on the comment period and the public hearings, if conducted, and a full, final text version of the new (or amended) standard is reported in the *Federal Register*. Accompanying the text is an explanation of the standard and a rationale for its implementation. The date the standard becomes effective also is reported. OSHA also must publish whether the determination resulted in the decision that no standard or amendment was needed.

Under certain conditions, OSHA can authorize an emergency temporary standard. Such standards become effective immediately and remain in effect until a permanent standard is enacted. OSHA must determine that workers are in grave danger and need immediate protection. Emergency standards are published in the *Federal Register* and serve as proposed permanent standards, which undergo the usual review process. Emergency and permanent standards may be challenged in court.

STATE SAFETY AND HEALTH PROGRAMS

State plans are OSHA-approved job safety and health programs operated by individual states instead of the federal OSHA. The Occupational Safety and Health Act of 1970 encourages states to develop and operate their own job safety and health plans and precludes state enforcement of OSHA standards unless the state has an approved plan. OSHA approves and monitors all state plans.

Once a state plan is approved under Section 18(b) of the act, OSHA funds up to 50% of the operating costs of the program. State plans must provide standards and enforcement programs and voluntary compliance activities that are at least as stringent as the federal program. State plans covering the private sector also must cover state and local

government employees. OSHA rules also permit states to develop plans that cover only public sector (state and local government) employees. In these cases, private sector employment remains under federal OSHA jurisdiction.

Twenty-five states, plus Puerto Rico and the Virgin Islands operate approved plans, with six plans covering only the public sector. These states are listed at the following OSHA Web site (http://www.osha.gov/dcsp/osp/index.html) and in Appendix A.

States with approved plans cover most private sector employees and state and local government workers in the state. Federal OSHA continues to cover federal employees and certain other employees specifically excluded by a state plan; for example, those who work in maritime industries and on military bases.

DEPARTMENT OF LABOR 2011-2016 STRATEGIC PLAN

In 2010, the DOL undertook a strategic planning effort focused on developing performance measures and strategies to support a vision of good jobs for everyone. That vision was further defined by 5 strategic goals with 14 outcomes.

1. Goal 1: Prepare workers for good jobs and ensure fair compensation.
   - Increase workers' incomes and narrow wage and income inequality.
   - Assure skills and knowledge that prepare workers to succeed in a knowledge-based economy, including in high growth and emerging industry sectors like "green" jobs.
   - Help workers who are in low wage jobs or out of the labor market find a path into middle class jobs.
   - Help middle class families remain in the middle class.
   - Secure wages and overtime.
   - Foster acceptable work conditions and respect for workers' rights in the global economy to provide workers with a fair share of productivity and protect vulnerable people.
2. Ensure workplaces are safe and healthy.
   - Secure safe and healthy workplaces, particularly in high-risk industries.
3. Assure fair and high quality work-life environments.
   - Break down barriers to fair and diverse workplaces so that every worker's contribution is respected.
   - Provide workplace flexibility for family and personal caregiving.
   - Ensure worker voice in the workplace.
4. Secure health benefits, and for those not working, provide income security.
   - Facilitate return to work for workers experiencing workplace injuries or illnesses who are able to work.
   - Ensure income support when work is impossible or unavailable.
   - Improve health benefits and retirement security for all workers.

5. Produce timely and accurate data on the economic conditions of workers and their families.
   • Provide sound and impartial information on labor market activity, working conditions, and price changes in the economy for decision making, including support for the formulation of economic and social policy affecting virtually all Americans.

STRATEGIC CHALLENGES

Since OSHA was created in 1971, the workplace fatality rate among employees has decreased by 60% and occupational injury and illness rates have declined by 40%. At the same time, private sector employment in the United States and the number of workplaces have doubled.

Today, OSHA oversees 135 million workers at 8.9 million establishments.

The decrease in fatalities, injuries, and illnesses across such an expanding population of workers indicates remarkable progress. However, there were 1202 employee deaths in 2010-2011, a slight increase from the 2009-2010 total of 1193. Fatalities related to highway incidents and homicides increased, whereas deaths related to falls decreased.

Safety and health hazards exist in varying degrees and forms throughout the population. Some occupations, such as construction and manufacturing, are inherently more hazardous than others. However, less-obvious hazards, such as injuries caused by ergonomic factors and exposure to dangerous substances, pose subtle yet serious threats in a wider cross-section of occupations and industries.

SELECTED READINGS

Department of Labor: *Strategic Plan for Fiscal Years 2011-2016*, at http://www.dol.gov/_sec/stratplan/. accessed April 2012.

Miller CH: Complying with OSHA, *Dent Prod Rep* 41:82, 84, 86, 88. 2007.

Occupational Safety and Health Administration: *All about OSHA, Occupational Safety and Health Administration*, http://osha.gov/about.html. accessed April 2012.

Occupational Safety and Health Administration: *Regional federal and state fatality/catastrophe weekly report ending September 24, 2011*, http://www.osha.gov/dep/fatcat/fatcat_regional_rpt_09242011.html. accessed April 2012.

Palenik CJ, Miller CH: All about OSHA, part I, *Dent Asepsis Rev* 18:1–2, 1997.

Palenik CJ, Miller CH: All about OSHA, part II, *Dent Asepsis Rev* 18:1–4, 1997.

REVIEW QUESTIONS

Multiple Choice

1. How many states have approved OSHA plans?
   a. 6
   b. 10
   c. 16
   d. 26
   e. 39

2. The Occupational Safety and Health Administration was created in
   a. 1959
   b. 1965
   c. 1971
   d. 1980
   e. 1986

3. Can an interested party, like a dental assistant, start the process through which OSHA promulgates standards?
   a. Yes
   b. No

4. The Occupational Safety and Health Administration funds up to what percent of each state-approved plan?
   a. 5%
   b. 15%
   c. 50%
   d. 75%
   e. 100%

5. Since OSHA was created in 1971, the workplace occupational injury and illness rates have declined by:
   a. 5%
   b. 10%
   c. 20%
   d. 40%
   e. 80%

Please visit http://evolve.elsevier.com/Miller/infectioncontrol/ for additional practice and study support tools.

OUTLINE

LEARNING OBJECTIVES

After completing this chapter, the learner should be able to:

1. Describe OSHA's legal mandate to protect employees in the workplace and its inspection priorities.
2. List the OSHA standards that apply to dentistry.
3. Outline why and how OSHA conducts workplace inspections and describe the possible outcomes of an inspection.
4. Identify ways that dental offices can proactively prepare for an OSHA inspection.

KEY TERMS

Abatement

Catastrophes and Fatal Accidents

Complaints and Referrals

De minimis Violation

Failure to Abate Violation

Follow-up Inspections

General Duty Clause

Imminent Danger

Notice of Intent to Contest

Occupation Safety and Health Administration (OSHA)

Occupational Safety and Health Act of 1970 (The Act)

Organization for Safety, Asepsis and Prevention (OSAP)

Other-than-serious Violation

Programmed Inspections

Repeated Violation

Serious Violation

Standards

Willful Violation

ABOUT OSHA

Under the Occupational Safety and Health Act of 1970 (The Act), the Occupational Safety and Health Administration (OSHA) is authorized to conduct workplace inspections and investigations to determine whether employers are complying with standards issued by the agency for safer and healthier workplaces. OSHA monitors the safety and health of almost all workers in the United States. More information about OSHA is given in Chapter 23.

OSHA performs its duties by promulgation of legally enforceable standards. Standards may describe conditions or the use of practices, means, methods, or processes that are reasonably necessary and appropriate to protect employees in the workplace. Standards are often performance based—mandating achievement of a specific goal. For example, it is the responsibility of an employer to protect employees from patient body fluids in dental environments. The employer is challenged to protect the employees as much as possible.

One section of The Act, often referred to as the General Duty Clause, is a broad statement designed to cover all events and locations. The General Duty Clause requires employers to "furnish to each of his employees employment and a place of employment which is free from recognized hazards that are causing or are likely to cause death or serious physical harm to his employees." The General Duty Clause requires employers to "comply with occupational safety and health standards promulgated under this Act" and for each employee to comply with occupational safety and health standards and all rules, regulations, and orders issued pursuant to this Act that are applicable to their actions and conduct.

INSPECTION PRIORITIES

In OSHA's system of inspection priorities, the worst situations go first. OSHA priorities are listed in the following order:

- **Imminent danger**. The first priority investigates the reasonable certainty that a danger exists that could cause death or serious physical harm unless eliminated.
- **Catastrophes and fatal accidents**. The second priority goes to investigations of fatalities and accidents resulting in a death or hospitalization of three or more employees.
- **Complaints and referrals**. The third priority deals with formal employee complaints of unsafe or unhealthy working conditions and referrals from any source (including patients) about a workplace hazard.
- **Programmed inspections**. The fourth priority is aimed at specific high-hazard industries, workplaces, and occupations or health substances or other industries identified in OSHA's current inspection procedures.
- **Follow-up inspections**. The fifth priority determines if an employer has corrected previously cited violations.

APPLICABLE STANDARDS FOR DENTISTRY

There are currently no specific standards for dentistry. However, exposure to numerous biological, chemical, environmental, physical, and psychological workplace hazards that may apply to dentistry are addressed in specific standards for the general industry. For more extensive information, visit http://www.osha.gov/SLTC/dentistry/index.html.

The following standards, in order, were the most frequently cited by the federal OSHA from October 2010 through September 2011, in the Offices and Clinics of Dentists Industry Group (NAICS Code 621210):

1. Bloodborne pathogens
2. Hazard communication
3. Electrical, general requirements
4. Personal protective equipment, general requirements
5. Medical services and first aid
6. Wiring methods, components, and equipment for general use
7. Eye and face protection
8. Portable fire extinguishers
9. Forms
10. Formaldehyde

The following standards, in order, were the most frequently cited by the federal OSHA from October 2010 through September 2011, in the Medical and Dental Laboratories Industry Group (NAICS Code 621511):

1. Bloodborne pathogens
2. Hazard communication
3. Forms
4. General recording criteria
5. Walking–working surfaces, general requirements
6. Maintenance, safeguards, and operational features for exit routes
7. Formaldehyde
8. Guarding floor and wall openings and holes
9. Eye and face protection
10. Electrical, general requirements

WHAT DOES THE INSPECTION PROCESS INVOLVE?

The Complaint

The Act gives employees the right to file complaints about workplace safety and health hazards. Furthermore, The Act gives complainants the right to request that employers do not know their names. OSHA takes complaints from employees and their representatives seriously. Other interested parties (such as patients) can also make a formal complaint about a dental office concerning any OSHA standard.

To report hazards at a worksite to OSHA, or to report possible discrimination against an employee based on safety and health issues, the following options are available:

- File a complaint online at http://www.osha.gov/pls/osha7/eComplaintForm.html. *Note:* Most online complaints go through OSHA's phone/fax system. An OSHA-7 form will need to be completed. The issues presented may be resolved informally over the phone with the employer (off-site investigation). If the person reporting the complaint is concerned about confidentiality, the complaint should be filed from a home computer or a computer in the local library.
- Download and print the OSHA *complaint form,* complete it, and then fax or mail it to the local OSHA *regional office.* A person can also contact the local OSHA office to receive a copy of the complaint form. When completing the form, the persons filing the complaint must be sure to include their names, addresses, and telephone numbers so that OSHA can contact them. The OSHA regional office staff can address any complaints and respond to any questions.
- Written, signed complaints submitted to OSHA are more likely to result in on-site OSHA inspections. Complaints from workers in states with OSHA-approved plans also involve the state agency.
- A discrimination complaint should be filed if an employer has punished an employee for exercising any *employee rights* established under the OSHA Act

or for *refusing to work* when faced with an imminent danger of death or serious injury and there is insufficient time for OSHA to inspect. A complaint can be filed by calling the local OSHA regional office. In states with approved state plans, employees may file a complaint with both the state and federal OSHA.

In the event of an emergency or if the hazard is immediately life threatening, the local OSHA regional office or 1-800-321-OSHA should be contacted.

OSHA Responds to the Complaint

Depending on the circumstances, OSHA will respond in one of three ways to the complaint. OSHA will:

1. stage no inquiry,
2. stage an inquiry, or
3. conduct an on-site inspection.

Before beginning an inspection, the OSHA staff must be able to determine from the complaint that there are reasonable grounds to believe that a violation of an OSHA standard or a safety or health hazard exists. If OSHA has information indicating the employer is aware of the hazard and is correcting it, the agency may not conduct an inspection after obtaining the necessary documentation from the employer.

Complaint inspections are generally limited to the hazards listed in the complaint, although citation of other violations in plain sight may occur as well. The inspector may decide to expand the inspection based on the inspector's professional judgment or on conversations with workers.

Inspections of complaints do not occur on a "first come, first served" basis. OSHA ranks complaints based on the severity of the alleged hazard and the number of employees exposed. That is why review of lower-priority complaints uses the phone/fax method rather than on-site inspections.

On-site Inspection

The Act authorizes OSHA to conduct workplace inspections to enforce standards. Usually, on-site inspections occur unannounced. Inspections often involve failure by an employer to provide an adequate response to an inquiry from OSHA. Inspections are the last option, and OSHA considers any inspection to be a serious issue.

Prior to an inspection, involved OSHA personnel will become familiar with as many important facts as possible about the workplace, such as its inspection history, the nature of the business, and the particular standards that might apply. OSHA compliance officers are professionally educated in safety and industrial hygiene. An OSHA inspection involves an opening conference, a walk-through review, and a closing conference.

OSHA usually does not have a warrant for an inspection when its inspectors first arrive. If challenged, OSHA will not conduct a warrantless inspection without the employer's permission, but the OSHA representative will return with a warrant or its equivalent based on administrative probable cause.

If an OSHA inspector arrives to conduct an inspection, the inspector will likely follow the procedures listed here.

- Before an inspection, the inspector will conduct an opening conference during which the purpose of the visit and what to expect during the inspection are explained.
- The inspector will ensure that an employee representative is present at the opening conference.
- After the opening conference, the inspector will conduct a walk-through inspection for safety and health hazards.
- A workplace representative must accompany the inspector during the walk-through.
- After the inspection, the inspector conducts a closing conference with office personnel during which the inspector will provide a copy of *Employer Rights and Responsibilities Following an OSHA Inspection, OSHA 3000-08R* (http://www.osha.gov/Publications/osha3000.pdf).
- The closing conference will also include a discussion of all unsafe or unhealthy conditions observed during the inspection and citations that may result. Finally, the inspector explains the appeals process.
- After the closing conference, workplace personnel should meet to discuss what events occurred and to plan for action as needed.

During an Inspection

There are several things to keep in mind during an unannounced OSHA inspection, including the following:

- Ask the inspector for credentials (a badge or identification card) specifying that the person is an agent of OSHA.
- Ensure the inspector has a warrant.
- Answer all questions truthfully, without directly admitting guilt.
- Never knowingly give false information or intentionally mislead an inspector. If you cannot answer a question, explain that you are uncertain and will look for an answer.
- Stay with the inspector at all times.
- Photographically record all areas inspected.
- Correct all identified violations immediately if possible.
- Do not offer information unless asked.
- Do not talk about accidents or incidents that have occurred in the past, unless specifically asked to do so.
- Be courteous. Do not be rude to or argue with the inspector.
- Ask the inspector for a receipt for any documents provided.
- Take notes of any problems identified by the inspector and record any abatement procedures.

WHAT ARE THE POSSIBLE OUTCOMES OF AN INSPECTION?

After the OSHA inspector reports his or her findings to the office, the area director will determine what violations, if any, were present. If the director determines violations are present, OSHA will issue citations and give the employer a reasonable time for abatement of the violations. Employers have the right to contest a citation.

If an employer agrees with the citation, the employer must correct the situation by the date set and pay the penalty (if any). Employers who do not agree with the citation must submit a written petition (Notice of Intent to Contest) within 15 days of the citation to the OSHA Review Commission. The Notice must identify which of the following is being addressed: disagreement with the citation, penalty, or abatement. Some hazards take quite a while to resolve, so the complainant can at this time ask to have more abatement time (90 days or more).

More than 90% of OSHA inspections of dental offices involve complaints about the Blood-borne Pathogens and Hazard Communication Standards. Table 24-1 identifies the standards cited by federal OSHA for dental offices and clinics during the period from October 2010 through September 2011. Citations exceed inspections because violations can come from different components of the same standard. Inspections involved 41 locations, but often for more than 1 standard violation.

The following general information defines the types of violations and explains the action an office may take if receiving a citation because of an inspection.

- **Willful violation.** The employer knew that a hazardous condition (which violated a standard) existed but made no reasonable effort to eliminate it.
- **Serious violation.** A violation is categorized as "serious" when a workplace hazard exists that could cause injury or illness that would most likely result in death or serious physical harm, unless the employer did not know or could not have known of the violation.
- **Other-than-serious violation.** A situation in which the most serious injury or illness that would most

TABLE 24-1   **Standards Cited by Federal OSHA for Dental Offices and Clinics During the Period From October 2010 Through September 2011**

Standard Type	Number of Inspections*	Number of Citations†	Penalties ($)‡
Bloodborne pathogens	36	141	155,743
Hazard communication	16	36	28,915
General requirements, electrical	4	6	9275
Medical services and first aid	3	3	3202
Posting of notices, availability of The Act	1	1	0
Guarding the floor and wall opening and holes	1	1	1530
Eye and face protection	3	3	4790
Wiring problems, components, and equipment for general use	2	3	2800
Walking–working surfaces	2	2	0
General requirement, personal protection equipment	4	5	9000
Portable fire extinguishers	1	2	900
Forms	3	3	0
Formaldehyde	1	2	1428
Hand protection	1	1	0
General requirement, all machines	1	1	2550
General duty	2	2	2380
Totals	41	212	222,531

*Inspections represent the number of inspections in which the specified standard was cited. For the total line, it represents the number of inspections in which one or more citations were issued. Note that the total is not the sum of the number of inspections associated with each standard cited; multiple standards may be cited in one inspection.
†Number of citations represents the number of times the specified standard was cited. The number in the total line is the sum of the number of citations for each standard.
‡The penalty represents the total penalty amount, in dollars, currently assessed for the specified citations. The number in the total line is the sum of the penalty for each standard. The amounts reflect what exists at the current time, taking into consideration any settlement action adjustments that may have occurred.
Adapted from http://www.osha.gov/pls/imis/citedstandard.sic?p_esize=&p_state=FEFederal&p_sic=8021.

likely occur from the hazardous condition cannot reasonably cause death or serious illness.

- *De minimis* violation. Violations that have no direct or immediate relationship to safety or health.
- Failure to abate violation. Exists when the employer has not corrected a violation for which OSHA has issued a citation and the abatement date has passed or was covered under the settlement agreement.
- Repeated violation. Repeated violations can occur when a preciously cited condition exists upon a revisit.

Violation types have penalty guidelines. Sometimes after, or other times concurrently with the issuance of a citation and within reasonable time after the inspection, the local OSHA director will inform the employer of the proposed penalty. In some cases, there is no penalty. OSHA reserves the right to assign penalties even if there has been a prompt abatement by the employer.

PROACTIVE THINKING

There are steps to prepare (or even better, prevent) a workplace for an unexpected visit from an OSHA inspector. The steps include:

- Establish regular office meetings to discuss safety and health and to seek employee feedback cornering OSHA-related issues.
- Join the Organization for Safety, Asepsis and Prevention (OSAP) (http://www.osap.org or telephone: 800-298-6727), a nonprofit organization dedicated to helping dental professions with their infection control and occupational safety and health needs. OSAP offers training, answers to technical questions, print materials, a comprehensive website, and much more (see Appendix D).
- Make sure the required OSHA poster, Job Safety and Health Protections—It's the Law, OSHA Poster 3165 (http://www.osha.gov/Publications/poster.html) is displayed in an area accessible to all employees.
- Identify, make available, and review all OSHA standards that apply to the employees.
- Ensure that all required written programs, documents, and employee records are current.
- Monitor safety and health compliance in-house.
- Designate a workplace safety coordinator.
- Identify the person who needs to be present if there is an OSHA inspection.
- Make sure that employee training concerning OSHA standards is current, recorded, and correct.
- Regularly review employee records required by OSHA.
- Designate duties for all employees in the event of an inspection.

SELECTED READINGS

Miller CH: Standard procedure: complying with OSHA, *Dent Prod Rep* 41:82, 84, 86 and 88. 2007.

Occupational Safety and Health Administration: *Dentistry—OSHA standards*, http://www.osha.gov/SLTC/dentistry/index.html. accessed April 2012.

Occupational Safety and Health Administration: *OSHA inspections*, http://www.osha.gov/Publications/osha2098.pdf. accessed April 2012.

Occupational Safety and Health Administration: *Fact sheet-OSHA inspections*, http://www-.osha.gov/OshDoc/data_General_Facts/fact sheet-inspections.pdf. accessed April 2012.

Occupational Safety and Health Administration: *How to file a complaint with OSHA*, http://www.osha.gov/as/opa/worker/complain.html. accessed April 2012.

Occupational Safety and Health Administration: *Standards cited for SIC 802 (dental offices and clinics of dentists), all sizes, federal—OSHA standards*, http://www.osha.gov/pls/imis/citedstandard.sic?p_esize=&p_state=FEFederal&p_sic=802. accessed June 2008.

Palenik CJ: Complying with OSHA standards, *Inside Dent* 2:78–81, 2006.

REVIEW QUESTIONS

Multiple Choice

1. Which of the following best describes an OSHA standard?
   a. A strong recommendation
   b. A regulation (law)
   c. Involves only health care workplaces
   d. Does not apply in all states

2. Which of the following has the top priority concerning OSHA inspections?
   a. Serious violation
   b. Willful violation
   c. Imminent danger violation
   d. Catastrophes and fatal accidents

3. What standard causes the greatest number of OSHA inspections of dental offices?
   a. Hazard communication
   b. Sanitation
   c. General duty clause
   d. Bloodborne pathogens

4. Can an OSHA inspection not result in a penalty?
   a. Yes
   b. No

5. Who can file a complaint with OSHA about a dental office?
   a. Only employees
   b. Only patients
   c. Any interested party
   d. Only employers

Please visit http://evolve.elsevier.com/Miller/infectioncontrol/ for additional practice and study support tools.

Management of the Office Safety Program

OUTLINE

LEARNING OBJECTIVES

After completing this chapter, the student should be able to do the following:

1. Describe the position and duties of an office safety coordinator.
2. Describe the importance of and give examples of written step-by-step safety procedures and list the safety documents, policy statements, and records needed by a dental office.
3. Design a program to evaluate infection control in the office.
4. Describe the general nature of a checklist that can be used to organize and assess infection control procedures in the office.

KEY TERMS

Safety Coordinator

Exposure Control Plan

Infection Control Overkill

Material Safety Data Sheets

Office Safety Coordinator

Practicing infection control procedures, managing hazardous materials and regulated medical waste, and ensuring safety against fire and storms are referred to collectively as office safety. The office safety aspects of dentistry are expanding rapidly, with new and revised regulations and recommendations appearing frequently. New asepsis or other safety products and equipment continually appear on the market, and advances in research are bringing new concepts and approaches to controlling the spread of disease agents.

Today, dental practices face the challenge of finding a way to maintain and implement an effective, efficient, and affordable office safety program.

SAFETY COORDINATOR

Management of the multifaceted office safety program is facilitated if the employer identifies one person in the office to organize and supervise office safety. Such a **safety** coordinator works under the guidance of the employer and could be a hygienist or a dental assistant.

The safety coordinator must have a basic understanding of microbiology and the modes of disease spread in the office, infection prevention and other safety procedures, and products and equipment used with these procedures, and also must know the related state and federal regulations. Extra training may be necessary at the time of initial assignment to the position, and continuing education is important so that the person can keep up with changes. The safety coordinator also should possess good written and verbal communication skills and good organizational skills, and must be given time to perform the duties related to office safety.

MANAGEMENT DUTIES

Box 25-1 lists duties involved in managing the office safety program. Although the employer is responsible for all of these duties, most, if not all, can be delegated to the safety coordinator. Chapter 8 provides a review of steps to take to comply with the Occupational Safety and Health Administration (OSHA) Bloodborne Pathogens Standard.

The office safety coordinator and employer should develop a written personnel health program for the office workers that includes policies, procedures, and guidelines for education and training; immunizations; exposure prevention and postexposure management; medical conditions, work-related illnesses, and associated work restrictions; contact dermatitis and latex allergy; and maintenance of records, data management, and confidentiality.

DEVELOPMENT OF STEP-BY-STEP PROCEDURES

Establishing written step-by-step procedures, much like those presented in some chapters of this book, help to ensure compliance with and understanding of office safety procedures. Writing down the steps allows proper organization of the procedures, documents their existence, and enhances learning by providing material that one may review periodically in the office, particularly dust on horizontal surfaces in the operating and waiting rooms.

Chapter 19 gives an example of an overall clinical asepsis protocol that describes step-by-step procedures to be performed before seating the patient, during patient care, and after patient care. The protocol presented may not apply to all practices and should be changed to relate specifically to each office.

Review Regulations and Advances

After reviewing all of the current regulations from local, state, and federal agencies, the office safety coordinator should maintain continuing education in this and related areas. The coordinator should establish contacts with or review educational material from organizations such as

---

BOX 25-1

Office Safety Management Duties

- Continually review infection control, hazardous materials, and other office safety regulations.
- Prepare, review, and update the office exposure control plan, infection control procedures manual, hazard communication program, personnel health program, tuberculosis infection control plan, and other safety procedures for the office.
- Develop protocols that provide step-by-step procedures to follow in practicing office safety.
- Provide new and continuing team members with initial and updated training on all office safety policies and procedures.
- Ensure that the janitorial staff has received proper training related to personal protection during office cleaning procedures.
- Monitor compliance with office safety procedures and related regulations.
- Organize and manage procedures for hepatitis B vaccination of new team members and procedures for postexposure medical evaluation and follow-up.
- Review circumstances surrounding exposure incidents.
- Evaluate, select, and maintain the stock of products and equipment needed to accomplish office safety.
- Ensure proper maintenance, availability, cleaning, and disposal of personal protective equipment and all other items needed for office safety.
- Perform spore-testing and mechanical and chemical monitoring of office sterilizers.
- Manage disposal of regulated medical waste.
- Check equipment for decontamination and label contaminated portions before shipping for repair.
- Organize and maintain safety data sheets, proper labeling, the inventory list, and proper storage for all hazardous chemicals in the office.
- Maintain eyewash stations.
- Maintain smoke alarms and fire extinguishers and monitor electric cords and connections.
- Keep exit doors and evacuation routes clear and ensure other compliance with local fire safety codes.
- Maintain certification of radiographic equipment.
- Maintain appropriate documents and records.
- Ensure that all members of the dental team have a constant opportunity to voice concerns about and suggest improvements in office safety.
- Conduct and document routine evaluations of the office infection control program.
- Communicate with patients regarding safety procedure practices in the office.

the American Dental Association; Organization for Safety, Asepsis and Prevention; Centers for Disease Control and Prevention; American Dental Hygienists Association; American Dental Assistants Association; state dental associations; and a local school of dentistry (see Appendix A).

The Centers for Disease Control and Prevention (CDC) recommendations are published in their own journal called *Morbidity and Mortality Weekly Report Recommendations and Reports* (MMWR RR). Federal laws are published in the *Federal Register*; state laws are published in state registers. These publications are available in law schools and some public libraries, or one may obtain copies of regulations by contacting the respective federal or state agency (see Appendix A).

Enhance Communication

Among the Dental Team

Office policies and procedures and details of regulations and compliance must be communicated periodically to members of the dental team during the required training on bloodborne pathogens and management of hazardous materials. Also, a key aspect of employee satisfaction is open communication among all members of the dental team. The entire team

should participate in developing the total office safety program (see Chapter 18), and lines of communication should be established for constructive criticism and suggestions for improvement. An internal mechanism to resolve employee complaints is best.

Small posters with one-liners placed in strategic areas can be helpful in reinforcing infection prevention (Table 25-1). Infection prevention communication among the staff also is enhanced if each staff meeting includes a topic on safety. Box 25-2 shows some suggested topics.

With Patients

Communication with patients regarding their safety while in the office is also important for establishing trust and ensuring return visits. Patients have varying degrees of knowledge about infection control and routes of disease spread. Today, patients are asking an increasing number of questions about their safety in the office because of news media coverage of issues in dentistry, such as the safety of amalgam fillings, the incident in Florida in which a dentist apparently infected six of his patients with human immunodeficiency virus in the late 1980s, and the concern about disease transmission through dental handpieces in the early 1990s, and, more recently, contaminated dental unit water. These and other issues can erode public confidence in dentistry. Patients must be made aware of office procedures designed for their protection, many of which are conducted "behind the scenes." Box 25-3 lists suggestions for instilling trust in patients regarding the care taken in the office for patient protection.

TABLE 25-1 Examples of Safety Signs and Where to Place Them

Sign	Placement
Spore Test This Friday	Sterilization Room
Hot – Don't Touch	
Contaminated	
Dirty	
Clean	
Sterile	
Not Ready	
Change Solution on: ____ Date	
Prepared on: ____ Date	
Expiration Date: ____ Date	
Look Before You Reach	
Recap Safely	Staff Bulletin Board
Check Your Gloves	
Report Exposures	
Get Your Flu Shot	
Be Careful	
Remove Your Personal Protective Equipment	Lunch Room
For Food Only (Refrigerator)	
Decontaminate Your Hands	
Contaminated	Laboratory
Disinfected	
Ready to Ship	
Decontaminate Your Hands	
Wash Hands Before Leaving	Restrooms
No Food in This Refrigerator	Storage Room

BOX 25-2

Examples of Safety Topics for Staff Meetings

- List the various ways exposures may occur.
- Ask for tips on how to prevent injuries.
- Remind everyone where the safety data sheets are kept and the location of eyewash stations.
- Review steps to take if an exposure occurs.
- Ask for post-it slogans about sharps safety or other safety topics.
- Ask for comments about the infection control products being used.
- Ask if anyone has heard of new infection control products or equipment.
- Review sections of OSHA's Bloodborne Pathogens Standard.
- Review section of OSHA's Hazard Communication Standard.
- Review sections of the CDC's infection control guidelines for dental facilities.
- Review recent articles on infection control in dentistry.

Maintain Office Safety Documents

Documents and records must be prepared, maintained in proper form, and made readily available to dental team members (Box 25-4).

Develop Responses to Emergencies

The office safety coordinator should develop mechanisms for rapid responses to body fluid exposures, hazardous material exposures, medical emergencies, fire, and storms. As regards body fluid exposure, the procedure must involve a medical evaluation and follow-up as described in Chapter 8. The employer should maintain medical emergency kits, smoke alarms, and fire extinguishers; should identify an evacuation route in case of fire; and should identify procedures for protection in case of tornadoes, hurricanes, or earthquakes.

Procure and Manage Safety Products and Equipment

The employer should purchase, maintain, clean, and dispose of all products and equipment needed for infection control, management of hazardous materials, and other office safety procedures (Box 25-5). The costs of providing office safety can be difficult to recover; consequently, management of the supplies inventory, preventive maintenance

of equipment, and avoiding of infection control overkill can be important.

Evaluate Products and Equipment

Although adequate supplies need to be maintained, overstocking is a problem. Overstocking prolongs changing to another supply item of better quality or lower cost until current supplies have been used. The employer should evaluate products

---

BOX 25-3

Developing Patient Trust Regarding Infection Control Procedures in the Office

- Establish all infection control procedures.
- Let patients observe you washing your hands at the beginning of their care and especially when you return after being away from chairside.
- Let patients observe gloving, especially the use of fresh gloves when you return after being away from chairside.
- Let patients see you unwrap the sterile instruments that will be used so they will know that those instruments have been prepared carefully and protected.
- Know the facts about infection control procedures and encourage questions.
- Provide patients with brief written information about the infection control procedures used.
- Offer tours of the office and the sterilizing room to new or returning patients.
- Maintain general cleanliness; particularly dusting of horizontal surfaces in the operatory and waiting room.

Adapted from Miller CH: Make a lasting positive impression with infection control procedures, *RDH* 13:36, 1993.

BOX 25-4

Examples of Office Safety Documents and Records

Regulatory Documents
- OSHA Bloodborne Pathogens Standard
- OSHA Hazard Communication Standard
- State, local, or other regulatory documents that may apply (e.g., instrument sterilization, sterilization monitoring, and waste disposal)

Policy Documents
- OSHA written exposure control plan for the office
- OSHA written hazard communication program for the office
- CDC personal health program
- CDC tuberculosis infection control plan
- Management of fire and other emergencies*
- Policies not covered by OSHA standards (e.g., state regulations on instrument sterilization, sterilization monitoring, and waste disposal)
- OSHA poster (Form 3165) "Job Safety and Health"

Records
- OSHA bloodborne pathogens and hazard communication training records
- OSHA written schedule for cleaning and disinfecting areas in the office
- OSHA employee medical records†
- Hepatitis B vaccination refusal forms
- Written opinion from physician on vaccination of employees
- Exposure incident reports
- Written opinion from physician on postexposure medical evaluation and follow-up
- Sterilizer spore testing mechanical monitoring and chemical monitoring results
- Radiographic equipment certification
- Fire extinguisher certification
- Manifests from regulated medical waste haulers
- Verification of on-site treatment of regulated medical waste
- Safety data sheets of hazardous chemicals

*Written Emergency Action Plan and Fire Protection Plan are required if the facility has more than 11 employees.
†Employee medical records are confidential.

BOX 25-5

Examples of Supplies and Equipment for Office Safety

- Alcohol-based hand rub
- Antimicrobial hand wash
- Biohazard bags
- Biohazard labels and signs
- Biological indicators
- Cardiopulmonary resuscitation ventilation devices
- Chemical indicators
- Chemical safety cabinets
- Cleaning solution
- Disposable items
- Exit signs
- Eyewash stations
- Face shields
- Fire extinguishers
- First-aid kit
- Handpiece cleaner/lubricant
- Heat sterilizers
- High-volume evacuation
- Instrument cassettes
- Latex-free kit
- Liquid sterilant
- Masks
- Medical emergency kit
- Mercury management kit
- Oxygen
- Patient care gloves
- Preprocedure mouth rinse
- Protective clothing
- Protective eyewear
- Radiation badges
- Rubber dam
- Safety signs
- Sharps containers
- Smoke alarms
- Sterilization packaging
- Surface covers
- Surface disinfectant
- Ultrasonic cleaner and basket
- Utility gloves
- Water quality improvement system

carefully and request samples before ordering and should let the entire dental team assist in the evaluation to ensure proper use when the item is purchased. The employer should make sure an item purchased will be appropriate for the desired use and should not purchase unproven substitutes or otherwise compromise appropriate quality for low cost. The employer should ensure that written and especially verbal claims about products have been documented appropriately with testing or peer-reviewed, published, scientific evaluation.

Use and Maintain Products and Equipment Correctly

The employer should make sure that dental team members read, understand, and follow all labels and operating manuals for products and equipment. Misuse of products and equipment can lead to compromises in disease prevention or personal safety, damage to the equipment or surface related to product use, or damage to the equipment itself. Maintenance of equipment such as sterilizers, ultrasonic cleaners, vacuum traps, radiographic machines, smoke alarms, and fire extinguishers is particularly important so that they will work properly and have maximum use-life.

Periodically the employer should check and replace protective equipment such as utility gloves, eyewear, face shields, and reusable protective clothing when necessary. An inventory of all incoming chemicals ensures the availability of material safety data sheets and the presence of proper labels. The employer should ensure that disinfectants, sterilants, or other items with a specific shelf-life or use-life are replaced when indicated and should ensure that sharps containers are located where needed and that they are replaced before they overflow.

Infection Control Overkill

Examples of infection control overkill that can be time-consuming and costly are routinely hand scrubbing and ultrasonically cleaning instruments; routinely cleaning and disinfecting surfaces after removal of surface covers; using more than one layer of sterilization wrap during packaging; routinely disinfecting instruments before sterilization; using thick rather than thin plastic as surface covers; using sterile gloves for routine procedures; and using special disposal mechanisms for items that are not considered as regulated medical waste.

EVALUATION OF THE INFECTION CONTROL PROGRAM

Evaluation of the office infection control program is an effective way to improve procedures so they are useful, feasible, ethical, and accurate. A successful evaluation program depends on the following:

- Developing standard operating procedures
- Evaluating practices
- Documenting adverse outcomes and work-related illnesses
- Monitoring health care–associated infections in patients

The strategies used for the evaluation include the use of checklists to document that procedures are in place (see the following discussion), documentation that written procedures are in place and are available to all in the office, and direct observation of work activity to make sure procedures are performed correctly. One should take care about the validity of passive evaluation procedures such as secondhand verbal information obtained from staff interviews.

TABLE 25-2   **Measure the Effectiveness of an Infection Control Program**

Desired Outcomes	Examples to Measure
1. Infection control procedures have been learned.	Has appropriate training occurred?
2. The office is assessing up-to-date infection control information.	Is the office following the 2003 CDC infection control guidelines?
3. Infection control procedures are being performed correctly.	Does surface asepsis include precleaning prior to disinfection?
4. Appropriate infection control products and equipment are being used.	Is the surface disinfectant used to clean up visible blood and saliva an intermediate-level disinfectant?
5. The particular infection control product or equipment is being used correctly.	Does the timing of the dry heat sterilizer start after the unit has reached the sterilizing temperature?
6. The office infection control program is compliant with laws and recommendations.	Is the OSHA-required annual infection control training provided to all staff?

Adapted from Miller, CH: Don't wait, evaluate, *Dent Prod Rep* 39:142, 2006.

TABLE 25-3   **Examples of What to Evaluate in a Dental Office Infection Control Evaluation Program**

What to Evaluate	How to Evaluate
Immunizations of the office staff	Conduct an annual review of staff records to ensure up-to-date immunizations.
Occupational exposures to infectious materials	Report the exposures. Document and review the steps that occurred around the exposure and plan how it could be prevented in the future.
Postexposure management and follow-up	Ensure the postexposure management plan is understood by all office staff and that the exposure evaluation procedures are available at all times.
Hand hygiene procedures	Observe and document circumstances of appropriate and inappropriate hand hygiene. Review findings in a staff meeting.
Use of personnel protective barriers	Observe and document the use of barrier precautions and careful handling of sharps. Review findings in a staff meeting.
Monitoring the sterilization process	Compare the paper log of mechanical monitoring (time/temperature) and chemical monitoring (temperature strips) of each sterilizer load with the weekly biological monitoring (spore testing) results. Document that appropriate procedures are in place and are performed when sterilization failure occurs.
Evaluating safety devices	Conduct an annual review of the exposure control plan for documentation of new developments in safety devices.
Microbial quality of dental unit water	Monitor the microbial content of water exiting the dental units to determine compliance with the Environmental Protection Agency drinking water standard of no more than 500 colony-forming unites per milliliter (CFU/mL) of heterotrophic bacteria.

Adapted from Kohn WG, Collins AS, Cleveland JL, et al; Centers for Disease Control and Prevention: Guidelines for infection control in dental health-care settings–2003, *MMWR Recomm Rep* 52(RR-17):37, 2003.

Direct observation and documentation are usually more reliable. Table 25-2 gives six suggestions on how to determine the effectiveness of an infection control program. CDC examples of procedures one could evaluate in the office and how to evaluate them are given in Table 25-3.

Preparation of standard operating procedures will document the correct way of doing something. Direct observation of work activity ensures that the dental team understands how properly to perform procedures and use equipment. Problems with compliance may indicate that further training is needed. The person performing a procedure may use a checklist when direct observation is not possible.

CHECKLIST FOR THE INFECTION CONTROL PROGRAM

One can use the following checklist to organize, review, and update an infection control program for the office.

Exposure Control Plan and Other Written Documents

1. A written **exposure control plan** (as required by OSHA) for the office is available and contains the following:
   a. The exposure determination
   b. The schedule and method of implementation of the methods of compliance, the hepatitis vaccination, the postexposure medical evaluation and follow-up, the communication of biohazards, and the record keeping related to the OSHA Bloodborne Pathogens Standard
   c. The procedures for evaluating the circumstances surrounding an exposure incident
   d. The methods used and the results of the evaluation of new safety devices for use in the office
2. The exposure control plan is updated at least annually and whenever changes occur in the laws; in modes of exposure; or in procedures, equipment, or supplies used to prevent the spread of disease agents.
3. A copy of the exposure control plan is made available to all involved employees.
4. A written personnel health program (recommended by the CDC) for the office staff exists that includes policies, procedures, and guidelines for education and training; immunizations; exposure prevention and postexposure management; medical conditions, work-related illness, and associated work restrictions; contact dermatitis and latex hypersensitivity; and maintenance of records, data management, and confidentiality.
5. A written tuberculosis infection control plan based on CDC recommendations is available to all office staff and is followed.
6. The office infection control program is evaluated routinely.

Training of the Office Staff

1. The OSHA-required bloodborne pathogens training of appropriate office staff is provided on initial employment at no cost to the staff at a reasonable time and place by a person knowledgeable about the subjects and about the dental office environment. It includes the following:
   a. A description of the cause, symptoms, epidemiology, spread, and prevention of bloodborne diseases and tuberculosis
   b. Details of the exposure control plan for the office
   c. The selection, use, limitations, and management of equipment or supplies used to prevent spread of disease agents in the office
   d. The description, safety, efficacy, administration, and benefits of hepatitis B vaccination and immunity
   e. What to do if an exposure to blood or saliva occurs
   f. An explanation of biohazard/color code communication used in the office
   g. The availability of a copy and an explanation of the OSHA Bloodborne Pathogens Standard and other applicable infection control laws
   h. An opportunity for the trained employees to have questions immediately answered
2. Updated training of all involved office staff is given at least annually and whenever changes occur in the laws; in modes of exposure; or in procedures, equipment, or supplies used to prevent the spread of disease agents.

Hepatitis B Vaccination

1. The hepatitis B vaccination series is offered free of charge at a reasonable time and place by a licensed physician or nurse practitioner within 10 days of employment of a new person who has received proper training (see the previous discussion) about the vaccine.
2. The physician's office involved has a copy of the OSHA Bloodborne Pathogens Standard.
3. Prescreening for immunity to hepatitis B is not a condition of employment.
4. Employees not accepting the vaccination offer must read and sign the specific vaccination refusal statement given at the end of the OSHA Bloodborne Pathogens Standard.
5. Written confirmations are received from the physician indicating that each involved employee has been evaluated/vaccinated.
6. Employees are tested for antibody to hepatitis B surface antigen 1 to 2 months after the third inoculation, and nonresponders are evaluated and counseled.

Postexposure Medical Evaluation and Follow-up

1. A medical evaluation and follow-up is offered free of charge at a reasonable time and place by a licensed physician or nurse practitioner to all employees who experience an occupational exposure to blood or saliva.
2. Identifiable patients involved in such exposures are requested to be evaluated for their hepatitis B and human immunodeficiency virus disease status.
3. The physician's office involved has a copy of the OSHA Bloodborne Pathogens Standard.
4. Written confirmations are received from the physician indicating that each involved employee has been informed of the results of the evaluations and of any medical conditions resulting from the exposure that require further evaluation or treatment.

General Methods and Aseptic Techniques

1. Standard precautions are practiced (OSHA still refers to universal precautions related to bloodborne diseases).
2. Handwashing facilities and handwashing agents are available to staff.
3. Hand hygiene is performed after removal of gloves or other protective barriers and whenever contaminated with blood, saliva, or other body fluid.

4. Eating, drinking, smoking, and applying cosmetics, contacts, or lip balm are not done in areas where blood or saliva may be spread from patients.
5. Spattering or spraying of blood or saliva during patient treatment is minimized.
6. Preprocedure mouth rinsing is used.
7. Dental unit water is not used to irrigate surgical sites.
8. Dental unit water quality does not exceed 500 colony-forming units per milliliter (CFU/mL) of heterotrophic bacteria.
9. Water and air are flushed for a minimum of 20 seconds between patients through all devices that are connected to the dental unit water system.
10. Antiretraction valves in the dental unit water line system (if present) are maintained properly.
11. Unit dosing is used or an aseptic retrieval system (e.g., sterile forceps) is used with every patient if a supply type item must be obtained from a bulk container.
12. Disposable items (e.g., plastic air/water syringe tips, evacuation tips, ejector tips, prophylactic cups, and prophylactic angles) are not cleaned and reused on other patients.
13. A one-way cardiopulmonary resuscitation airway or oxygen with bagging is available for staff qualified to use such devices.
14. Sterilized instrument packages are inspected just before being opened, and if the package integrity has been compromised, the instruments are not used but are repackaged and resterilized.
15. The employer identifies, evaluates, and selects devices with engineered safety features (e.g., safety syringes) as they become available on the market and at least annually. The employer enters the evaluation results and an explanation of the decision to use or not to use an evaluated device in the exposure control plan.
16. Patients are asked not to close their lips around and spit into saliva ejector tips.
17. Medication is not administered to multiple patients from a single syringe unless the syringe is sterilized between uses.
18. Single-dose vials for parenteral medications are used when possible, and multiple-dose vials are used only with appropriate aseptic techniques.
19. Single-use (disposable) devices are used for only one patient and then are discarded.

Protective Barriers

1. Appropriate gloves, mask, protective eyewear, and protective clothing are made available and are used properly when the potential exists for exposure to patient's blood or saliva or to other contaminated surfaces or items.
2. Gloves, mask, protective eyewear, and protective clothing are removed before leaving the clinical work area and are not worn in lunch areas or out of the office.

3. Gloves, mask, protective eyewear, and protective clothing are cleaned properly, laundered, maintained, or discarded.
4. Alternative items are provided to those who may have adverse reactions to the normal barriers.
5. Sterile surgeon's gloves are worn when performing surgical procedures.
6. Patients are screened for latex allergy.
7. Latex-free kits are available at all times.
8. Fingernails are kept short, and those who wear patient care gloves do not wear artificial nails.
9. Hand lotions are used at the end of the day to prevent skin dryness associated with hand hygiene.
10. Lotions with petrolatum or other oil emollients are not used along with latex gloves.
11. Hand-care products are stored in closed containers that are disposable or can be washed and dried before refilling.
12. Soap or lotion is not added to partially empty dispensers.
13. Contaminated, reusable, protective clothing is containerized properly and laundered in the office or by a laundry service and is not taken home by employees for laundering.
14. Proper containers/bags are used for handling contaminated laundry.
15. Contaminated laundry is identified properly by a biohazard symbol/color coding that is recognizable by the office staff.

Management of Regulated Waste

1. Proper barriers, procedures, and containers are used for safe handling of sharps, nonsharp waste, liquid waste, and human tissue, including teeth.
2. Regulated waste is identified properly by a biohazard symbol/color coding and, where required, name and address labels.
3. Recapping of needles is accomplished by a safe technique.
4. Sharps containers are located where sharps are used or may be found.
5. Sharps containers are not overfilled and are closed when being transported.
6. Tongs are available for picking up broken glass, needles, scalpel blades, and other sharps.
7. Everyone is instructed to never reach blindly to pick up or move a sharp item.
8. Specimens of human tissue, blood, saliva, or other body fluids are placed in proper containers and are identified properly by a biohazard symbol/color coding during collecting, handling, processing, storing, or transporting.
9. Regulated waste is treated properly and discarded or transported for final disposal.

Decontamination

1. Appropriate personal protective equipment is used during decontamination of instruments or operatory surfaces.

2. Equipment and instruments are decontaminated properly before servicing or shipping, and if they contain sites that are incompletely contaminated, these sites are identified before servicing or shipping.

3. Operatory or other surfaces involved in patient treatment are covered with protective barriers that are changed for every patient, or contaminated surfaces involved in patient treatment are cleaned and then disinfected between patients.

4. A written schedule of decontamination of the various work areas is maintained.

5. Reusable containers contaminated with body fluids are cleaned and disinfected after use.

6. Liquid chemical sterilants are not used for surface disinfection or as an instrument holding solution.

7. Floors, walls, and sinks are cleaned routinely, and blinds and window curtains in patient care areas are cleaned when they are visibly dusty or soiled.

8. Carpeting and cloth-covered furnishings are not used in dental operatories.

Instrument Processing

1. Containers of contaminated reusable sharps (e.g., sharp instruments) are labeled properly with a biohazard symbol/color coding, are closed on transport, and do not require one to reach inside without being able to see the sharps.

2. A central area for instrument processing is designated and divided physically or spatially by signage into the following:
   a. Cleaning and decontamination
   b. Packaging
   c. Sterilization and storage

3. Contaminated instruments are mechanically cleaned routinely (rather than hand scrubbed) before rinsing and packaging for sterilization.

4. Cleaned and rinsed instruments are dried and packaged before sterilization.

5. Packaging materials designed for use in sterilizers and the proper procedures for sealing packages are used.

6. Cleaned and packaged reusable instruments, handpieces, handpiece attachments, and other items are sterilized between use on patients.

7. Equipment identified by its manufacturer as a sterilizer is used for sterilization.

8. Cleaned reusable items that melt in heat sterilizers are sterilized by a low-temperature procedure (e.g., glutaraldehyde) between use on patients.

9. The use and functioning of each sterilizer is spore-tested with biological indicators at least weekly.

10. Every package processed through the sterilizer contains an internal chemical indicator (e.g., temperature strip)

and an external chemical indicator if the internal indicator cannot be seen from the outside of the package.

11. Every sterilizer run is monitored mechanically (recording of time and temperature conditions achieved).

12. Sterilized instrument packages and cassettes are allowed to dry inside the sterilizer before being handled.

13. Proper procedures are performed if sterilization monitoring detects a sterilization failure.

14. Sterilized packages are handled and stored properly and managed on a date- or event-related basis.

Laboratory Asepsis

1. Items contaminated with oral fluids are sterilized when possible but at least are rinsed and disinfected before being taken into the in-office laboratory or sent to a commercial laboratory.

2. Items from in-office or commercial laboratories are:
   a. Disinfected and rinsed
   b. Confirmed to have been disinfected
   c. Known to be uncontaminated before being placed into patients' mouths

Radiographic Asepsis

1. X-ray films or digital x-ray sensors are protected with plastic surface covers before being placed in the patient's mouth or are rinsed and disinfected or handled aseptically after removal from the patient's mouth.

2. The sleeves of daylight loaders do not come in contact with contaminated gloves or films.

Record Keeping

1. Medical records (name, Social Security number, written confirmation about hepatitis B evaluation for vaccination, any vaccination refusal statement, written confirmation about postexposure medical evaluation and follow-up) for each employee who may have the potential to be exposed occupationally to body fluids are maintained (to comply with OSHA and some other state requirements) in confidentiality for the duration of employment plus 30 years.

2. Records of staff training (names and job classifications of trainees, date and contents of training, name and qualifications of the trainer) are maintained (to comply with OSHA and some other state requirements) for at least 3 years.

3. Records of spore-testing results (identification of the specific sterilizer tested, dates of the testing, results, and who performed the tests) are maintained according to state and local requirements.

4. Records for the treatment or transport and final disposal of regulated waste are maintained.

SELECTED READINGS

Miller CH: Don't wait, evaluate, *Dent Prod Rep* 39:142, 2006.

Miller CH: Double check your office asepsis procedures, *Dent Prod Rep* 7:94–97, 2003.

Miller CH: Safety coordinator's duties go beyond casual organization of safety plans, *RDH* 17:52, 1997.

Runnells RR, Powell L: Managing infection control, hazard communication, and infectious waste disposal, *Dent Clin North Am* 35: 299–308, 1991.

Stibich M: *Guidelines for evaluating new technologies for infection control*, http://www.infectioncontroltoday.com/articles/2010/11/guidelines-for-evaluating-new-technologies-for-infection-control.aspx. accessed January 2012.

REVIEW QUESTIONS

Multiple Choice

1. Which of the following cannot be a responsibility of the office safety coordinator?
   a. Review infection control laws and recommendations.
   b. Monitor the sterilization process.
   c. Evaluate the office infection control program.
   d. Pay for hepatitis B vaccination of new office staff.

2. Which of the following is infection control overkill?
   a. Cleaning and then disinfecting a contaminated dental operatory surface
   b. Cleaning and then sterilizing hand instruments
   c. Hand scrubbing and then ultrasonically cleaning contaminated instruments

3. Which of the following strategies should not be used to evaluate the office infection control program?
   a. Confirming the presence of written infection control policy documents
   b. Using secondhand information from personnel interviews
   c. Direct observation of work activities

4. The Centers for Disease Control and Prevention publishes its recommendations in the:
   a. *Journal of the American Dental Association*
   b. *Morbidity and Mortality Weekly Report Recommendations and Reports*
   c. *Federal Register*
   d. *Assistant*
   e. *RDH*

5. Which of the following is known as the infection control education organization?
   a. Environmental Protection Agency
   b. Organization for Safety, Asepsis and Prevention
   c. American Dental Association
   d. Centers for Disease Control and Prevention
   e. American Dental Assistants Association
   f. American Dental Hygienists Association

Please visit http://evolve.elsevier.com/Miller/infectioncontrol/ for additional practice and study support tools.

Managing Chemicals Safely

OUTLINE

LEARNING OBJECTIVES

After completing this chapter, the student should be able to do the following:

1. Define the goal of a hazard communication program and the terms that are important in the development of a hazard communication program.
2. Describe the process by which OSHA monitors and helps improve safety conditions in the workplace and provide a description of their Hazard Communication Standard.
3. Develop a method to determine the hazard potential of chemicals.
4. Design and maintain a written hazard communication program.
5. Describe additional safety requirements used to manage hazardous chemicals, including inventory, labels, other forms of warning, and safety data sheets.

6. Outline an employee information and training program for dealing with hazardous chemicals in the workplace.
7. Identify the four ways "OSHA solves a problem."
8. List the seven sections/components of maintaining compliance with the Safe Use of Chemicals in the Laboratory Standard.
9. Describe the general principles for working with laboratory chemicals, including prudent practices.
10. List employee chemical hygiene responsibilities, describe the chemical hygiene safety requirements in laboratory facilities, and design and maintain a written chemical hygiene plan.

KEY TERMS

Chemical Distributors
Chemical Hygiene Officer
Chemical Hygiene Plan
Chemical Importers
Chemical Manufacturers
Employees
Employers
Engineering Controls
Hazard Communication Program

Hazard Communication Standard
    (HazCom Standard, HazMat
    Program, "Employee Right
    to Know")
Hazardous Chemical
Health Hazard
Safety Data Sheets (SDSs)
Occupational Exposure to Blood-
    borne Pathogens Standard

Performance Standards
Personal Protective Equipment (PPE)
Physical Hazard
Prudent Practices
Work Practice Controls
Written Hazard Communication
    Program (WHCP)

HAZARD COMMUNICATION PROGRAM

The U.S. Department of Labor Occupational Safety and Health Administration (OSHA) has estimated that more than 32 million workers are exposed to 650,000 hazardous chemical products in more than 3 million American workplaces. This exposure poses a serious problem for workers and their employers.

The basic goal of a hazard communication program is to be sure employers and employees know about work hazards and how to protect themselves; this knowledge should help reduce the incidence of chemical source illness and injuries.

If one were to ask most dental practitioners about their personal risk of experiencing an occupationally related injury, their responses most likely would include incidents such as needlestick accidents, allergies, burns, abrasions, or muscle strains. Being injured on the job while using or handling a hazardous material, such as a skin exposure to an acid solution, often would not be mentioned. Most health care workers consider topics such as safer use of chemicals in the workplace to be problems primarily associated with large manufacturing facilities, such as oil refineries, chemical manufacturers, steel mills, coal mines, and metal fabrication shops. Unfortunately, a significant number of workers in dental environments are exposed to and injured each year by hazardous materials while performing normal clinical and laboratory duties.

STATEMENT OF THE PROBLEM

Millions of workers in the United States are occupationally at risk for exposure to one or more hazardous chemicals (Table 26-1). Almost 650,000 chemicals can be purchased in the United States, and literally thousands of new chemicals are introduced each year. The risk of exposure is increasing continually, and workplace use of toxic chemicals is commonplace.

Adverse exposure to chemicals can have serious health consequences. Heart, kidney, liver, and lung tissues could be damaged. The result could be a variety of diseases that range from short-term discomfort (e.g., burns or rashes) to life threatening (e.g., cancer, sterility, or organ failure). Preventing exposure to hazardous chemicals is the ultimate goal. Also important is the proper response when an exposure does occur.

OCCUPATIONAL SAFETY AND HEALTH ADMINISTRATION

For more than 40 years, OSHA has monitored and helped to improve safety conditions in the workplace. The greatest initial need (numbers of employees and severity of injuries), as one would expect, was (and remains) based in large and naturally dangerous worksites. Through a process of improving engineering controls and changing work practice controls (see Table 26-1), OSHA's work has begun to reduce the number of workplace injuries.

In time, OSHA issued comprehensive standards that held the weight of law. Noncompliance, even in the absence of injury, could result in citations, fines, and even temporary closure for the employer. OSHA also began to describe the required performance standards (see Table 26-1) expected from various pieces of work equipment (e.g., ladders, pipes, and electric service). Then, OSHA applied Environmental Protection Agency (EPA) standards for maximum workplace exposure to chemicals, such as gases and volatile chemicals, radioactivity, and even heat and sound.

Finally, OSHA generated standards for the development, use, and review of personal protective equipment (PPE) and devices (see Table 26-1). In dental offices, examples of PPE include gloves, masks, respirators, glasses, and uniforms for employees.

The overall goal was to minimize the chances of occupationally related injuries through several mechanisms. Success of such efforts is based on a number of interrelated factors. Of course, issuance of reasonable and reliable standards by OSHA is the guiding force. However, employers must make themselves knowledgeable of what is required and create within their environments as safe a workplace as possible. Employees also must be aware of the required standards and be active participants in the process. Although employers must provide proper safe working environments, employees must comply with implementation and performance of the processes.

Over the past 15 years, dental workers have become aware of OSHA activities. For example, without the emergence of human immunodeficiency virus/acquired immunodeficiency syndrome in the United States and the involvement of OSHA in health care settings, this book probably would not have

TABLE 26-1   **Important Definitions for a Hazard Communication Program**

Term	Definition
Chemical	Any element, chemical compound, or mixture of elements and compounds
Chemical distributors	A business, other than a chemical manufacturer or importer, that supplies hazardous chemicals to other distributors or to employer
Chemical manufacturers and importers	An employer with a workplace where chemical(s) are produced for use or distribution
Employee	A worker who may be exposed to hazardous chemicals under normal operating conditions or in foreseeable emergencies; some workers, such as office workers or bank tellers, encounter hazardous chemicals only in nonroutine, isolated instances and are not covered by the Hazard Communication Standard
Employer	A person engaged in a business where chemicals are used, distributed, or produced for use or distribution, including a contractor or subcontractor
Engineering controls	Procedures and materials that help prevent employee exposure to hazardous chemicals. Examples include changing a chemical to a less problematic form or subcontracting a process to another location or facility
Exposure ("exposed")	Subjection of an employee to a hazardous chemical in the course of employment through any route of entry (inhalation, ingestion, skin contact, absorption), including potential (e.g., accidental or possible) exposure
Hazardous chemicals	A chemical for which statistically significant evidence based on a scientifically designed and conducted study indicates the acute or chronic health effects that may occur to exposed employees; many chemicals used within dental offices/clinics are considered hazardous
Hazard warning	Words, pictures, symbols, or combinations thereof appearing on a label or other appropriate form of warning that convey the specific physical or health hazard(s), including target organ effects, of the chemical(s) present in a container
HazCom compliance officer	An employee responsible for clinic/office compliance with the HazCom Standard; the person is responsible for listing all hazardous chemicals, collection of matching safety data sheets (SDSs), preparation of labels and warning signs, and the transfer of necessary safety information and training employees
Written HazCom program (WHCP)	A compliance process for the Hazard Communication Standard that includes a written clinic/office program manual, container labeling, and other forms of information transfer and warnings and employee training; best if administered by a HazCom compliance officer (see Table 26-2)
HazCom Standard	The Hazard Communication Standard (aka "Employee Right to Know") that has the goal of preventing employee exposures to hazardous chemicals; information from manufacturers of hazardous chemicals must be conveyed by employers to employees; facilities are responsible to ensure that the information is received and understood; facilities enhance safety through their HazCom program
Health hazard warnings	Words, pictures, symbols, or combinations appearing on a label or other appropriate form of warning that conveys the specific physical or health hazard(s), including target organ effects, of the chemical(s) present in a container
Label	Any written, printed, or graphic material displayed on or affixed to containers of hazardous chemicals that provides necessary information
Safety data sheets (SDSs)	Written or printed material concerning a hazardous chemical; an SDS for each hazardous chemical listed within a facility must be obtained
Performance standard	A combination of procedures and materials (work practices, engineering controls, personal protective equipment, and training) to comply with an OSHA standard; OSHA does not usually dictate what process is to be followed; rather, it describes the outcome of some behavior, for example, keeping exposures within some limit; how well this is done can be called proper performance or proper achievement (level of compliance)
Personal protective equipment and devices	Specialized clothing or equipment worn by an employee for protection against a hazard; general work clothes usually are not designed or intended to prevent exposure to hazardous chemicals
Physical hazard	A chemical for which scientifically valid evidence indicates that it is a combustible liquid, a compressed gas, explosive, flammable, an organic peroxide and oxidizer, pyrophoric, unstable (reactive), or water reactive
Work practice controls	Means that reduce the likelihood of exposure by altering the manner in which a task is performed; for example, the use of a fume hood or vacuum evacuation

Adapted from Occupational Safety and Health Administration: Hazard communication; final rule, 29 CFR Part 1910.1030, *Fed Regist* 59:6126, 1994; and US Department of Labor, Occupational Safety and Health Administration: *Chemical hazard communication* (OSHA 3084), Washington, DC, 1995, US Government Printing Office.

been written. Before 1986, an overall interest in infection control, hazardous materials handling, and waste management was modest. This lack of concern negatively affected employee safety. However, with the growing epidemic of acquired immunodeficiency syndrome, the interests of health care professionals and the general population grew. A heightened awareness of an increased need for patient and practitioner safety quickly developed.

HAZARD COMMUNICATION STANDARD

The main directive of OSHA is the protection of employees. The response of OSHA to current needs involves development of new standards and broadening the scopes of others. Most dental workers are acutely aware of the OSHA Occupational Exposure to Bloodborne Pathogens Standard (issued December 6, 1991). In fact, the majority of interest, effort, and resources in dental environments involves infection control. Conversely, relatively little attention is paid to other OSHA standards. One particularly deficient area is the OSHA Hazard Communication Standard (HCS), CFR 29.1910.1200 (also known as HazCom Standard, HazMat Program, "Employee Right to Know"; see Table 26-1).

On September 23, 1987, OSHA, in an attempt to promote safer use of hazardous materials, began to require chemical manufacturers, chemical importers, and chemical distributors to provide safety data sheets (SDSs) (see Table 26-1) with their shipments of all hazardous chemicals.

Initially, the center of activity involved manufacturing locations. However, with continued evidence of employee injuries, OSHA on May 23, 1988, began to require that employers from the nonmanufacturing sector (including health care facilities) comply with all provisions of the HCS. Even though the standard has been in effect for almost 10 years, compliance by dental clinics/offices is less than universal. Such deficiencies could be related to heightened concern about (and overemphasis on) infection control issues or lack of interest or awareness of the HCS. In any case, dental clinics and offices must comply with all tenets of the standard. A significant proportion of OSHA inspections involves complaints associated with injuries or the potential for injury involving the handling, use, storage, and disposal of hazardous materials.

Original Hazard Communication Standard Updated in 2012

The HCS was updated in 2012 to align with the Globally Harmonized System of Classification and Labeling of Chemicals (GHS). In 2003, the United Nations (UN) adopted the GHS, which is an international approach to hazard communication. It includes criteria for the classification of health, physical, and environmental hazards, as well as specifying what information should be included on labels of hazardous chemicals and SDSs. The HCS was updated to be consistent with the GHS and provides a common and coherent approach to classifying chemicals and communicating hazard information on labels

and SDSs. The regulatory text of the current HCS is provided in Appendix H. The major changes in the new standard include:

- **Hazard classification:** Provides specific criteria for classification of health and physical hazards, as well as classification of mixtures.
- **Labels:** Chemical manufacturers and importers are required to provide a label that includes a harmonized signal word, pictogram (see Figure 26-1), and hazard statement for each hazard class and category. Precautionary statements must also be provided.
- **SDSs:** Formerly known as Material Safety Data Sheets, now have a specified 16-section format (see Table 26-3).
- **Information and training:** Employers are required to train workers on the new label elements and SDSs format to facilitate recognition and understanding.

The effective dates for implementation of the updated standard are as follows:

- employers must train employees regarding the new label elements and SDSs format by December 1, 2013;
- chemical manufacturers, importers, distributors, and employers must be in compliance with all modified provisions no later than June 1, 2015, except:
  - after December 1, 2015, the distributor must not ship containers labeled by the chemical manufacturer or importer unless the label has been modified appropriately;
  - all employers must, as necessary, update any alternative workplace labeling used, update the hazard communication program, and provide any additional employee training on newly identified physical or health hazards no later than June 1, 2016;
- chemical manufacturers, importers, distributors, and employers may comply with either the old or the current version of this standard, or both during the transition period.

Purpose of the Hazard Communication Standard

The purpose of the HCS is to ensure that hazards of all chemicals produced or imported be evaluated and that employers transmit the information concerning such hazards directly to employees. Information is conveyed through a comprehensive hazard communication program (see Table 26-1). The program includes a written clinic/office program manual, container labeling, and other forms of warning, SDSs, and employee training.

Users of hazardous materials are not in a position to easily evaluate the potential hazards associated with the chemicals. Logically, this responsibility falls to the chemical manufacturer or importer and eventually to the chemical distributors. The responsibility of employers is to inform and train their employees (see Table 26-1) concerning all safety materials provided, including all warnings, required personal protective devices, and safer handling and disposal methods.

OSHA has a variety of materials and publications to help employers and employees develop and implement effective

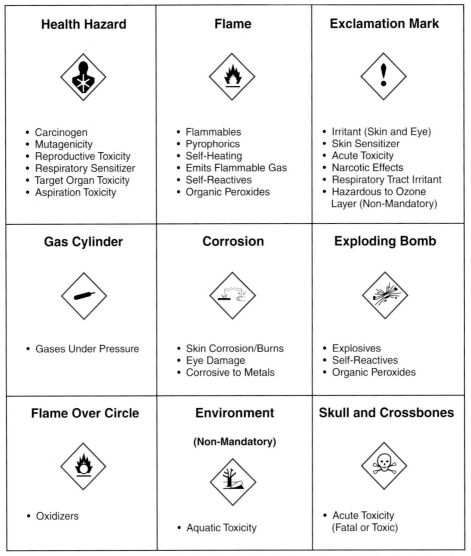

Health Hazard

- Carcinogen
- Mutagenicity
- Reproductive Toxicity
- Respiratory Sensitizer
- Target Organ Toxicity
- Aspiration Toxicity

Flame

- Flammables
- Pyrophorics
- Self-Heating
- Emits Flammable Gas
- Self-Reactives
- Organic Peroxides

Exclamation Mark

- Irritant (Skin and Eye)
- Skin Sensitizer
- Acute Toxicity
- Narcotic Effects
- Respiratory Tract Irritant
- Hazardous to Ozone Layer (Non-Mandatory)

Gas Cylinder

- Gases Under Pressure

Corrosion

- Skin Corrosion/Burns
- Eye Damage
- Corrosive to Metals

Exploding Bomb

- Explosives
- Self-Reactives
- Organic Peroxides

Flame Over Circle

- Oxidizers

Environment

(Non-Mandatory)

- Aquatic Toxicity

Skull and Crossbones

- Acute Toxicity (Fatal or Toxic)

FIGURE 26-1 HCS pictograms and hazards. As of June 1, 2015, the Hazard Communication Standard requires pictograms on labels to alert users of the chemical hazards to which they may be exposed. Each pictogram consists of a symbol on a white background framed within a red border and represents a distinct hazard(s). The pictogram on the label is determined by the chemical hazard classification.

hazard communication programs. One can obtain brochures on related topics by contacting the Department of Labor, OSHA/OSHA Publications, P.O. Box 37535, Washington, DC, 20013-7535 (Box 26-1). One can obtain single copies at no charge by sending a self-addressed mailing label with the request. More extensive information kits are available for a fee from the U.S. Government Printing Office at Superintendent of Documents, U.S. Government Printing Office, 732 N. Capitol St., NW, Washington, DC, 20401, or by calling (202) 512-0000. Some items are available as downloads from the Internet.

Scope and Application of the Hazard Communication Standard

As previously stated, chemical manufacturers and importers are charged to assess the hazards associated with the use of their products. Distributors also must inform their clients of the hazards. In turn, employers must inform their employees. The HCS covers any workplace that employs workers (even one).

Hazardous chemicals involved in the standard are limited to those present in the workplace to which employees may be exposed under normal working conditions and in the case of a foreseeable emergency (e.g., an employee may not directly use a chemical but must be informed and trained about the proper procedures to follow if another employee were to drop and break open a jar of the chemical).

Technically, OSHA considers most health care facilities, including dental clinics or offices, to be "laboratories." Employers must ensure that employees are informed and trained considering the types and amounts of hazardous materials present, the labeling system and warning signs utilized, the location and use of SDSs, and procedures to be followed in case of emergencies.

Some chemicals are exempt from the standard. These chemicals include tobacco and tobacco products; wood and wood products; and food, drugs, cosmetics, or alcoholic beverages packaged and sold for consumer use. Foods, drugs, or cosmetics intended for personal consumption by employees while at work are also exempt. Consumer products (e.g., glass cleaner) used in a manner similar to those used by persons at home (applications, amounts used, and duration and frequency of use) generally are considered as not being hazardous. Finally, any chemical defined as a "drug" by the Federal Food, Drug, and Cosmetic Act when present in its solid, final form, ready for direct administration to patients (e.g., aspirin) is exempt.

Before reviewing the details of the various parts of the HCS, a brief review of its design may be helpful. This standard is different from other OSHA standards in that it covers all hazardous chemicals (not just those associated with a certain type of workplace). The rule incorporates a "downstream flow of information." Producers must inform distributors, who then tell employers, who must transmit information to their employees.

HAZARD CLASSIFICATION

The standard requires workplaces to have a list of hazardous chemicals as part of the written hazard communication program (WHCP). The list eventually will serve as an inventory of everything for which an SDS must be maintained.

The quality of a hazard communication program depends on the adequacy and accuracy of the hazard assessment. A hazardous chemical is any chemical that is a physical hazard or a health hazard (see Table 26-1). The EPA specifically designates which chemicals are hazardous. The EPA considers a chemical as hazardous if it can catch fire, if it can react or explode when mixed with other substances, if it is corrosive, or if it is toxic. Included are chemicals that are flammable, spontaneously ignitable, explosive, oxidizing agents, corrosive, toxic, or radioactive.

The EPA estimates that the average American house with a garage holds about 30 gallons of materials that can be considered hazardous. Consumers readily use many of these items, including gasoline, fertilizers, pesticides, strong acids or bases, lubricants, paint and varnishes, drain cleaners, and engine coolants. Many chemicals can be considered hazardous for more than one reason (e.g., gasoline is flammable, explosive, and toxic and at times can ignite spontaneously). Although the volume of hazardous materials in a dental clinic/office may not exceed that of many households, the number and forms of potentially harmful chemicals is usually far greater. Of course, the standard regulates safety in the workplace, not within residences.

The identification, evaluation, and notification of any chemical as being hazardous are the initial responsibility of its manufacturer or importer. These entities may generate their own scientific data, or when appropriate, they may cite previously published information. Distributors are required to pass along this information to their clients. Hazardous means any chemical that has shown the capability of causing a physical or a health hazard. Toxicity and carcinogenicity are of significant importance. Although many chemicals have been tested, literally thousands of new compounds are produced each year. Many chemicals in common use have not been evaluated completely. Even if considered to be toxic or carcinogenic, debate on the status of a chemical can continue for an extended period. The stories associated with the investigation of dioxin, asbestos, chlorine, formaldehyde, and even the sweetener saccharin have proved legendary. When in doubt, one can consult federal chemical registries (e.g., The Registry of Toxic Effects of Chemical Substances produced by the National Institute for Occupational Safety and Health). Some hazardous materials are listed in the HCS itself.

For a single, pure chemical, such as ethanol, to be used in dental environments is uncommon. A more frequent event is the mixing of chemicals. Kits containing various chemicals are mixed to achieve the desired end product. Trituration of amalgam is a common example of chemical mixing in a dental clinic/office. The manufacturer or importer (and eventually the employer) of a chemical kit must identify the hazards associated with mixing. The combination of chemicals initially may involve more than one hazardous chemical. The result of such combinations can vary (Figure 26-2). Chemicals that are benign when separate can produce an end product of significant danger after being mixed. Warning information as to the type of hazard generated and procedures to handle, use, and store the mixture safely must be

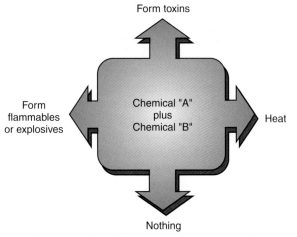

Form toxins

Form flammables or explosives

Chemical "A" plus Chemical "B"

Heat

Nothing

FIGURE 26-2 Potential outcomes of mixing chemicals.

provided. Warnings must include specific comments concerning the types of PPE that need to be worn and the procedures to be used for exposure or for disposal.

WRITTEN HAZARD COMMUNICATION PROGRAM

All workplaces where employees are exposed to hazardous chemicals must have a written plan that describes how the standard will be implemented in that facility.

The HCS commonly is referred to as the "Employee Right to Know Rule." Another way to look at the standard is as the "No Surprises Rule." The goal is that by training and the sharing of information, employee injuries involving hazardous chemicals can be kept to a minimum. Employers must develop, implement, and maintain at the workplace a written, comprehensive hazard communication program that includes provisions for container labeling, collection, and availability of SDSs, and an employee training program.

A central activity to meet this goal is the production of a WHCP (see Table 26-1). Although such efforts are usually modest (six to eight pages), they cannot be mere reiterations of the HCS. They are designed to be manuals that reflect the type and size of the dental practice. Table 26-2 presents an outline of a generic WHCP. Task identification and proper responses follow.

Employers are required to develop, implement, and maintain (monitor) a WHCP for their workplaces. Minimal contents include a list of all known hazardous materials present, the labeling and warning sign system used, the location and use of SDSs, emergency procedures, and the nature and frequency of employee information and training. The WHCP helps explain how the clinic/office complies with the various criteria of the standard.

The overall purpose of a WHCP is to provide for the implementation of the requirements of the standard in the workplace and to serve as a reference for employers' or employees' questions about official clinic/office policies. Because great differences exist even among clinics/offices in

the same general locale, the WHCP must be "personalized" to reflect what actually is being performed.

Writing the WHCP involves nine stages or steps.

1. *Provide copies of the HCS to each employee.* Familiarity with the standard increases compliance. Employers may devise a modest examination to ensure that employees have read and understood the basic tenets of the standard.
2. *Determine who is responsible for implementing the WHCP.* The most effective way for a clinic/office to comply with the standard is to identify, train, empower, and reward the HazCom compliance officer (see Table 26-1). A single individual can complete many, if not all, of the various activities associated with HCS compliance. Compliance is especially important when considering the listing of the hazardous chemicals and the collection of the required SDSs. The process is improved if a single individual performs all transactions. This person's name and title must be listed formally. A backup officer (e.g., the dentist) should be identified also.
3. *List all chemicals used or produced in the workplace.* Specific guidelines on the development of the required list appear later. The compliance officer must review the list often because new chemicals are brought into the clinic/office regularly. The goal is to generate and maintain a complete list and location of all hazardous chemicals.
4. *Describe the methods to be used to inform employees of the hazards of nonroutine tasks.* Cleaning or repair of some pieces of equipment is an example of nonroutine tasks. Sometimes chemical hazards are released during such processes. In other cases, hazardous chemicals are used during the cleaning or repair. Some office or clinic employees also perform work that does not normally place them at risk for exposure to hazardous chemicals. Such individuals require less information and training.
5. *Describe methods used to inform contract employees of the hazardous chemicals to which they could be exposed.* Part-time employees or persons hired to clean or repair must be extended the same level of protection as permanent, full-time employees. Contract employees who bring hazardous materials as part of their work into the clinic/office environment must provide appropriate SDSs.
6. *Describe methods used to label containers.* This step has three phases.
   a. Provide the name and title of the person responsible for the proper labeling of all containers.
   b. Describe the labeling system used. (A proper label must contain the identity of the chemical, the name and address of the chemical manufacturer or importer, and appropriate hazard warnings.)
   c. Describe the clinic/office procedures for reviewing and updating labeling information.
7. *Collect and maintain SDSs.* Use of SDSs is described later. However, SDSs are the central element for information concerning hazardous materials. The WHCP must describe who is responsible for collecting the SDSs for each hazardous material and the method used to maintain the SDS collection (e.g., in notebooks and their locations).

TABLE 26-2   **Generic Written Hazard Communication Program**

Step	Required Action
Provide copies of the HazCom Standard to each employee.	☑ Indicate that the written hazard communication plan (WHCP) includes the standard, introductory comments, a written manual that describes the procedures to be used in the facility, and some definitions.
	☑ Provide individual copies of the HazCom Standard.
	☑ Discuss in general the materials shared.
	☑ Use examinations to ensure employee review of the standard.
Determine who is responsible for implementing the WHCP.	☑ Indicate the WHCP date of preparation/review.
	☑ Indicate that the subject of the WHCP is to comply with the Hazard Communication Program for General Industry (OSHA 29 CFR 1910.1200).
	☑ Prepare a rationale for workplace compliance (a paragraph or two describing that workplace injuries and infections can occur; these can be gleaned from the standard).
	☑ Acknowledge the responsibility of the facility to determine the hazards associated with all chemicals present and that hazard information and appropriate use of protective measures will be transmitted to employees.
	☑ Identify the HazCom compliance officer of the facility by name and title; establish a trained backup officer.
	☑ Ensure that the compliance officer will maintain and review at least annually the WHCP, including a written manual, chemical inventory, information dissemination (including safety data sheets [SDSs], labels, and warnings), and employee training.
List all chemicals used or produced in the workplace.	☑ Identify, list, and provide the locations of hazardous chemicals present in the workplace as part of the WHCP (best done by one individual).
	☑ Use a listing scheme (alphabetic, alphanumeric, or numeric) that all employees understand and can use readily.
	☑ Inform employees of the locations of the hazardous chemicals list.
	☑ Obtain SDSs for each listed chemical, and use the SDSs and the list to prepare labels and when necessary warning signs for each hazardous chemical.
Describe methods to be used to inform employees of the hazards of nonroutine tasks.	☑ Ensure that employees are not asked to perform nonroutine tasks for which they may not be fully trained.
	☑ Discuss all nonroutine tasks before initiation (includes training).
	☑ Record the processes used and place within the WHCP.
Describe methods used to inform contract employees of the hazardous chemicals to which they could be exposed.	☑ Assign task to the compliance officer of the facility.
	☑ Ensure that part-time or contract employees are aware of the chemical hazards associated within their specific work areas.
	☑ Ensure that if such workers bring hazardous chemicals into the facility that they are fully trained regarding their use, storage, and disposal and that they bring appropriate information and hazard signs and SDSs.
Describe methods used to label containers.	☑ Ensure that incoming chemicals are properly labeled, placed on the hazardous chemical list, and have an associated SDS.
	☑ Complete labeling for improperly or unmarked containers so that the name and title of the person responsible for labeling are present and a description of the labeling system used (must contain the identity of the chemical, the name and address of the chemical manufacturer or importer, and appropriate hazard warnings, including proper personal protective equipment) is present.
	☑ List and train employees concerning the procedures for reviewing and updating labeling and location information.
	☑ Keep all hazardous chemicals separate from foods or beverages; this may include processes such as using two refrigerators.
Collect and maintain SDSs.	☑ Collect an appropriate SDS for every chemical that is on the list of hazardous chemicals at the facility.
	☑ Maintain two collections: one in office storage and another where employees have easy access.
	☑ Train employees concerning the location and proper use of SDSs.

Continued

TABLE 26-2   Generic Written Hazard Communication Program—cont'd

Step	Required Action
Describe employee information transmission and training schemes.	☑ List the training coordinator (and backup) of the facility by name and title.
	☑ Describe procedures used to train employees.
	☑ Describe procedures used to inform employees of the HazCom Standard, operations that use hazardous chemicals, location of the WHCP, list of hazardous chemicals, and location of SDSs.
	☑ Collect an appropriate SDS for every chemical that is on the list of hazardous chemicals at the facility.
	☑ Train employees concerning the written emergency and postexposure protocols of the facility.
Train employees in use of chemicals that involve trade secrets.	☑ Identify chemicals containing "secret ingredients."
	☑ Design a protocol for postexposure activities for "secret chemicals" in which a medical emergency exists.
	☑ Design a protocol for postexposure activities for "secret chemicals" in which no immediate health hazard exists.

Adapted from U.S. Department of Labor, Occupational Safety and Health Administration: *Chemical hazard communication* (OSHA 3084), Washington, DC, 1995, US Government Printing Office; and from U.S. Department of Labor, Occupational Health and Safety Administration: Hazard communication; final rule, 29 CFR 1910.1030, *Fed Regist* 59:6126-6184, 1994.

Also to be listed are how employees can access SDSs and how the list of SDSs is kept current.

8. *Describe employee information transmission and training.* This step has the following five phases:
   a. Provide name and title of the person responsible for employee training.
   b. Describe the procedures used to train employees.
   c. Describe the procedures for informing employees of the HCS, the operations that use hazardous materials, the location of the WHCP, a list of hazardous chemicals, and the location of the SDSs.
   d. Describe the training program, including hazardous materials monitoring, all physical or health hazards present, and measures used to protect employees.
   e. Provide details of the WHCP, including an explanation of the labeling system used and how the employees are trained to use SDSs.
9. *Use of chemicals that involve trade secrets.* Some chemical manufacturers are reluctant to share information concerning their products because they think that some trade secret could be gleaned. Although the ratios or percentages of the component chemicals can be withheld, the manufacturer/importer has the responsibility to inform the user of the hazardous chemicals. This information includes specific comments as to which protective equipment or processes should be used when handling their product.

After preparation of the WHCP, the compliance office must review it regularly. New employees need to review the WHCP as soon as possible.

INVENTORY AND LISTING OF HAZARDOUS CHEMICALS

Each facility is required to inventory holdings of any hazardous chemicals. Inventories of chemicals can be organized in several ways. Some clinics/offices prefer to use an alphabetic

listing; others use a numeric listing in which a chemical is given the next available number. Another method is to organize the chemicals by hazard category. Such divisions usually include corrosive, flammable, reactive, and toxic. No matter which listing process one uses, it must be understood and used properly by employees.

The list can include scientific and common chemical names and even associated hazards. To create an additional column for the PPE and other safety processes to be used for each hazardous chemical is wise. Listing where various hazardous chemicals are located throughout the facility is also useful. Of course, the preparation date (and updates) of the list should be noted prominently. The clinic/office HazCom coordinator should generate and maintain the list. If all purchases and disposals are handled by this individual, there will be little chance that a hazardous chemical will be present but not listed.

Completing a chemical inventory provides an excellent opportunity to discard unwanted chemicals. Such chemicals might be items never used, past expiration, samples, and those no longer having clinical value. To learn the volume of unwanted chemicals that are present is always a surprise. One always should contact the local environmental regulatory agency concerning proper disposal procedures.

Chemical inventory lists are valuable. All listed chemicals must be cross-referenced to their own SDSs. Lists are also important in the generation of informative signs and warnings and should be used for employee training. All employees must know the location of the list of hazardous chemicals and be able to interpret the information present.

LABELS AND OTHER FORMS OF WARNING

In-house containers of hazardous chemicals must be labeled, tagged, or marked with the identity of the material and appropriate hazard warnings.

Chemical manufacturers and importers and their distributors are required by the HCS to label properly all products considered hazardous. The minimal acceptable label includes:

- Product identifier
- Signal word (e.g., Danger, Warning, Asphyxiant)
- Hazard statement(s) (describes the nature of the hazard)
- Pictogram(s) (Figure 26-1)
- Precautionary statement(s) and, name, address, and telephone number of the chemical manufacturer, importer, or other responsible party

Ideally, the sources of the chemical will label all their containers of hazardous chemicals properly. If an employer determines that a container is labeled properly, the container requires no additional information. Unfortunately, some chemicals (especially dental materials kits) are not labeled properly by their sources. In such cases, the clinic/office must complete the labeling process. The clinic/office also must act when a hazardous chemical is removed from properly labeled containers to an improperly (possibly even blank) container. For example, iodophor surface disinfectant is purchased in a concentrated form and then is diluted to its working concentration and placed within spray bottles. The new containers must be labeled with (1) the identity of the hazardous chemical(s), (2) appropriate hazard warning (including target organs/tissues and applicable PPE and procedures), and (3) the name and address of the chemical manufacturer, importer, or responsible party.

No official labeling system exists. Clinics/offices can photocopy the label from the original container and affix it to the new containers. Several other labeling schemes are available. The most important factors are that the system is easy to use and that employees are trained properly to understand and use the system.

Safe use of hazardous chemicals involves other activities in addition to container labels. Employers can use signs, placards, posted operating procedures, and other written or pictorial information (e.g., pictograms). Such signage must be in English, and when necessary, in an alternative language. Warning signs are readily available from many commercial sources. They also, however, can be handmade. The goal is not artistic beauty but simplicity, ease of use, and conveyance of the desired information.

SAFETY DATA SHEETS (FORMERLY KNOWN AS MATERIAL SAFETY DATA SHEETS)

Few safety constructs are more valuable than SDSs. These are written reports prepared by manufacturers or importers that describe an individual chemical or a group collection of chemicals. Valuable information includes the chemicals present, the associated hazards, handling and cleanup procedures, and special PPE that needs to be in place.

Chemical manufacturers and importers must obtain or develop an SDS for each product containing hazardous chemicals. This rule applies to single chemicals and multiple-chemical kits. The employer must obtain an SDS specific for each hazardous chemical present in the workplace. If a clinic/office uses three types of amalgam, three specific (unique) SDSs are needed. Generic SDSs are not acceptable. Safety data sheets contain phone numbers that are answered 24 hours a day, 7 days a week. These contacts are trained to offer highly specific and useful information about the product. Photocopies of SDSs are acceptable.

Unfortunately, some chemical sources are reluctant, unable, or unwilling to distribute SDSs, but this does not diminish the requirement of employers to obtain SDSs for all their hazardous chemicals. Clinics/offices can obtain SDSs other than from the manufacturer or importer in several ways. Again, a photocopy of an SDS is as good as an original. In fact, many SDSs sent with products are actually copies. A small degree of networking among local dental practices (e.g., local study club) can result in a "master list" of SDSs that can be shared by participants. Many SDSs are now available on the Internet.

Another difficulty facing clinics/offices is that SDSs are sometimes incomplete or inaccurate; that is, not all of the sections are filled out. One reason is the reluctance of suppliers to describe all chemicals present in their products. Another reason is that if common domain information is not available about a hazardous chemical, the manufacturer or importer must pay to have the product evaluated by a laboratory. Clinics/offices when presented with an incomplete SDS should write the source for more specific information.

SDSs must be readily accessible to employees. Ideally, two copies of an SDS could be kept in notebooks. One set could remain in an office file cabinet; the other could be placed in a general work area, such as the laboratory or instrument recycling room. SDSs are essential to a successful clinic/office HazCom program.

Chemical information presented in SDSs is essential for the generation of proper labeling and the development of correct warning signs, and notices are present in an SDS. Table 26-3 describes the 16 required sections of the SDS.

EMPLOYEE INFORMATION AND TRAINING

Employers must provide employees with information and training on all hazardous chemicals present in the workplace, even if an employee does not use some of them in the course of normal work. The employer must provide information and training at the time of an employee's initial assignment (no matter how experienced or trained the employee may be) or whenever a new hazard is introduced into the work area. To maintain proper clinic/office awareness of hazardous chemicals, annual training sessions are expected.

Employees must be informed of (1) the requirements of the HCS, (2) any and all operations in the work area where hazardous chemicals are present or are used, and (3) the location and availability of the WHCP, including the required list of hazardous chemicals and collection of SDSs. As previously

TABLE 26-3   **Minimum Information for an SDS**

	Heading	Subheading
1.	Identification	(a) Product identifier used on the label; (b) Other means of identification; (c) Recommended use of the chemical and restrictions on use; (d) Name, address, and telephone number of the chemical manufacturer, importer, or other responsible party; (e) Emergency phone number.
2.	Hazard(s) identification	(a) Classification of the chemical in accordance with paragraph (d) of §1910.1200*; (b) Signal word, hazard statement(s), symbol(s) and precautionary statement(s) in accordance with paragraph (f) of §1910.1200. (Hazard symbols may be provided as graphical reproductions in black and white or the name of the symbol, e.g., flame, skull and crossbones); (c) Describe any hazards not otherwise classified that have been identified during the classification process; (d) Where an ingredient with unknown acute toxicity is used in a mixture at a concentration = 1% and the mixture is not classified based on testing of the mixture as a whole, a statement that X% of the mixture consists of ingredient(s) of unknown acute toxicity is required.
3.	Composition/information on ingredients	Except as provided for in paragraph (i) of §1910.1200 on trade secrets: For Substances (a) Chemical name; (b) Common name and synonyms; (c) CAS number and other unique identifiers; (d) Impurities and stabilizing additives which are themselves classified and which contribute to the classification of the substance. For Mixtures In addition to the information required for substances: (a) The chemical name and concentration (exact percentage) or concentration ranges of all ingredients which are classified as health hazards in accordance with paragraph (d) of §1910.1200 and (1) are present above their cut-off/concentration limits; or (2) present a health risk below the cut-off/concentration limits. (b) The concentration (exact percentage) shall be specified unless a trade secret claim is made in accordance with paragraph (i) of §1910.1200, when there is batch-to-batch variability in the production of a mixture, or for a group of substantially similar mixtures (See A.0.5.1.2) with similar chemical composition. In these cases, concentration ranges may be used.For All Chemicals Where a Trade Secret is Claimed Where a trade secret is claimed in accordance with paragraph (i) of §1910.1200, a statement that the specific chemical identity and/or exact percentage (concentration) of composition has been withheld as a trade secret is required.
4.	First-aid measures	(a) Description of necessary measures, subdivided according to the different routes of exposure, i.e., inhalation, skin and eye contact, and ingestion; (b) Most important symptoms/effects, acute and delayed. (c) Indication of immediate medical attention and special treatment needed, if necessary.
5.	Fire-fighting measures	(a) Suitable (and unsuitable) extinguishing media. (b) Specific hazards arising from the chemical (e.g., nature of any hazardous combustion products). (c) Special protective equipment and precautions for firefighters.
6.	Accidental release measures	(a) Personal precautions, protective equipment, and emergency procedures. (b) Methods and materials for containment and cleaning up.
7.	Handling and storage	(a) Precautions for safe handling. (b) Conditions for safe storage, including any incompatibilities.
8.	Exposure controls/personal protection	(a) OSHA permissible exposure limit (PEL), American Conference of Governmental Industrial Hygienists (ACGIH) threshold limit value (TLV), and any other exposure limit used or recommended by the chemical manufacturer, importer, or employer preparing the safety data sheet, where available. (b) Appropriate engineering controls. (c) Individual protection measures, such as personal protective equipment.

TABLE 26-3   **Minimum Information for an SDS—cont'd**

Heading	Subheading
9. Physical and chemical properties	(a) Appearance (physical state, color, etc.); (b) Odor; (c) Odor threshold; (d) pH; (e) Melting point/freezing point; (f) Initial boiling point and boiling range; (g) Flash point; (h) Evaporation rate; (i) Flammability (solid, gas); (j) Upper/lower flammability or explosive limits; (k) Vapor pressure; (l) Vapor density; (m) Relative density; (n) Solubility(ies); (o) Partition coefficient: n-octanol/water; (p) Autoignition temperature; (q) Decomposition temperature; (r) Viscosity.
10. Stability and reactivity	(a) Reactivity; (b) Chemical stability; (c) Possibility of hazardous reactions; (d) Conditions to avoid (e.g., static discharge, shock, or vibration); (e) Incompatible materials; (f) Hazardous decomposition products.
11. Toxicological information	Description of the various toxicological (health) effects and the available data used to identify those effects, including: (a) Information on the likely routes of exposure (inhalation, ingestion, skin and eye contact); (b) Symptoms related to the physical, chemical, and toxicological characteristics; (c) Delayed and immediate effects and also chronic effects from short- and long-term exposure; (d) Numerical measures of toxicity (such as acute toxicity estimates); (e) Whether the hazardous chemical is listed in the National Toxicology Program (NTP) Report on Carcinogens (latest edition) or has been found to be a potential carcinogen in the International Agency for Research on Cancer (IARC) Monographs (latest edition), or by OSHA.
12. Ecological information (nonmandatory)	(a) Ecotoxicity (aquatic and terrestrial, where available); (b) Persistence and degradability; (c) Bioaccumulative potential; (d) Mobility in soil; (e) Other adverse effects (such as hazardous to the ozone layer).
13. Disposal considerations (nonmandatory)	Description of waste residues and information on their safe handling and methods of disposal, including the disposal of any contaminated packaging.
14. Transport information (nonmandatory)	(a) UN number; (b) UN proper shipping name; (c) Transport hazard class(es); (d) Packing group, if applicable; (e) Environmental hazards (e.g., Marine pollutant [Yes/No]); (f) Transport in bulk (according to Annex II of MARPOL 73/78 and the IBC Code); (g) Special precautions which a user needs to be aware of, or needs to comply with, in connection with transport or conveyance either within or outside their premises.
15. Regulatory information (nonmandatory)	Safety, health, and environmental regulations specific for the product in question.
16. Other information, including date of preparation or last revision	The date of preparation of the SDS or the last change to it.

From OSHA: *Hazard communication standard, appendix D*, http://www.osha.gov/dsg/hazcom/ghs-final-rule.html.

*1910.1200 refers to the Hazard Communication Standard presented in Appendix H.

stated, for better compliance, each employee must receive a copy of at least the regulatory text of the actual standard.

Training is an essential component of a successful HCS program. Training is required at the time of hiring, when a new hazard is introduced, and annually for all continuing employees. Training has five major components.

1. *How the HCS is implemented in the workplace.* Employees must be trained in the reading and interpretation of labels and SDSs and how they can obtain and use the available hazard information.

2. *Physical and health hazards present.* Employees are to be trained about the physical and health hazards associated with hazardous chemicals. The use of SDSs, container labels, and other forms of warning signs reinforce this process.

3. *Personal protective devices.* Employees must be informed of and provided with all the PPE needed to protect them while using hazardous chemicals.

4. *Site-specific information.* The employer must convey details of the clinic/office WHCP, including an explanation of the labeling system and the SDS collection, to the employees and must inform employees as to how they can obtain and use appropriate hazard information. Protection includes physical pieces of equipment and specific posted procedures such as appropriate engineering controls, work practice changes, and emergency procedures.

5. *Methods and observations.* This part of training involves knowledge of the appearance and smell of hazardous chemicals, which helps employees limit exposures to chemicals. This section also assumes that the clinic/office has designed and practiced an emergency plan.

TRADE SECRETS

Chemical manufacturers and importers may withhold specific chemical information, including the chemical name or other specific data that could help identify a hazardous chemical on its SDS. The central argument is the claim by the source that the information withheld is indeed a trade secret. The rationale is that publication of such information negatively affects market share.

The HCS attempts to strike a balance between the need to protect exposed employees and a manufacturer's need to maintain the confidentiality of a bona fide trade secret. Balance is achieved by the source providing, under specified need and confidentiality, limited disclosure to health professionals who are furnishing medical or other occupational health services to exposed employees, employee representatives, or contract workers.

Chemical manufacturers, importers, and in some cases employers must disclose immediately the specific chemical identity of a hazardous chemical to a treating physician or nurse when the information is needed for prompt emergency or first-aid treatment. Companies can request the treating physician or nurse to prepare a written statement of need and to complete a confidentiality agreement after the emergency has abated.

When the case is a nonemergency, the issue can become protracted. A health care professional (e.g., physician, industrial hygienist, toxicologist, epidemiologist, or occupational health nurse) must write the source company, describing the circumstances surrounding the petition.

HOW THE OCCUPATIONAL SAFETY AND HEALTH ADMINISTRATION SOLVES A PROBLEM

Of interest is the examination of the thought processes used to solve potentially complex interpersonal problems within the workplace. Successful resolution of questions concerning OSHA compliance and other employee health and safety issues is no exception. For example, an employee on the job for a few weeks begins to complain about feeling ill at work. The employee could state, "I don't know. Something smells funny in here, and I'm starting to get headaches." How should this person's employer best handle the complaint?

Employers must take all employee complaints seriously. Most employees are reluctant to report problems, especially if they seem to involve only themselves. The employer has the responsibility to establish an environment in which employee safety is paramount and in which open communication is the rule. Dismissing out of hand an employee complaint is unfair and unwise. Employees who think their reasonable requests are not being addressed properly are far more likely to seek an answer outside of the office or clinic. In other words, the chances of them reporting the case to a regulatory agency are greatly increased.

The first action the employer should take is to determine whether a request is reasonable. This is probably more difficult than it sounds. Some employees at times make and maintain unreasonable requests. Fortunately, such cases are the exception. However, separation may be the only viable answer in extreme situations. A guiding rule as to whether a request or a policy, procedure, or piece of equipment has validity is to subject it to three challenges: "Is it reasonable?" "Is it necessary?" and "Is it appropriate?"

Employers must do what is required and proper, but they are not obligated to provide more than what is necessary. Regular clinic/office meetings at which compliance issues are discussed in an open manner are central to clinic/office morale and compliance. After such discussions, a decision should be made quickly. If the answer is "no," the logic behind the position should be presented. Because the employer is responsible for employee safety, the employer makes the final decision. However, employees usually expect and wish to be active participants in the process. Employers must provide a working environment that is safe; the employees have the responsibility to comply with established clinic/office procedures.

If after careful review an employer decides that an employee complaint has merit, remedial action is required. This does not mean necessarily that just because an odor is present, the odor is causing the employee's headaches or that it is indeed even potentially harmful. The employer has an obligation to investigate the matter further. Of course, the first temptation is to provide personal protective devices, such as masks. When presented with such a scenario, OSHA would consider its resolution to be a four-step process that progresses from more effective actions to those less effective. The steps are as follows:

1. *Determine whether a problem exists.* The presence of an odor may or may not indicate a potential problem. Of course, some dangerous chemical vapors have little or no odor. Some types of monitoring devices, such as air samplers attached to color change chemicals or spectrophotometric devices, may be required. Other chemicals can be monitored easily with the use of inexpensive badges. Persistent problems may require consultation with an industrial hygienist or the local health or air quality department. Fortunately, in most cases, no problem exists or it is solved readily. Problems, of course, can involve issues such as air quality, sound, heat, and lighting (e.g., curing lights).

2. *Engineering controls.* Engineering controls are measures designed to isolate or remove the chemical hazard from a workplace. If a problem exists, OSHA indicates that the most effective and efficient method of resolution is to remove or change the chemical used or somehow to use it differently. A common dental example is a glutaraldehyde solution. All sterilizing chemicals are harsh at room temperature and easily can generate irritating fumes, which could cause allergies. Direct contact with unprotected skin or mucous membranes likely would lead to complaints and possible injury. If an employee complains about the use of glutaraldehydes, the best option is to change how reusable instruments and equipment are sterilized. This change could include a change to a heat treatment process such as autoclaving. If the items are heat sensitive, other glutaraldehyde solutions are commercially available. A change in the chemical used could help eliminate the problem.

3. *Work practices.* Work practice controls are methods that reduce the likelihood of exposure by altering the manner in which a chemical is used. If engineering controls cannot be used because the chemical is absolutely necessary, the employer should investigate using work practice controls. Again, using glutaraldehyde as an example, such solutions usually can be used safely when present in small amounts and when held within tightly sealed containers. Ideally, removing or changing the chemical is the most effective process. However, if the chemical must be used, workplace practices may have to be changed significantly. Of course, an increase in ventilation, such as using a fume hood, is always beneficial.

4. *PPE.* PPE includes specialized clothing or equipment worn by an employee for protection against a chemical hazard. General work clothes usually are not sufficiently protective. For several reasons, PPE is

considered to be the least-effective and least-efficient method of preventing employee exposures. One major deficiency is the lack of universal application. One cannot expect that employees always will wear the proper equipment whenever the hazard is present, including accidents. Obviously, PPE must be in place whenever any risk of exposure exists. Another fault of PPE involves the physical nature of barriers. Eventually all barriers fail. With newer designs and fabrication, materials have improved the longevity of some PPE. Technological advances also have helped to improve overall barrier performance. Unfortunately, personal protective barriers will never be as effective as removing or changing a hazardous chemical or the use of improved handling methods.

OCCUPATIONAL EXPOSURE TO HAZARDOUS CHEMICALS IN LABORATORIES

OSHA has promulgated a safety standard (29 CFR Part 1450, Occupational Exposure to Hazardous Chemicals in Laboratories) that helps protect employees engaged in the laboratory use of hazardous chemicals (Table 26-4).

In many ways, dental offices and clinics function as laboratories. Although carcinogenic, radioactive, or extremely toxic materials are rarely present, dental workplaces contain significant amounts and varying types of hazardous chemicals. Employees routinely prepare, use, store, and dispose of these materials, in addition to being exposed daily to infectious agents and physical methods of harm (e.g., heat, sound, light, and air quality).

The major objective of the standard is to limit employee exposures to specific permissible levels when working in laboratories. For some chemicals, other OSHA and EPA standards apply that are stricter. In some cases, absolutely no exposure is permitted. Some chemicals, however, are exempt. These include chemicals that have no potential for employee exposure; for example, (1) procedures that use chemically impregnated test media (dipsticks) that are placed into liquid specimens and then the amount of color changed is observed and (2) commercial kits in which all the reagents needed to conduct a test are contained within the kit (a pregnancy test is an example).

Limits are not known for all individual chemicals or for groups of chemicals mixed to create a new end product. However, complaints about odors, headaches, runny noses and eyes, nausea, or skin hypersensitivities are common. The initial response is to determine whether a problem actually exists.

COMPLIANCE

Compliance with the Safe Use of Chemicals in the Laboratory Standard involves seven sections or components: (1) general principles, (2) responsibilities, (3) laboratory facility, (4) components of the chemical hygiene plan, (5) general

TABLE 26-4   **Important Definitions for a Chemical Hygiene Plan**

Term	Definition
Action plan	Includes concentrations designated in 29 CFR part 1910 for a specific substance as being safe, calculated on an 8-hour average exposure. Action plan usually is constructed in response to a complaint or is part of the regular review program of the facility. Appropriate responses include exposure monitoring and medical surveillance.
Chemical hygiene officer	An employee who is designated by the employer and who is qualified by training or experience to provide technical guidance in the development and implementation of a chemical hygiene plan. For clinical dentistry, the position is similar to the office infection control hazard communication officer.
Chemical hygiene plan	A written program developed and implemented by the employer that sets forth procedures, equipment, personal protective equipment, and work practices that (1) are capable of protecting employees from health hazards presented by hazardous chemicals used in a particular workplace and (2) involve the application of the tenets of "prudent practice."
Emergency	Any occurrence such as equipment failure, rupture of containers, or failure of control equipment that results in the uncontrolled release of a hazardous chemical into the workplace.
Hazardous chemical	A chemical for which statistically significant evidence based on a scientifically designed and conducted study indicates the acute and chronic health effects that may occur to exposed employees. Many of the chemicals used within dental offices/clinics are considered hazardous.
Prudent practices	Originally developed in 1981 by the National Research Council, this plan is useful for preparing a workplace chemical hygiene plan. The plan helps to organize identified hazards better and offers recommendations for each type of hazard and deals with safety and chemical hazards; the Laboratory Standard is concerned primarily with chemical hazards.

Adapted from Occupational Safety and Health Administration: *29 CFR Part 1450: Occupational exposure to hazardous chemicals in laboratories standard and Standard Appendixes A and B*, Washington, DC, 1990, US Government Printing Office.

principles of working with chemicals, (6) safety recommendations, and (7) SDSs. This organization of topics corresponds to sections in the standard and the recommendations made in Appendices A and B of the standard. Compliance is mandatory for the standard; however, the materials presented in Appendices A and B do not have to be followed exactly as presented. These appendices offer valuable organizational help and make valid suggestions. Reviewing (and possibly using) these materials may help any clinic/office compliance program greatly.

GENERAL PRINCIPLES FOR WORKING WITH LABORATORY CHEMICALS

Each workplace must develop an appropriate chemical hygiene plan (see Table 26-4). No official form or format exists. However, information given in Appendices A and B of the Laboratory Standard helps make compliance an easier and more effective process.

Many of the recommendations offered follow those provided by the National Research Council (1981). These recommendations often are called Prudent Practices for Handling Hazardous Chemicals in Laboratories or simply prudent practices (see Table 26-4). The practices actually are an assessment of risk and a listing of recommendations that have the ultimate goal of limiting workplace exposure to harmful chemicals. Prudent practices have a broader scope or intent than the Laboratory Standard. Prudent practices

deal with safety and chemical hazards, whereas the Laboratory Standard is concerned primarily with chemical hazards.

Minimization of all exposures to chemicals is prudent. General precautions for the use of chemicals should be developed and implemented effectively. Written general precautions are usually more valuable than the generation of specific guidelines for particular chemicals. An analogy is the concept of universal precautions. In this case, the objective is to prevent contact of health care workers with patient body fluids. The combination of engineering controls, work practices, and PPE selected should protect against any infectious agent present in blood and other body fluids.

One should not underestimate risk. Even for chemicals that seem to have little or no toxicity, exposure always should be kept to a minimum. Of course, chemicals known to cause problems require special handling. Information on use may come from the manufacturer/importer and is present on the SDSs. OSHA also can provide lists of chemicals that indicate their relative toxicity and acceptable levels of employee exposures. Minimization of exposure also involves an action plan (see Table 26-4) that is a determination of the levels of chemicals present in the workplace over a specific time and then the generation of an appropriate response.

One of the most effective ways to minimize employee exposure is to limit release and to dilute with air any emissions. Adequate ventilation must be provided and may include fume hoods and other ventilation devices.

A central activity for compliance with the Laboratory Standard is the mandatory preparation of a chemical hygiene plan designed to minimize exposures. This plan always should be considered "as a work in progress," should address all salient issues, and should be in writing.

CHEMICAL HYGIENE RESPONSIBILITIES

Every person working at a location is responsible for chemical hygiene. The chief executive officer is ultimately responsible; however, all employees must understand the Laboratory Standard and comply with its tenets.

One way to deal with the requirements is to appoint a chemical hygiene officer (see Table 26-4) who can serve as liaison between employees and management. Responsibilities include (1) monitoring procurement, use, and disposal of laboratory chemicals; (2) maintaining lists of chemicals present; (3) being aware of current exposure limits for the chemicals present; and (4) working with management continually to improve the chemical hygiene plan.

The chemical hygiene officer in a dental office or clinic also may serve as laboratory supervisor. The responsibilities of this individual include (1) ensuring that workers know and follow chemical hygiene rules, (2) ensuring that proper PPE and other types of protective equipment are present and in working order, (3) performing necessary inspections, (4) keeping up to date on current legal requirements concerning regulated substances, (5) evaluating and selecting protective apparel and equipment, and (6) ensuring that the facility and the workers are prepared (usually through training) for the use of a new chemical.

Workers are responsible for planning and conducting each operation according to the chemical hygiene procedures of the office/clinic, which usually involves a "safety first" philosophy. Workers must comply with the tenets of the Laboratory Standard as presented in the written plan of the facility.

LABORATORY FACILITIES

Laboratories should have an adequate general ventilation system. In some cases, special air exhaust equipment (e.g., ventilation hood) is needed. Personal protective equipment more commonly is required. Proper air circulation is needed in all areas of the facility. The best setup is to have an eye-face wash fountain and a sink readily available when handling hazardous chemicals (Figure 26-3). Having more than one fountain or sink may be necessary. Each facility also should have a formal procedure for the disposal of waste chemicals.

To have the ventilation, exposure control, and PPE materials functioning properly, significant attention must be paid to their maintenance, performance, and applicability. Having the equipment and materials checked by an outside sales and service company may be necessary.

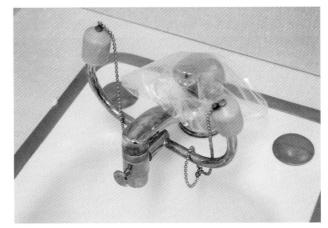

FIGURE 26-3 Eyewash station.

CHEMICAL HYGIENE PLAN

A chemical hygiene plan is the central element for compliance with the Laboratory Standard. The plan should be in writing and begins with a listing of the basic rules and procedures to be used in a facility (Table 26-5). Specific comments on chemical procurement, distribution, and storage and disposal of chemicals follow.

Regular instrument monitoring usually is not required. However, such tests can help determine whether a problem exists and what changes are needed.

Proper housekeeping, regular maintenance, and periodic inspections need to be performed. Clean floors and surfaces enhance safety. Inspections can identify needed maintenance. For example, eye-face wash fountains should be inspected every 3 months. Other pieces of equipment also can be inspected at regular intervals. Methods of egress and access to emergency equipment and utility controls in the event of an emergency (see Table 26-5) must be available. Passageways, stairways, and hallways must not be used as chemical storage areas.

Each office or clinic must be prepared to provide a medical program, which may involve regular surveillance. More commonly present is the need for first aid, which includes in-house and emergency room activities. Protective apparel and equipment needed include PPE that is compatible with the required degree of protection for the substances being handled, an eye-face wash fountain, fire extinguishers, respiratory protection (including dust), fire alarms, emergency phone numbers, and any other items chosen by the chemical hygiene officer.

Certain records need to be kept to be in compliance. A written record of all accidents must be retained. Because federal and state agencies differ on how long such records need to be kept, one should consider their storage as permanent. The office or clinic plan should be reviewed regularly and changed when necessary. Chemical inventory and use records for hazardous chemicals also should be completed.

TABLE 26-5   **Components of a Chemical Hygiene Plan**

Component	Required Action
Basic rules and procedures	Put everything in writing. List environmental preventive methods and procedures. List PPE and uses. Outline actions when confronting a spill, accident, or emergency.
Chemical procurement, distribution, and storage	List procurement procedures. Follow established processes concerning introduction of chemicals to the collection of a facility. Store chemicals properly. Distribute chemicals throughout the facility safely.
Environmental monitoring	Do not regularly monitor for chemicals. Do monitor if required by regulatory agency or if a problem appears to exist.
Housekeeping, maintenance, and inspections	Ensure cleanliness. Inspect equipment and safety materials regularly. Maintain safety items as per inspection or need. Allow for easy egress and access to safety and emergency equipment and utility controls.
Medical program	Provide safety and medical surveillance. Discover potential exposure outcomes with proper authorities. Provide necessary first aid.
Protective apparel and equipment (PPE)	Provide environmental safety equipment such as fire extinguishers, fire alarms, and adequate ventilation. Ensure that PPE such as eye-face wash fountains, respirators and masks, and special clothing are readily available. Prohibit eating, drinking, smoking, application of cosmetics, and the use of contact lenses in the presence of chemicals.
Records	Maintain written records concerning all accidents. Establish and maintain a list of all hazardous chemicals present and their uses. Keep any required medical records in accordance with federal state regulations.
Signs and labels	Post emergency phone numbers. Label properly all containers holding hazardous chemicals as to content, hazard, and methods/modes of protection. Show through signage the locations of safety equipment and materials.
Spills and accidents	Ensure that all employees are aware of the written plan and its tenets. Plan for accidents; establish procedures. Analyze the causes of all spills or accidents.
Information and training programs	Provide information concerning chemical hazards present. Train employees as to proper preventive measures. Train employees concerning postexposure or accident procedures.
Waste disposal programs	Identify methods to collect, segregate, and transport waste hazardous chemicals. Follow federal/state mandates for disposal. Regularly dispose of waste chemicals.

Adapted from Occupational Safety and Health Administration: *29 CFR Part 1450: Occupational exposure to hazardous chemicals in laboratories standard and Standard Appendixes A and B*, Washington, DC, 1990, US Government Printing Office.

One of the most effective safety processes is the placement of signs and labels. Such items need to be posted prominently; the four categories are (1) emergency telephone numbers (in-house and community rescue), (2) labels that show the contents of containers (including waste receptacles) and associated hazards, (3) location signs for eye-face wash fountains and other safety and first-aid equipment and areas where food and beverage consumption and storage are permitted (e.g., refrigerators), and (4) warnings at locations where special or unusual hazards are present.

Accidents and spills should be uncommon events. However, planning and practice of the plan should minimize employee exposure to harmful chemicals. The written chemical hygiene plan must be communicated to each employee and provide procedures for evacuation, medical care, incident reporting, clean up (spill control), and drill. Some type of alarm system is helpful. The purpose of a training program is to ensure that all individuals at risk are informed adequately about working in the laboratory, its risks, and what to do if an accident occurs, including first aid and the use of special chemical abatement equipment.

A proper waste disposal system helps ensure minimal harm to persons, other organisms, and the environment from the disposal of waste laboratory chemicals, including collection, segregation, and transportation. An office or clinic must follow local regulations when disposing of chemicals. Waste should be removed regularly. Indiscriminate disposals, such as pouring down a drain or mixing of chemicals with other refuse and placement in landfills, are unacceptable.

WORKING WITH CHEMICALS

A chemical hygiene plan requires workers to know and follow safety rules and procedures. Methods designed to avoid chemical contact must be followed regularly. In the event of an exposure, prompt action is necessary. Extended flushing of eyes with water (usually for 10 to 15 minutes) followed by medical attention is an example. Water rinsing and removal of soiled clothing helps minimize skin contact. Obviously, planning for accidents is essential. One must assume that exposures will occur, and an effective and efficient response is essential.

Preventive behaviors are also helpful. Personnel must avoid eating, smoking, drinking, gum chewing, and applying of cosmetics in the presence of hazardous laboratory chemicals. Segregation of chemicals from foodstuffs is imperative. Having two refrigerators, one for food and the other for chemicals, may be necessary. Some types of contact lenses adsorb chemical vapors. One should avoid the use of contacts unless necessary.

SAFETY RECOMMENDATIONS

Safety is a two-part equation: prevention and proper handling of accidents and emergencies. If precautions fail, the chances of exposures increase. Working hard to prevent injuries is always better than managing exposures.

SELECTED READINGS

Indiana Department of Labor, Bureau of Safety Education and Training: Guidelines for developing a written hazard communication program, Indianapolis, 1992, State of Indiana.

Indiana Department of Labor, Bureau of Safety Education and Training: How to read and understand a material safety data sheet, Indianapolis, 1991, State of Indiana.

Meyer E: *Chemistry of hazardous materials*, ed 2, Englewood Cliffs, NJ, 1989, Prentice-Hall.

Miller CH: Chemical reactions, *Dent Prod Rep* 41(110):112–114, 2007.

Miller CH, Palenik CJ: Sterilization, disinfection and asepsis in dentistry. In Block SS, editor: *Disinfection, sterilization and preservation*, ed 5, Philadelphia, 2001, Lippincott Williams & Wilkins, pp 1049–1068.

Office of the Federal Register, National Archives and Records Administration: CFR 29 Part 1900-1910.99, Washington, DC, 1996, US Government Printing Office.

Palenik CJ, Miller CH: All about OSHA, part I, *Dent Asepsis Rev* 18(6):1–2, 1997.

U.S. Department of Labor: *Occupational Safety and Health Administration: Chemical hazard communication (OSHA 3084)*, Washington, DC, 1998, US Government Printing Office. Also available from http://www.osha.gov/Publications/osha3084.pdf, 1998. accessed April 2012.

U.S. Department of Labor: *Occupational Safety and Health Administration: Hazard communication standard/globally harmonized system of classification and labeling of chemicals and appendices*. http://www.osha.gov/dsg/hazcom/ghs-final-rule.html. accessed April 2012.

REVIEW QUESTIONS

Multiple Choice

1. Chemical-resistant gloves are an example of:
   a. a work practice control
   b. an engineering control
   c. personal protection equipment
   d. a material safety data sheet
   e. a hazard warning

2. Who determines the hazards of a chemical?
   a. Employers
   b. Employees
   c. Manufacturers
   d. Distributors

3. The four major changes in the 2012 update of the Hazard Communication Standard involved Hazard Classification, Material Safety Data Sheets, Information and Training and:
   a. the Exposure Control Plan
   b. the Postexposure Medical Follow-up
   c. Labels
   d. Required vaccinations

4. Safety data sheets have _____ sections.
   a. 4
   b. 5
   c. 9
   d. 16

5. According to the Occupational Safety and Health Administration, the most effective way to solve a problem is:
   a. a work practice control
   b. an engineering control
   c. personal protection equipment
   d. a safety data sheet

Please visit http://evolve.elsevier.com/Miller/infectioncontrol/ for additional practice and study support tools.

Employee Fire Prevention and Emergency Action Plans

CHAPTER 27

OUTLINE

29 CFR Parts 1910.38 and 1910.39
Fire Prevention Plans
Emergency Action Plans
Alcohol-Based Hand Rub Solutions

LEARNING OBJECTIVES

After completing this chapter, the student should be able to do the following:
1. Design a practice fire prevention plan.
2. Design an employee emergency plan.
3. Define a procedure for using and storing alcohol-based hand rubs.

KEY TERMS

Alcohol-based Hand Rubs
Emergency Action Plan (EAP)

Fire Prevention Plan
Fire Safety Standard

Occupational Safety and Health
Administration (OSHA)

29 CFR PARTS 1910.38 AND 1910.39

The **Occupational Safety and Health Administration (OSHA)** has safety plans that specifically address fire prevention and emergencies in general (Department of Labor, OSHA, 29 CFR Part 1910.38, Emergency Action Plans and Part 1910.39, Fire Prevention Plans). These plans are a combination of preventive actions and courses of action for anticipated emergencies and are designed to support other OSHA standards that require written emergency action plans. The most important standards for dentistry include the bloodborne pathogens (see Chapter 8 and Appendix G), hazard communication (see Chapter 26 and Appendix H), and safe use of chemicals in the laboratory standards (see Chapter 26 and Appendix H).

FIRE PREVENTION PLANS

Workplace fire safety is important. National Safety Council data indicate that fires and explosions in the United Sates accounted for 4% of all occupational fatalities in 2006.

When OSHA conducts a workplace inspection, it monitors employee compliance with the **Fire Safety Standard**. OSHA also checks whether the employer has provided adequate methods of egress, firefighting equipment, and employee training to reduce (even to the point of prevention) deaths and injuries.

The best way to comply with the Fire Safety Standard is to generate and use a written office/clinic plan. The written fire safety plan must include a minimum of nine elements.

- A list of major workplace fire hazards
- Proper use, storage, and disposal of potential ignition sources
- Types of fire protection equipment or systems present
- Procedures to control accumulations of flammable and combustible waste materials
- Procedures for regular maintenance of safeguards installed on heat-producing equipment to prevent the accidental ignition of combustible materials
- Names or regular job titles of persons responsible for equipment/systems maintenance
- Names or regular job titles of persons responsible for control of fuel source hazards
- Policing of flammable and combustible materials to minimize fire (housekeeping)
- Employee training

An employer must review with each employee on initial assignment all parts of the fire safety plan that the employee must know to protect coworkers (and patients) in the event of an emergency. A written plan must be present in the work environment and must be made available for employee review. For worksites with fewer than 10 employees, the plan may be communicated orally, and the employer is not required to maintain a written plan. However, a written plan offers several advantages, including establishment of a formal office/clinic policy, plan implementation to be used in training and training updates, and more effective communication to employees of any changes in the plan.

Clinical dentistry does not pose the same risk for fire as do many other work environments. However, the employer still must establish a fire emergency plan and a fire prevention plan.

An emergency evacuation action plan must list the expected activities of each employee during a fire, including accounting for all employees to ensure their escape. If some employees are impaired physically, the employer will have to develop special procedures. If employees must remain temporarily behind (e.g., to shut off utilities or close files), the plan must describe their actions fully.

Employee notification of a problem must be part of the fire safety plan. An alarm system may be a voice communication or a sound signal such as bells, whistles, or horns. Employees must know the signal and help patients and coworkers vacate the premises.

Training is essential. Employees first must become knowledgeable about the plan, especially newly assigned employees. The employer must contact all employees if the plan is altered. Practicing of responses helps to ensure that employees take the correct actions.

Fire exits are essential for efficient vacating of a workplace. Each workplace must have at least two means of escape. The exits should be as distant from each other as possible. If fire doors are present, they must not be blocked or locked when employees are in the work area. Exit routes must be marked clearly and must be free of obstructions. Office/clinic signs must match those used in the rest of the building.

Each workplace must have a full complement of the proper types of extinguishers for the fire hazards present. Several large ABC-type extinguishers in a dental office/clinic should be adequate. The presence of portable fire extinguishers indicates that some employees will remain to fight small fires. Those expected or anticipated to use fire extinguishers must receive instruction concerning firefighting and proper use of the equipment.

Employers should use only approved fire extinguishers and must keep them in good working order. The best option may be to hire a fire protection company to estimate the fire prevention needs of an office or clinic and then to maintain and inspect the equipment. Employers also may consider fire suppression systems such as sprinklers. These choices are the responsibility of the employer.

Employers need to develop a written fire prevention plan to complement the fire evacuation plan so as to minimize the frequency of evacuation. Fire prevention is always preferable to firefighting. The employees must review such plans.

Fire prevention is assisted by proper housekeeping procedures for storage, use, and cleanup of flammable materials and proper disposal of flammable waste. Any source of heat, especially open flames, must be monitored and controlled, including correct maintenance of equipment.

All employees must be knowledgeable of the fire prevention and fire emergency plans of their office or clinic. Again, the employer has the responsibility to develop the plans and to ensure that employees are trained.

EMERGENCY ACTION PLANS

An emergency action plan (EAP) describes the actions employees should take to ensure their safety if a fire or other emergency situation occurs. Well-developed emergency plans and proper employee training (such that employees understand their roles and responsibilities within the plan) result in fewer and less severe employee injuries and less structural damage to the facility during emergencies. A poorly prepared plan likely will lead to a disorganized evacuation or emergency response, resulting in confusion, injury, and property damage.

An EAP is a written document required by particular OSHA standards. The purpose of an EAP is to facilitate and organize employer and employee actions during workplace emergencies.

The elements of the plan must include at least the following:

- Procedures for reporting a fire or other emergency
- Evacuation procedures and emergency escape route assignments
- Procedures employees are to follow who remain to operate critical plant operations before they evacuate
- Procedures to account for all employees after an emergency evacuation has been completed
- Rescue and medical duties for those employees who are to perform them
- Names or job titles of persons who can be contacted for further information or explanation of duties under the plan

Each office must generate escape procedures and designate escape routes for any emergency. An emergency plan can be incorporated into the written plans of an applicable standard, such as the Hazard Communication Standard. Each employee must know and follow assigned duties and escape routes. In an emergency, some employees will be asked to remain to activate safety equipment or to perform critical operations (e.g., shut off utilities and machinery). Which employees will remain, what they will do, and when they must leave is situational and will need to be described well. During an emergency, an accounting of all employees is essential. The written EAP must include a method to ensure that all employees are outside the affected work areas. An established meeting place is one way to meet this requirement. In some situations, employees will perform rescue and medical duties, and the employer needs to establish which employees and what actions. Each workplace must establish a method by which emergencies, including fires, are reported to the proper authorities. The employer also must determine official contacts and the names and titles of the cadre of employees.

To implement the EAP properly, employees must receive training about the types of emergencies that could occur and the written protocol of response activities, including emergency evacuations. Additional training is needed if employee responsibilities or designated areas are changed. Practicing emergency activities regularly increases the probability that employees will respond properly if an actual emergency occurs. Table 27-1 is a checklist that can help dental practices establish, maintain, and monitor the EAP.

An employer must review with each employee on initial assignment all parts of the emergency plan or with all employees when the plan is changed. A written plan needs to be present in the work environment and made available for employee review. For work sites with fewer than 10 employees, the plan may be communicated orally and the employer is not required to maintain a written plan. A written plan, however, is considered the superior communication method. The written plan offers several advantages, including the establishment of a formal office policy, the ability to be used in training and training updates, and the ability to be modified easily, with changes being communicated more effectively to employees.

TABLE 27-1   **Emergency Action Plan Checklist**

General Issues	Explanations
☑ Does the plan consider all potential natural or manmade emergencies that could disrupt your workplace?	Common sources of emergencies identified in emergency action plans include fires, explosions, floods, hurricanes, tornadoes, toxic material releases, radiological and biological accidents, civil disturbances, and workplace violence.
☑ Does the plan consider all potential internal sources of emergencies or chemical hazards that could disrupt your workplace?	Conduct a hazard assessment of the workplace to identify any physical or chemical hazards that may exist and could cause an emergency.
☑ Does the plan consider the impact of these internal and external emergencies on the workplace's operations, and is the response tailored to the workplace?	Brainstorm worst case scenarios, asking yourself what you would do and what would be the likely impact on your operation, and devise appropriate responses.
☑ Does the plan contain a list of key personnel with contact information as well as contact information for local emergency responders, agencies, and contractors?	Keep your list of key contacts current and make provisions for an emergency communications system such as a cellular phone, a portable radio unit, or other means so that contact with local law enforcement, the fire department, and others can be swift.
☑ Does the plan contain the names, titles, departments, and telephone numbers of individuals to contact for additional information or an explanation of duties and responsibilities under the plan?	List names and contact information for individuals responsible for implementation of the plan.
☑ Does the plan address how rescue operations will be performed?	Unless you are a large employer handling hazardous materials and processes or have employees regularly working in hazardous situations, you will probably choose to rely on local public resources, such as the fire department, whose personnel are trained, equipped, and certified to conduct rescues. Make sure any external department or agency identified in your plan is prepared to respond as outlined in your plan. Untrained individuals may endanger themselves and those they are trying to rescue.
☑ Does the plan address how medical assistance will be provided?	Most small employers do not have a formal internal medical program and make arrangements with medical clinics or facilities close by to handle emergency cases and provide medical and first-aid services to their employees. If an infirmary, clinic, or hospital is not close to your workplace, ensure that onsite person(s) has(have) adequate training in first aid. The American Red Cross, some insurance providers, local safety councils, fire departments, or other resources may be able to provide this training. Treatment of a serious injury should begin within 3 to 4 minutes of the accident. Consult with a physician to ensure there are appropriate first-aid supplies for emergencies. Establish a relationship with a local ambulance service so transportation is readily available for emergencies.
☑ Does the plan identify how or where personal information on employees can be obtained in an emergency?	In the event of an emergency, it could be important to have ready access to important personal information about your employees. This includes their home telephone numbers, the names and telephone numbers of their next of kin, and medical information.

Continued

TABLE 27-1   **Emergency Action Plan Checklist—cont'd**

General Issues	Explanations

EVACUATION POLICY AND PROCEDURE

General Issues	Explanations
☑ Does the plan identify the conditions under which an evacuation would be necessary?	The plan should identify the different types of situations that will require an evacuation of the workplace. This might include a fire, earthquake, or chemical spill. The extent of evacuation may be different for different types of hazards.
☑ Does the plan identify a clear chain of command and designate a person authorized to order an evacuation or shutdown of operations?	It is common practice to select a responsible individual to lead and coordinate your emergency plan and evacuation. It is critical that employees know who the coordinator is and understand that this person has the authority to make decisions during emergencies. The coordinator should be responsible for assessing the situation to determine whether an emergency exists requiring activation of the emergency procedures, overseeing emergency procedures, notifying and coordinating with outside emergency services, and directing shutdown of utilities or plant operations if necessary.
☑ Does the plan address the types of actions expected of different employees for the various types of potential emergencies?	The plan may specify different actions for employees depending on the emergency. For example, employers may want to have employees assemble in one area of the workplace if it is threatened by a tornado or earthquake but evacuate to an exterior location during a fire.
☑ Does the plan designate who, if anyone, will stay to shut down critical operations during an evacuation?	You may want to include in your plan locations where utilities (such as electrical and gas utilities) can be shut down for all or part of the facility. All individuals remaining behind to shut down critical systems or utilities must be capable of recognizing when to abandon the operation or task and evacuate themselves.
☑ Does the plan outline specific evacuation routes and exits, and are these posted in the workplace where they are easily accessible to all employees?	Most employers create maps from floor diagrams with arrows that designate the exit route assignments. These maps should include locations of exits, assembly points, and equipment (such as fire extinguishers, first-aid kits, spill kits) that may be needed in an emergency. Exit routes should be clearly marked and well lit, wide enough to accommodate the number of evacuating personnel, unobstructed and clear of debris at all times, and unlikely to expose evacuating personnel to additional hazards.
☑ Does the plan address procedures for assisting people during evacuations, particularly those with disabilities or who do not speak English?	Many employers designate individuals as evacuation wardens to help move employees from danger to safe areas during an emergency. Generally, one warden for every 20 employees should be adequate, and the appropriate number of wardens should be available at all times during working hours. Wardens may be responsible for checking offices and bathrooms before being the last person to exit an area as well as ensuring that fire doors are closed when exiting. Employees designated to assist in emergency evacuation procedures should be trained in the complete workplace layout and various alternative escape routes. Employees designated to assist in emergencies should be made aware of employees with special needs (who may require extra assistance during an evacuation), how to use the buddy system, and any hazardous areas to avoid during an emergency evacuation.
☑ Does the plan identify one or more assembly areas (as necessary for different types of emergencies) where employees will gather and a method for accounting for all employees?	Accounting for all employees following an evacuation is critical. Confusion in the assembly areas can lead to delays in rescuing anyone in the building, or unnecessary and dangerous search-and-rescue operations. To ensure the fastest, most accurate accounting of your employees, consider taking a head count after the evacuation. The names and last known location of anyone not accounted for should be passed on to the official in charge.
☑ Does the plan address how visitors will be assisted in evacuation and accounted for?	Some employers have all visitors and contractors sign in when entering the workplace. The hosts and/or area wardens, if established, are often tasked with helping these individuals evacuate safety.

REPORTING EMERGENCIES AND ALERTING EMPLOYEES IN AN EMERGENCY

General Issues	Explanations
☑ Does the plan identify a preferred method for reporting fires and other emergencies?	Dialing 911 is a common method for reporting emergencies if external responders are utilized. Internal numbers may be used. Internal numbers are sometimes connected to intercom systems so that coded announcements may be made. In some cases, employees are requested to activate manual pull stations or other alarm systems.

Continued

TABLE 27-1   Emergency Action Plan Checklist—cont'd

General Issues	Explanations
☑ Does the plan describe the method to be used to alert employees, including disabled workers, to evacuate or take other action?	Make sure alarms are distinctive and recognized by employees as a signal to evacuate the work area or perform other actions identified in your plan. Sequences of horn blows or different types of alarms (bells, horns, etc.) can be used to signal different responses or actions from employees. Consider making available an emergency communications system, such as a public address system, for broadcasting emergency information to employees. Ideally, alarms will be able to be heard, seen, or otherwise perceived by everyone in the workplace, including those who may be blind or deaf. Otherwise floor wardens or others must be tasked with ensuring all employees are notified. You might want to consider providing an auxiliary power supply in the event of an electrical failure.

EMPLOYEE TRAINING AND DRILLS

☑ Does the plan identify how and when employees will be trained so that they understand the types of emergencies that may occur, their responsibilities and actions as outlined in the plan?	Training should be offered employees when you develop your initial plan and when new employees are hired. Employees should be retrained when your plan changes because of a change in the layout or design of the facility, when new equipment, hazardous materials, or processes are introduced that affect evacuation routes, or when new types of hazards are introduced that require special actions. General training for your employees should address the following: • Individual roles and responsibilities; • Threats, hazards, and protective actions; • Notification, warning, and communications procedures; • Emergency response procedures; • Evacuation, shelter, and accountability procedures; • Location and use of common emergency equipment and emergency shutdown procedures. You may also need to provide additional training to your employees (e.g., first-aid procedures, portable fire extinguisher use, etc.) depending on the responsibilities allocated employees in your plan.
☑ Does the plan address how and when retraining will be conducted?	If training is not reinforced, it will be forgotten. Consider retraining employees annually.
☑ Does the plan address if and how often drills will be conducted?	Once you have reviewed your emergency action plan with your employees and everyone has had the proper training, it is a good idea to hold practice drills as often as necessary to keep employees prepared. Include outside resources such as fire and police departments when possible. After each drill, gather management and employees to evaluate the effectiveness of the drill. Identify the strengths and weaknesses of your plan and work to improve it.

ALCOHOL-BASED HAND RUB SOLUTIONS

Over the last few years, **alcohol-based hand rubs** have become popular in the United States (see Chapter 10). Such products have been used successfully for more than 30 years in Europe. Extensive research indicates that such products are more effective for standard hand hygiene or hand asepsis by health care personnel than soap or anti-microbial-containing soap products. The ease of use also increases rates of compliance for handwashing (e.g., after removing gloves).

However, such alcohol-based products are flammable. Two of the more common formulations used in the United States are equal to or greater than 60% ethyl alcohol or isopropyl alcohol by volume. One can hardly conceive that something that one would rub routinely on the hands could pose such a fire hazard. However, genuine concerns exist as to the installation of dispensers and the storage of the product.

The American Society for Healthcare Engineering has reviewed the situation and determined that (1) installing hand rub dispensers is acceptable in corridors and suite locations and (2) placing dispensers at or near each patient room entrance is not a significant risk.

The society has also issued a set of important recommendations including the following:

• Single containers installed in an egress corridor should not exceed a maximum capacity of 1.2 liters (L) for alcohol-based rub solutions in gel/liquid form.
• Single containers installed in a suite (or a dental operatory) should not exceed a maximum capacity of 2.0 L for alcohol-based rub solutions in gel/liquid form.

- Dispensers should not be installed over electric receptacles or near other potential sources of ignition.
- Dispensers that project more than 3.5 inches into the corridors should be noted in the fire plan and training program of the facility.
- All storage of replacement alcohol-based hand rub containers on patient floors, regardless of the quantity, should be within an approved flammable liquid storage cabinet.
- The quantity of replacement alcohol-based hand rub containers stored and used on any floor, including bulk storage in central supply rooms, should not exceed the maximum quantity permitted by the local prevailing building and fire codes.

SELECTED READINGS

American Society for Healthcare Engineering: *NFPA 101 Life Safety Code. Alcohol-based hand rubs.* http://www.ashe.org/advocacy/organizations/NFPA/nfpa101lsc2005commentcloses. accessed April 2012.

Boyce JM, Pearson ML: Low frequency of fires from alcohol-based hand rub dispensers in healthcare facilities, *Infect Control Hosp Epidemiol* 24:618–619, 2003.

Boyce JM, Pittet D: Healthcare Infection Control Practices Advisory Committee; HICPAC/SHEA/APIC/IDSA Hand Hygiene Task Force: Guideline for hand hygiene in health-care settings. Recommendations of the Healthcare Infection Control Practices Advisory Committee and the HICPAC/SHEA/APIC/IDSA Hand

Hygiene Task Force. Society for Healthcare Epidemiology of America/Association for Professionals in Infection Control/Infectious Diseases Society of America, *MMWR Recomm Rep* 51(RR-16):1–45, 2002.

Occupational Safety and Health Administration: *Evacuation plans and procedures: what is an emergency action plan*http://www.osha.gov/SLTC/etools/evacuation/eap.html. accessed April 2012.

Occupational Safety and Health Administration: *Fire prevention plans —1910.39*http://www.osha.gov/pls/oshaweb/owadisp.show_document?p_table=STANDARDS&p_id=12887. accessed April 2012.

Occupational Safety and Health Administration: *Fire safety in the workplace*http://www.osha.gov/OshDoc/data_General_Facts/FireSafetyN.pdf. accessed April 2012.

Occupational Safety and Health Administration: *Safety and health topics: fire safety*http://www.osha.gov/SLTC/firesafety/index.html. accessed April 2012.

Office of the Federal Register: *National Archives and Records Administration: 29 CFR Part 1900-1910.99*, Washington, DC, 1996, US Government Printing Office.

Palenik CJ, Miller CH: All about OSHA, part I, *Dent Asepsis Rev*181–182, 1997.

Palenik CJ, Miller CH: All about OSHA, part II, *Dent Asepsis Rev* 18:1–4, 1997.

REVIEW QUESTIONS

Multiple Choice

1. An emergency action plan may be communicated orally if the workplace has fewer than _____ employees.
   a. 3
   b. 5
   c. 7
   d. 10

2. Workplace fires and burns accounted for what percent of all occupational fatalities?
   a. 0.25%
   b. 1.25%
   c. 4.00%
   d. 7.85%
   e. 14.50%

3. Should workplace violence be addressed in your emergency action plan?
   a. Yes
   b. No

4. What is the maximum volume that a single container of alcohol-based hand rub solution placed within a dental operatory can legally have?
   a. 250 mL
   b. 500 mL
   c. 1.0 L
   d. 2.0 L
   e. 5.0 L

Please visit http://evolve.elsevier.com/Miller/infectioncontrol/ for additional practice and study support tools.

Infection Control Concerns During Remodeling or Construction

OUTLINE

LEARNING OBJECTIVES

After completing this chapter, the student should be able to do the following:
1. Describe some infection control concerns during times of construction or remodeling.
2. Outline a construction plan that is sensitive to infection control and human safety and health requirements.
3. Create construction policies with the contractor and practice personnel and describe the construction and remodeling process.
4. Develop a transition plan for taking possession of the new areas.

KEY TERMS

Construction
Construction-related Outbreaks
Contractors
Design

Environmental Airborne Contaminants
Nosocomial Infections
Preconstruction
Primary Contractor

Renovation
Retrofitting
Subcontractors
Transitional Days

Many of us dream about remodeling an area in our dental practices or even just adding on some additional space. The hope may be for additional chairs, easier patient flow, more storage, a new entrance, a bigger laboratory, and even better lighting. No matter the eventual goal, reality includes money, planning, money, interruptions, money, hassles, and even more money.

One not-so-obvious concern is the role infection control may play during demolition and construction. Too often the infection control component of the equation is minimized or even forgotten. This possible shortsightedness likely could lead to potentially expensive, yet preventable, mistakes, sometimes in the interest of just saving remodeling expenses.

STATEMENT OF THE PROBLEM

Important issues surround construction and renovation. Construction is the act or process of constructing a structure, such as a building, framework, or model, that is fashioned or devised systematically. Renovation is the process of improving a structure, as by repairing or remodeling.

One element central to construction and renovation is preventing transmission of infectious agents to potentially at-risk patients and to practitioners, visitors, and families. Environmental spread of microorganisms, resulting in nosocomial infections, has been well described. Generally, nosocomial infections include those acquired by being in a health care facility or from treatment in a facility. Infections often involve fungi and water-loving, environmentally resistant bacteria. Nosocomial infections cause substantial morbidity and mortality, prolong the hospital stay of affected patients, and increase direct patient care costs. Environmental airborne contaminants and other infectious agents often are associated with water and moisture-related conditions and thus affect any construction activity. Many examples exist of construction-related outbreaks of disease. A number of fungal genera (*Aspergillus, Rhizopus, Penicillium,* and *Mucor*) and bacteria (*Legionella, Pseudomonas,* group A *Streptococcus,* and *Mycobacterium*) have been shown to be involved.

To affect significant change without informing practice personnel is never wise. Ideally, the employer will solicit and incorporate input from practice personnel. The goal is for all parties to feel involved and eventually to take ownership. Resistance, even strong resistance, to change can be expected.

Some general guidelines include the following:
- Widely communicate the potential need for change.
- Obtain as much feedback as practical from personnel.
- Develop and keep the goals associated with the change.
- Make plans for before, during, and after construction.
- Familiarize practice personnel with construction personnel.
- Coordinate the efforts of personnel to provide quality care under demanding circumstances.
- Assume that everything will take longer than expected and that alterations in some plans will have to be made.
- Manage change, not try to control it.
- Celebrate completion of the project and the important roles all parties played.

STRATEGIC PLANNING

Initial planning involves **design** and **preconstruction**. Design is to formulate or devise a plan usually in a systematic manner and often involving graphics. Preconstruction can involve a number of activities, including acquisition of materials, securing of building approvals, demolition, and external evacuation.

A number of important factors form an infection control risk assessment punch list, such as the following:
- Verifying contractor and subcontractor bonds and insurance policies
- Securing all necessary building permits and worker rights permissions
- Assessing the impact of disrupting essential services
- Estimating patient disruptions or even cancellations
- Positioning of important physical barriers
- Maintaining environmental services such as heating or cooling
- Isolating some areas to create a safer environment
- Maintaining aseptic procedures at the preconstruction levels

Professional handholding may be required. Consultation with infection control personnel would be valuable. Additional reading is required. The approach should be multidisciplinary and would involve knowledgeable architects, **contractors,** and engineers.

The staff of the practice also must be engaged. Putting together a viable planning team is essential. Input is especially valuable in the early stages of the project and when blueprints are being prepared. Good early coordination

should help identify construction elements designed to prevent and control airborne contamination, which should help minimize the chances of costly redesigning or reworking. Design challenges today include **retrofitting** older buildings into offices and clinical areas that require treatment areas, instrument processing rooms, laboratories, and storage. Often the rules and regulations in such cases are not empirical, and the talents of the planning team are needed to narrow any gaps.

MAKING CONSTRUCTION POLICY

Construction and renovation projects in health care facilities pose risks for certain patients, particularly those who are immunocompromised. The staff must take a proactive approach to limit construction-related nosocomial infections. This effort requires having a multidisciplinary team plan and implement preventive measures throughout the construction project. A person familiar with infection control plays a major role by providing education to personnel; ensuring that preventive measures are identified, initiated, and maintained; and carrying out surveillance for infections in patients. Ensuring that the appropriate preventive measures are in place and that clear lines of communication exist among the personnel enhances patient safety.

A comprehensive construction and renovation policy helps to strengthen the plan and to heighten understanding. The policy identifies and describes the players involved. The monitoring eye of infection control and prevention is thus present from start to completion of the project. Of course, final approval should be a group decision.

Many publications identify sets of elements associated with construction processes. One set of possibilities includes the following:
- Making the contractor responsible for area preparation and demolition, intraconstruction operations and maintenance, project completion, cleanup, and, finally, monitoring
- Cooperating as to the timing of events, especially those that affect patient treatment
- Handling of vital utilities
- Developing a "Plan B" in the event of delays
- Allowing for emergency work interruptions
- Sharing of information
- Ensuring the safety of all workers
- Creating traffic flow patterns for patients, practice personnel, workers, and visitors
- Disposing of waste properly (waste management)
- Backing up in the event of a major utility failure

Personnel must consider all activities in terms of their effects on infection control. Important questions include: How long will the dust and mess be around? How great will the distracting activity be? What types of patients will we be able to see? What types of procedures can be afforded? Will special infection control interventions be required? And if so, what will they be? Is everyone in agreement with the plan?

CONSTRUCTION AND REMODELING

The planning is over and now it is time to work. Any potential problem, items such as sharps containers, medicaments, patient/employee records, personal effects, and anything of value, should be well secured outside of the construction area.

Probably a variety of **subcontractors** and their employees will be involved. Subcontractors take part of the contract awarded to the **primary contractor**. Usually subcontractors perform some type of specialized work. Examples include electricity, plumbing, flooring, and heating/ventilation/air conditioning. Subcontractors also perform less-specialized work, such as demolition, jobsite cleanup, and security. The primary contractor often pays the subcontractors, unless the owner chooses to serve as the primary contractor.

The number of potential visitors may be great. Visitors also often need access to areas not being remodeled (e.g., utility switches, breaker boxes, and heating/ventilation/air conditioning equipment). The general contractor helps secure the areas directly affected. However, the practice staff have the responsibility to protect the contents of all other areas.

Practice personnel will have to be patient and understanding. Temporary barriers may have to be erected, and utility interruptions may occur. The situation will not be business as usual. Flexibility and a sense of humor are key.

The quality of patient care must not be affected perceivably, and this undoubtedly will require extra effort and additional time.

Construction area cleaning is usually the responsibility of the contractor and includes removal and disposal of demolition rubble. Contracts should specify clearly the responsibility and expectations for routine and terminal cleaning before opening of the newly renovated areas.

Reestablishment of all utilities must be ensured. A punch list may have to be generated. The hope is that the remodeling will end up as a simple turnkey operation.

Cleaning of nonconstruction areas likely will need to be more frequent and more extensive. Staff must take care to protect sensitive equipment and supplies. The practice must ensure that all remodeled areas are safe for patient exposure, including equipment, ceilings, floors, safety items, furniture, and water. Where needed, items such as handwashing facilities, eyewash stations, sinks, and evacuation systems must be present and fully operational.

MOVING IN

Transitional days are opportunities to reinforce infection control in the remodeled areas. Time must be given to move materials in and to make equipment operational. Some in-service training may be necessary because new equipment or work patterns may be involved.

The hope is for the construction to be completed in an aseptic manner. Planning and monitoring are central elements. Now, it is time to enjoy the new digs.

SELECTED READINGS

American Institute of Architects: *Guidelines for design and construction of health care facilities: 2006 edition,* Washington, DC, 2006, AIA.

Bartley J: *APIC infection control tool kit series: construction and renovation,* Washington, DC, 1999, Association for Professionalism in Infection Control and Epidemiology.

Bartley JM: APIC state-of-the-art report: the role of infection control during construction in health care facilities, *Am J Infect Control* 28:156–169, 2000.

Bartley J, Bjerke NB: Infection control considerations in critical care unit design and construction: a systematic risk assessment, *Crit Care Nurs* 24:43–58, 2001.

Beitler MA: *Strategic organizational change: a practitioner's guide for managers and consultants,* Milton Keynes, UK, 2003, Practitioner Press.

Black JS, Gregfersen HB: *Leading strategic change: breaking through the brain barrier,* Upper Saddle River, NJ, 2002, Prentice-Hall.

Boyce JM, Pittet D: Healthcare Infection Control Practices Advisory Committee; HICPAC/SHEA/APIC/IDSA Hand Hygiene Task Force: Guideline for hand hygiene in health-care settings. Recommendations of the Healthcare Infection Control Practices Advisory Committee and the HICPAC/SHEA/APIC/IDSA Hand Hygiene Task Force. Society for Healthcare Epidemiology of America/Association for Professionals in Infection Control/Infectious Diseases Society of America, *MMWR Recomm Rep* 51(RR-16):1–45, 2002.

Cheng SM, Streifel AJ: Infection control considerations during construction activities: land excavation and demolition, *Am J Infect Control* 29:321–328, 2001.

Finkelstein LE, Mendelson MH: Infection control challenges during hospital renovation, *Am J Nurs* 97:60–61, 1997.

Kidd F, Buttner C, Kressel AB: Construction: a model program for infection control compliance, *Am J Infect Control* 35:347–350, 2007.

Miller CH: Office design a key factor in maintaining infection control, *RDH* 14:24, 1994.

Miller MC: Infection control considerations when designing and equipping a dental office, *J Can Dent Assoc* 60:196–201, 1994.

Neskin GA, Peterson LR: Engineering infection control through facility design, *Emerg Infect Dis* 7:354–357, 2001.

REVIEW QUESTIONS

Multiple Choice

1. A plumber is an example of a:
   a. general contractor
   b. subcontractor
   c. primary contractor

2. Adding on a new room to a dental office is an example of:
   a. retrofitting
   b. renovation
   c. construction
   d. restoration

3. Demolition is an activity commonly associated with:
   a. design
   b. preconstruction
   c. jobsite security
   d. posting of safety signs

4. *Aspergillus* is an example of a species of:
   a. bacteria
   b. viruses
   c. protozoans
   d. fungi

Please visit http://evolve.elsevier.com/Miller/infectioncontrol/ for additional practice and study support tools.

Appendix A

Infection Control and Hazardous Materials Management Resource List

DENTAL-RELATED ORGANIZATIONS

American Dental Association
211 E Chicago Ave
Chicago, IL 60611
(800) 621-8091
http://www.ada.org
Recommendations, manuals, videotapes, brochures, *ADA News,* journal

American Dental Assistants Association
35 E Wacker, Suite 1730
Chicago, IL 60601
(312) 541-1550
http://www.dentalassistant.org
Member support services, journal

American Dental Hygienists Association
444 N Michigan Ave, Suite 3400
Chicago, IL 60611
(800) 243-2342
http://www.adha.org
Member support services, journal

Dental Assisting National Board, Inc.
444 N Michigan Ave, Suite 900
Chicago, IL 60611
(312) 642-3368
http://www.danb.org
Infection Control Examination

INFECTION CONTROL ORGANIZATIONS

Organization for Safety, Asepsis and Prevention
PO Box 6297
Annapolis, MD 21401
(800) 298-OSAP
http://www.osap.org
Educational conferences, recommendations, books, brochures, documents, audiotapes, videotapes, newsletter, member support services

Association for Professionals in Infection Control and Epidemiology, Inc.
1275 K Street NW, Suite 1000
Washington, DC 20005
(202) 789-1890
http://www.apic.org
Infection control organization for medicine

Association for the Advancement of Medical Instrumentation
Sterilization Standards Committee
4301 N Fairfax Drive, Suite 301
Arlington, VA 22203
(703) 525-4890
http://www.aami.org
Standards and recommended monitors, packaging material practices for use of sterilizers, decontamination procedures

OTHER INFECTION CONTROL WEB SITES

American Society for Microbiology: http://www.asm.org
Center for Biofilm Engineering: http://www.biofilm.montana.edu
Immunization Action Coalition: http://www.immunize.org/acip
Infectious Disease Society of America: http://www.idsociety.org/pg/toc.htm
Pan American Health Organization: http://www.paho.org
Society for Healthcare Epidemiology of America, Inc.: http://www.shea-online.org
World Health Organization: http://www.who.int

FEDERAL AGENCIES

Centers for Disease Control and Prevention (CDC)
1600 Clifton Rd, NE
Atlanta, GA 30333
(404) 488-4450
http://www.cdc.gov
Infection control recommendations, disease updates

CDC, Division of Oral Health
http://www.cdc.gov/oralhealth/index.htm
Voice information service on infection control in dentistry: (404) 332-4552

CDC, National Institute for Occupational Safety and Health
http://www.cdc.gov/niosh/homepage.html

CDC, *Morbidity and Mortality Weekly Report*
http://www2.cdc.gov/mmwr/mmwr.html

Environmental Protection Agency
http://www.epa.gov
Registration of germicides, solid waste management, water quality

Food and Drug Administration
10903 New Hampshire Avenue
Silver Springs, MD 20993
http://www.fda.gov
Regulates manufacturing and labeling of medical devices and accessories, handwashing agents, mouth rinses, drugs, food, sterilants

Occupational Safety and Health Administration (OSHA)
U.S. Department of Labor
200 Constitution Ave
Washington, DC 20210
http://www.osha.gov
Blood-borne Pathogens Standard and Hazard Communications Standard

National Institutes of Health
http://www.nih.gov

Regional OSHA Offices
  I. Boston, (617) 565-9860; Connecticut, Massachusetts, Maine, New Hampshire, Rhode Island, Vermont
 II. New York, (212) 337-2378; New Jersey, New York, Puerto Rico, Virgin Islands
III. Philadelphia, (215) 861-4900; District of Columbia, Delaware, Maryland, Pennsylvania, Virginia, West Virginia
IV. Atlanta, (678)237-0400; Alabama, Florida, Georgia, Kentucky, Mississippi, North Carolina, South Carolina, Tennessee
  V. Chicago, (312) 353-2220; Illinois, Indiana, Michigan, Minnesota, Ohio, Wisconsin
 VI. Dallas, (972) 850-4145; Arkansas, Louisiana, New Mexico, Oklahoma, Texas
VII. Kansas City, Missouri, (816) 283-8745; Kansas, Missouri, Nebraska, Iowa
VIII. Denver, (720) 264-6550; Colorado, Montana, North Dakota, South Dakota, Utah, Wyoming
 IX. San Francisco, (415) 625-2547; Arizona, California, Guam, Hawaii, Nevada
  X. Seattle, (206) 757-6700; Alaska, Idaho, Washington, Oregon

STATES WITH OSHA-APPROVED PROGRAMS

Alaska: Juneau, (907) 465-2700
Arizona: Phoenix, (602) 542-5795
California: Oakland, (510) 286-7000
Connecticut: Wethersfield, (203) 566-5123
Hawaii: Honolulu, (808) 586-9116
Indiana: Indianapolis, (317) 232-2378
Iowa: Des Moines, (515) 281-3469
Kentucky: Frankfort, (502) 564-0684
Maryland: Baltimore, (410) 767-2241
Michigan: Lansing, (517) 322-1817
Minnesota: St. Paul, (651) 284-5010
Nevada: Henderson, (702) 486-9020
New Jersey: Trenton, (609) 292-0501
New Mexico: Santa Fe, (505) 827-2855
New York: Albany, (518) 457-1263
North Carolina: Raleigh, (919) 733-7166
Oregon: Salem, (503) 378-3272
Puerto Rico: Hato Rey, (787) 754-2119
South Carolina: Columbia, (803) 896-7665
Tennessee: Nashville, (615) 741-2793
Utah: Salt Lake City, (801) 530-6901
Vermont: Montpelier, (802) 828-5084
Virgin Islands: St. Croix, (340) 772-1315
Virginia: Richmond, (804) 786-2377
Washington: Olympia, (360) 902-4805
Wyoming: Cheyenne, (307) 777-7786

Appendix B

Centers for Disease Control and Prevention Guidelines for Infection Control in Dental Health-Care Settings—2003

The following guidelines were prepared by:

William G. Kohn, DDS, Centers for Disease Control and Prevention

Amy S. Collins, MPH, Centers for Disease Control and Prevention

Jennifer L. Cleveland, DDS, Centers for Disease Control and Prevention

Jennifer A. Harte, DDS, U.S. Air Force, Retired

Kathy J. Eklund, MHP, The Forsyth Institute

Dolores M. Malvitz, DrPH, Centers for Disease Control and Prevention

Note: The background information, references, and tables are not included in this appendix. See the original publication for this information. Kohn WG, Collins AS, Cleveland JL, et al; Centers for Disease Control and Prevention: Guidelines for infection control in dental health-care settings–2003, *MMWR Recomm Rep* 52(RR-17):1-61, 2003. A link to the original publication can be found at http://www.cdc.gov/mmwr/preview/mmwrhtml/rr5217a1.htm.

RECOMMENDATIONS

Each recommendation is categorized on the basis of existing scientific data, theoretical rationale, and applicability. Rankings are based on the system used by the [Centers for Disease Control and Prevention] CDC and Healthcare Infection Control Practices Advisory Committee (HICPAC) to categorizing recommendations:

Category IA. Strongly recommended for implementation and strongly supported by well-designed experimental, clinical, or epidemiologic studies.

Category IB. Strongly recommended for implementation and supported by experimental, clinical, or epidemiologic studies and a strong theoretical rationale.

Category IC. Required for implementation, as mandated by federal or state regulation or standard. Whenever IC is utilized for a recommendation, a second rating category may be included to provide the basis of existing scientific data, theoretical rationale, and applicability.

Category II. Suggested for implementation and supported by suggestive clinical or epidemiologic studies or a theoretical rationale.

Unresolved Issue. No recommendation. Practices for which insufficient evidence or no consensus regarding efficacy exist.

I. Personnel Health Elements of an Infection-Control Program
  A. General Recommendations
    1. Develop a written personnel health program for [dental health-care personnel] DHCP that includes policies, procedures, and guidelines for education and training; immunizations; exposure prevention and postexposure management; medical conditions, work-related illness, and associated work restrictions; contact dermatitis and latex hypersensitivity; and maintenance of records, data management, and confidentiality (IB).
    2. Establish referral arrangements with qualified health-care professionals to ensure prompt and appropriate provision of preventive services, occupationally related medical conditions, and postexposure management with medical follow-up (IB, IC).
  B. Education and Training
    1. Provide DHCP (1) on initial employment, (2) when new tasks or procedures affect the employee's occupational exposure, and (3) at a minimum, annually, with education and training regarding occupational exposure to potentially infectious agents and infection control procedures/protocols appropriate for and specific to their assigned duties (IB, IC).
    2. Provide educational information appropriate in content and vocabulary to the educational level, literacy, and language of DHCP (IB, IC).
  C. Immunization Programs
    1. Develop a written comprehensive policy on immunizing DHCP, including a list of all required and recommended immunizations (IB).

2. Refer DHCP to a prearranged qualified health-care professional or to their own health-care professional to receive all appropriate immunizations based on the latest recommendations as well as their medical history and risk for occupational exposure (IB).

D. Exposure Prevention and Postexposure Management
   1. Develop a comprehensive postexposure management and medical follow-up program (IB, IC).
      a. Include policies and procedures for prompt reporting, evaluation, counseling, treatment, and medical follow-up of occupational exposures.
      b. Establish mechanisms for referral to a qualified health-care professional for medical evaluation and follow-up.
      c. Conduct a baseline tuberculin skin test (TST), preferably by using a two-step test, for all DHCP who might have contact with persons with suspected or confirmed infectious [tuberculosis] TB, regardless of the risk classification of the setting (IB).

E. Medical Conditions, Work-Related Illness, and Work Restrictions
   1. Develop and have readily available to all DHCP comprehensive written policies regarding work restriction and exclusion that include a statement of authority defining who may implement such policies (IB).
   2. Develop policies for work restriction and exclusion that encourage personnel to seek appropriate preventive and curative care and report their illnesses, medical conditions, or treatments that may render them more susceptible to opportunistic infection or exposures; do not penalize DHCP with loss of wages, benefits, or job status (IB).
   3. Develop policies and procedures for evaluation, diagnosis, and management of DHCP with suspected or known occupational contact dermatitis (IB).
   4. Seek definitive diagnosis by a qualified health-care professional for any DHCP with suspected latex allergy to carefully determine its specific etiology and appropriate treatment as well as work restrictions and accommodations (IB).

F. Maintenance of Records, Data Management, and Confidentiality
   1. Establish, and keep updated, a confidential medical record (e.g., any immunization records and documentation of tests received as a result of an occupational exposure) for all DHCP (IB, IC).
   2. Ensure that the practice complies with all applicable current federal, state, and local laws on medical record-keeping and confidentiality (IC).

II. Preventing Transmission of Bloodborne Pathogens
A. [Hepatitis B virus] HBV Vaccination
   1. Offer the HBV vaccination series to all DHCP who have potential occupational exposure to blood or other potentially infectious material (IA, IC).

2. Always follow current U.S. Public Health Service/CDC recommendations for hepatitis B vaccination, serologic testing, follow-up, and booster dosing (IA, IC).
3. Test DHCP for anti-HBs [hepatitis B surface antigen] 1 to 2 months after completion of the 3-dose vaccination series (IA, IC).
4. Complete a second 3-dose vaccine series or be evaluated to determine if they are [hepatitis B surface antigen] HBsAg-positive if no antibody response occurs to the primary vaccine series (IA) (IC).
5. Retest for anti-HBs at the completion of the second vaccine series. If no response to the second 3-dose series occurs, nonresponders should be tested for HBsAg (IC).
6. Counsel nonresponders to vaccination who are HBsAg-negative regarding their susceptibility to HBV infection and precautions to take (IA, IC).
7. Provide employees appropriate education about the risks of HBV transmission and the availability of the vaccine. Employees who decline the vaccination must sign a declination form to be kept on file with the employer (IC).

B. Preventing Exposures to Blood and Other Potentially Infectious Materials
   1. General recommendations
      a. Use Standard Precautions (OSHA's bloodborne pathogen standard retains the term universal precautions) for all patient encounters (IA, IC).
      b. Consider sharp items (e.g., needles, scalers, burs, lab knives, wires) that are contaminated with patient blood and saliva as potentially infective and establish engineering controls and work practices to prevent injuries (IB, IC).
      c. Implement a written, comprehensive program designed to minimize and manage DHCP exposures to blood and body fluids (IB, IC).
   2. Engineering and work practice controls
      a. Identify, evaluate, and select devices with engineered safety features as they become available on the market (e.g., safer anesthetic syringes, blunt suture needle, retractable scalpel, needleless [intravenous] IV systems) (IA, IC).
      b. Place used disposable syringes and needles, scalpel blades, and other sharp items in appropriate puncture-resistant containers located as close as feasible to the area in which the items are used (IA, IC).
      c. Do not recap used needles using both hands, or any other technique that involves directing the point of a needle toward any part of the body. Do not bend, break, or remove needles before disposal (IA, IC).
      d. Use either a one-handed "scoop" technique or a mechanical device designed for holding the needle cap when recapping needles (e.g., between multiple injections and prior to removing from a nondisposable aspirating syringe) (IA, IC).

3. Postexposure management and prophylaxis. Follow current CDC recommendations after percutaneous, mucous membrane, or nonintact skin exposure to blood or other potentially infectious material (IA, IC).

III. Hand Hygiene

A. General Considerations

1. Perform hand hygiene with either a nonantimicrobial or antimicrobial soap and water when hands are visibly dirty or contaminated with blood or other potentially infectious material. If hands are not visibly soiled, an alcohol-based hand rub may also be used. Follow the manufacturer's instructions (IA).

2. Indications for hand hygiene include:
   a. when hands are visibly soiled (IA, IC);
   b. after barehanded touching of inanimate objects likely to be contaminated by blood, saliva, or respiratory secretions (IA, IC);
   c. before and after treating each patient (IB);
   d. before donning gloves (IB); and
   e. immediately after removing gloves (IB, IC).

3. For oral surgical procedures, perform surgical hand antisepsis before donning sterile surgeon's gloves. Follow the manufacturer's instructions using either an antimicrobial soap and water, or soap and water followed by drying hands and application of an alcohol-based surgical hand scrub product with persistent activity (IB).

4. Store liquid hand-care products in either disposable closed containers or closed containers that can be washed and dried before refilling. Do not add soap or lotion to (i.e., top off) a partially empty dispenser (IA).

B. Special Considerations for Hand Hygiene and Glove Use

1. Use hand lotions at the end of the day to prevent skin dryness associated with handwashing (IA).

2. Consider the compatibility of lotion and antiseptic products and the effect of petroleum or other oil emollients on the integrity of gloves during product selection and glove use (IB).

3. Keep fingernails short, with smooth, filed edges, to allow thorough cleaning and prevent glove tears (II).

4. Do not wear artificial fingernails or extenders when having direct contact with patients at high risk (e.g., those in intensive care units or operating rooms) (IA).

5. Use of artificial fingernails is usually not recommended (II).

6. Do not wear hand or nail jewelry if they make donning gloves more difficult or compromise the appropriate fit and integrity of the glove (II).

IV. [Personal Protective Equipment] PPE

A. Masks, Protective Eyewear, Face Shields

1. Wear a surgical mask and eye protection with solid side shields or a face shield to protect mucous membranes of the eyes, nose, and mouth during procedures likely to generate splashing or spattering of blood or other body fluids (IB, IC).

2. Change masks between patients, or during patient treatment if the mask becomes wet (IB).

3. Clean with soap and water, or if visibly soiled, clean and disinfect reusable facial protective equipment (e.g., clinician and patient protective eyewear, face shield) between patients (II).

B. Protective Clothing

1. Wear protective clothing (e.g., reusable or disposable gown, laboratory coat, or uniform) that covers skin and personal clothing and skin (e.g., forearms) likely to be soiled with blood, saliva, or other potentially infectious materials (IB, IC).

2. Change protective clothing if visibly soiled; change immediately or as soon as feasible if penetrated by blood or other potentially infectious fluids (IB, IC).

3. Remove barrier protection, including gloves, masks, eyewear, and gowns before departing work area (e.g., dental patient care, instrument processing, or laboratory areas) (IC).

C. Gloves

1. Wear medical gloves when a potential exists for contacting blood, saliva, other potentially infectious materials or mucous membranes (IB, IC).

2. Wear a new pair of medical gloves for each patient, remove them promptly after use, and wash hands immediately to avoid transfer of microorganisms to other patients or environments (IB).

3. Remove gloves that are torn, cut, or punctured as soon as feasible and wash hands before regloving (IB, IC).

4. Do not wash surgeon's or patient examination gloves before use or wash, disinfect, or sterilize gloves for reuse (IB, IC).

5. Ensure that appropriate gloves in the correct size are readily accessible (IC).

6. Use appropriate gloves (e.g., puncture- and chemical-resistant utility gloves) when cleaning instruments and performing housekeeping tasks involving contact with blood or other potentially infectious materials (IB, IC).

7. Consult with glove manufacturers regarding the chemical compatibility of glove material and dental materials used (II).

D. Sterile Surgeon's Gloves and Double Gloving During Oral Surgical Procedures

1. Wear sterile surgeon's gloves when performing oral surgical procedures (IB).

2. No recommendation is offered regarding the effectiveness of wearing two pairs of gloves to

prevent disease transmission during oral surgical procedures. The majority of studies among health care personnel (HCP) and DHCP have demonstrated a lower frequency of inner glove perforation and visible blood on the surgeon's hands when double gloves are worn; however, the effectiveness of wearing two pairs of gloves in preventing disease transmission has not been demonstrated (Unresolved issue).

V. Contact Dermatitis and Latex Hypersensitivity
   A. General Recommendations
      1. Educate DHCP about the signs, symptoms, and diagnoses of skin reactions associated with frequent hand hygiene and glove use (IB).
      2. Screen all patients for latex allergy (e.g., take health history and refer for medical consultation when latex allergy is suspected) (IB).
      3. Ensure a latex-safe environment for patients and DHCP with latex allergy (IB).
      4. Have emergency treatment kits with latex-free products available at all times (II).

VI. Sterilization and Disinfection of Patient-Care Items
   A. General Recommendations
      1. Use only [Food and Drug Administration] FDA-cleared medical devices for sterilization and follow the manufacturer's instructions for proper use (IB).
      2. Clean and heat-sterilize critical dental instruments before each use (IA).
      3. Clean and heat-sterilize semicritical items before each use (IB).
      4. Allow packages to dry in the sterilizer before they are handled to avoid contamination (IB).
      5. Use of heat-stable semicritical alternatives is encouraged (IB).
      6. Reprocess heat-sensitive critical and semicritical instruments using FDA-cleared sterilant/high-level disinfectants or an FDA-cleared low-temperature sterilization method (e.g., ethylene oxide). Follow manufacturer's instructions for the use of chemical sterilants/high-level disinfectants (IB).
      7. Single-use disposable instruments are acceptable alternatives provided they are used once and disposed of properly (IB, IC).
      8. Do not use liquid chemical sterilants for surface disinfection or as holding solutions (IB, IC).
      9. Ensure that noncritical patient-care items are barrier-protected or cleaned, or if visibly soiled, cleaned and disinfected after each use with an [Environmental Protection Agency] EPA-registered hospital disinfectant. If visibly contaminated with blood, use an EPA-registered hospital disinfectant with a tuberculocidal claim (i.e., intermediate level) (IB).
    10. Inform DHCP of all [Occupational Safety and Health Administration] OSHA guidelines for

exposure to chemical agents used for disinfection and sterilization. With this information, identify the areas and tasks that have potential for exposure (IC).

   B. Instrument Processing Area
      1. Designate a central processing area. Divide the instrument processing area, physically or, at a minimum, spatially, into distinct areas for (1) receiving, cleaning, and decontamination; (2) preparation and packaging; (3) sterilization; and (4) storage. Do not store instruments in an area where contaminated instruments are held or cleaned (II).
      2. Train DHCP to employ work practices that prevent contamination of clean areas (II).

   C. Receiving, Cleaning, and Decontamination Work Area
      1. Minimize handling of loose contaminated instruments during transport to the instrument processing area. Use work-practice controls (e.g., carry instruments in a covered container) to minimize exposure potential (II). Clean all visible blood and organic contamination from dental instruments and devices before sterilization or disinfection procedures (IA).
      2. Use automated cleaning equipment (e.g., ultrasonic cleaner, washer-disinfector) to remove debris to improve cleaning effectiveness and decrease worker exposure to blood (IB).
      3. Use work practice controls that minimize contact with sharp instruments if manual cleaning is necessary (e.g., long-handled brush) (IC).
      4. Wear puncture- and chemical-resistant/heavy-duty utility gloves for instrument cleaning and decontamination procedures (IB).
      5. Wear appropriate personal protective equipment (e.g., mask, protective eyewear, and gown) when splashing or spraying is anticipated during cleaning (IC).

   D. Preparation and Packaging
      1. Use an internal chemical indicator in each package. If the internal indicator cannot be seen from outside the package, also use an external indicator. For unwrapped loads, place an internal chemical indicator among the instruments or items to be sterilized (II).
      2. Use a container system or wrapping compatible with the type of sterilization process used and that has received FDA clearance (IB).
      3. Before sterilization of critical and semicritical instruments, inspect instruments for cleanliness, then wrap or place them in containers designed to maintain sterility during storage (e.g., cassettes, organizing trays) (IA).

   E. Sterilization of Unwrapped Instruments
      1. Clean and dry instruments prior to the unwrapped sterilization cycle (IB).
      2. Use mechanical and chemical indicators for each unwrapped sterilization cycle (i.e., place an internal chemical indicator among the instruments or items to be sterilized) (IB).

3. Allow unwrapped instruments to dry and cool in the sterilizer before they are handled to avoid contamination and thermal injury (II).

4. Semicritical instruments that will be used immediately or within a short time frame can be sterilized unwrapped on a tray or in a container system, provided that the instruments are handled aseptically during removal from the sterilizer and transport to the point of use (II).

5. Critical instruments intended for immediate use can be sterilized unwrapped if the instruments are maintained sterile during removal from the sterilizer and transport to the point of use (e.g., transported in a sterile covered container) (IB).

6. Do not sterilize implantable devices unwrapped (IB).

7. Do not store critical instruments unwrapped (IB).

F. Sterilization Monitoring

1. Use mechanical, chemical, and biological monitors according to the manufacturer's instructions to ensure the effectiveness of the sterilization process (IB).

2. Monitor each load with mechanical (e.g., time, temperature, pressure) and chemical indicators (II).

3. Place a chemical indicator on the inside of each package. If it is not visible from the outside, also place an exterior chemical indicator on the package (II).

4. Place items/packages correctly and loosely into the sterilizer so as not to impede penetration of the sterilant (IB).

5. Do not use instrument packs if mechanical or chemical indicators suggest inadequate processing (IB).

6. Monitor sterilizers at least weekly using a biologic indicator with a matching control (i.e., biologic indicator and control from same lot number) (IB).

7. Use a biologic indicator for every sterilizer load that contains an implantable device. Verify results before using the implantable device, whenever possible (IB).

8. The following are recommended in case of a positive spore test:
   a. Remove the sterilizer from service and review sterilization procedures (e.g., work practices and use of mechanical and chemical indicators) to determine whether operator error could be responsible (II).
   b. Retest the sterilizer by using biological, mechanical, and chemical indicators after correcting any identified procedural problems (II).
   c. If the repeat spore test is negative, and mechanical and chemical indicators are within normal limits, put the sterilizer back in service (II).

9. The following are recommended if the repeat spore test is positive:
   a. Do not use the sterilizer until it has been inspected or repaired or the exact reason for the positive test has been determined (II).
   b. Recall (to the extent possible) and reprocess all items processed since the last negative spore test (II).
   c. Before placing the sterilizer back into service, rechallenge the sterilizer with biological indicator tests in three consecutive empty chamber sterilization cycles after the cause of the sterilizer failure has been determined and corrected (II).

10. Maintain sterilization records (i.e., mechanical, chemical, biological) in compliance with state and local regulations (IB).

G. Storage Area for Sterilized Items and Clean Dental Supplies

1. Implement practices based on date- or event-related shelf-life for the storage of wrapped, sterilized instruments and devices (IB).

2. Even for event-related packaging, at a minimum place the date of sterilization, and if multiple sterilizers are used in the facility, the sterilizer used, on the outside of the packaging material to facilitate the retrieval of processed items in the event of a sterilization failure (IB).

3. Examine wrapped packages of sterilized instruments before opening them to ensure the barrier wrap has not been compromised during storage (II).

4. Reclean, repack, and resterilize any instrument package that is compromised (II).

5. Store sterile items and dental supplies in covered or closed cabinets, if possible (II).

VII. Environmental Infection Control

A. General Recommendations

1. Follow the manufacturers' instructions for correct use of cleaning and EPA-registered hospital disinfecting products (IB) (IC).

2. Do not use liquid chemical sterilants/high-level disinfectants for disinfection of environmental surfaces (clinical contact or housekeeping) (IB) (IC).

3. Use personal protective equipment, as appropriate, when cleaning and disinfecting environmental surfaces. Such equipment might include gloves (e.g., puncture- and chemical-resistant utility), protective clothing (e.g., gown, jacket, lab coat), and protective eyewear/face shield, mask (IC).

B. Clinical Contact Surfaces

1. Use surface barriers to protect clinical contact surfaces, particularly those that are difficult to clean (e.g., switches on dental chairs) and change surface barriers between patients (II).

2. Clean and disinfect clinical contact surfaces that are not barrier-protected, by using an EPA-registered hospital disinfectant with a low- (i.e., [human immunodeficiency virus] HIV and HBV label claims) to intermediate-level (i.e., tuberculocidal claim) activity after each patient. Use an intermediate-level disinfectant if visibly contaminated with blood (IB).

C. Housekeeping Surfaces
  1. Clean housekeeping surfaces (e.g., floors, walls, sinks) with a detergent and water or an EPA-registered hospital disinfectant/detergent on a routine basis, depending on the nature of the surface and the type and degree of contamination, and as appropriate, based upon the location in the facility, and when visibly soiled (IB).
  2. Clean mops and cloths after use and allow to dry before reuse; or use single-use, disposable mop heads or cloths (II).
  3. Prepare fresh cleaning or EPA-registered disinfecting solutions daily and as instructed by the manufacturer (II).
  4. Clean walls, blinds, and window curtains in patient-care areas when they are visibly dusty or soiled (II).
D. Spills of Blood and Body Substances
  1. Clean spills of blood or other potentially infectious materials and decontaminate surface with an EPA-registered hospital disinfectant with low- (i.e., HBV and HIV label claims) to intermediate-level (i.e., tuberculocidal claim) activity depending on size of spill and surface porosity (IB, IC).
E. Carpet and Cloth Furnishings
  1. Avoid using carpeting and cloth-upholstered furnishings in dental operatories, laboratories, and instrument processing areas (II).
F. Regulated Medical Waste
  1. General Recommendations
    a. Develop a medical waste management program. Disposal of medical waste must follow federal, state, and local regulations (IC).
    b. Ensure that DHCPs who handle and dispose of potentially infective wastes are trained in appropriate handling and disposal methods and that they are informed of the possible health and safety hazards (IC).
  2. Management of Regulated Medical Waste in Dental Health-Care Facilities Constructed:
    a. Use a color-coded and labeled container that prevents leakage (e.g., biohazard bag) to contain nonsharp regulated medical waste (IC).
    b. Place sharp items (e.g., needles, scalpel blades, orthodontic bands, broken metal instruments, burs) in an appropriate sharps container (e.g., puncture-resistant, color-coded, leakproof). Close container immediately before removal or replacement to prevent spillage or protrusion of contents during handling, storage, transport, or shipping (IC).
    c. Pour blood, suctioned fluids, or other liquid waste carefully into a drain connected to a sanitary sewer system, provided that local sewage discharge requirements are met and that the state has declared this to be an acceptable method of disposal. Wear appropriate PPE while performing this task (IC).

VIII. Dental Unit Waterlines, Biofilm, and Water Quality
  A. General Recommendations
    1. Use water that meets regulatory standards set by the EPA for drinking water (500 [colony-forming units per milliliter] CFU/mL of heterotrophic water bacteria) for routine dental treatment output water (IB, IC).
    2. Consult with the dental unit manufacturer for appropriate methods and equipment to maintain the recommended quality of dental water (II).
    3. Follow recommendations for monitoring water quality provided by the manufacturer of the unit or waterline treatment product (II).
    4. Discharge water and air for a minimum of 20-30 seconds, after each patient, from any dental device connected to the dental water system that enters the patient's mouth (e.g., handpieces, ultrasonic scalers, air/water syringe) (II).
    5. Consult with the dental unit manufacturer on the need for periodic maintenance of antiretraction mechanisms (IB).
  B. Boil-water Advisories
    1. The following apply while a boil-water advisory is in effect:
      a. Do not deliver water from the public water system to the patient through the dental operative unit, ultrasonic scaler, or other dental equipment that uses the public water system (IB, IC).
      b. Do not use water from the public water system for dental treatment, patient rinsing, or handwashing (IB, IC).
      c. For handwashing, use antimicrobial-containing products that do not require water for use (i.e., alcohol-based hand rubs). If hands are visibly contaminated, use bottled water, if available, and soap for handwashing or an antiseptic towelette (IB, IC).
    2. The following apply when the boil-water advisory is cancelled:
      a. Follow guidance given by the local water utility on proper flushing of waterlines. If no guidance is provided, flush dental waterlines and faucets for 1-5 minutes before using for patient care (IC).
      b. Disinfect dental waterlines as recommended by the dental unit manufacturer (II).

IX. Special Considerations
  A. Dental Handpieces and Other Devices Attached to Air and Waterlines
    1. Clean and heat-sterilize handpieces and other intraoral instruments that can be removed from the air and waterlines of dental units between patients (IB, IC).
    2. Follow the manufacturer's instructions for the cleaning, lubrication, and sterilization of handpieces and other intraoral instruments that can

be removed from the air and waterlines of dental units (IB).

3. Do not surface-disinfect use liquid chemical sterilants or ethylene oxide on handpieces and other intraoral instruments that can be removed from the air and waterlines of dental units (IC).

4. Do not advise patients to close their lips around the tip of the saliva ejector to evacuate oral fluids (II).

B. Dental Radiology

1. Wear gloves when exposing radiographs and handling contaminated film packets. Use other personal protective equipment (e.g., protective eyewear, mask, gown) as appropriate if spattering of blood or other body fluids is likely (IA, IC).

2. Use heat-tolerant or disposable intraoral devices whenever possible (e.g., film-holding and positioning devices). Clean and heat-sterilize heat-tolerant devices between patients. At a minimum, high-level disinfect semicritical heat-sensitive devices, according to manufacturer's instructions (IB).

3. Transport and handle exposed radiographs in an aseptic manner to prevent contamination of developing equipment (II).

4. The following apply for digital radiography sensors:
   a. Use FDA-cleared barriers (IB);
   b. Clean and heat-sterilize, or high-level disinfect, between patients, barrier-protected semicritical items. If the item cannot tolerate these procedures, then at a minimum protect with an FDA-cleared barrier and clean and disinfect with an EPA-registered hospital disinfectant with intermediate-level (i.e., tuberculocidal claim) activity, between patients. Consult with the manufacturer for proper disinfection and sterilization methods of digital radiology sensors and for protection of associated computer hardware (IB).

C. Aseptic Technique for Parenteral Medications

1. Do not administer medication from a syringe to multiple patients even if the needle on the syringe is changed (IA).

2. Use single-dose vials for parenteral medications when possible (II).

3. Do not combine the leftover contents of single-use vials for later use (IA).

4. The following apply if multidose vials are used:
   a. Cleanse the access diaphragm with 70% alcohol before inserting a device into the vial (IA).
   b. Use a sterile device to access a multiple-dose vial and avoid touching the access diaphragm. Both the needle and syringe used to access the multidose vial should be sterile. Do not reuse a syringe even if the needle is changed (IA).
   c. Keep the multidose vials away from the immediate patient treatment area to prevent inadvertent contamination by spray or spatter (II).
   d. Discard the multidose vial if sterility is compromised (IA).

5. Use fluid infusion and administration sets (i.e., IV bags, tubings, and connections) for one patient only and dispose of appropriately (IB).

D. Single-Use (Disposable) Devices

1. Use single-use devices for one patient only and dispose of them appropriately (IC).

E. Preprocedural Mouth Rinses

1. No recommendation is offered regarding use of preprocedural antimicrobial mouth rinses to prevent clinical infections among DHCP or patients. Although studies have demonstrated that a preprocedural antimicrobial rinse (e.g., chlorhexidine gluconate, essential oils, or povidone-iodine) can reduce the level of oral microorganisms in aerosols and spatter generated during routine dental procedures and can decrease the number of microorganisms in the patient's bloodstream during invasive dental procedures, the scientific evidence is inconclusive that using these rinses prevents clinical infections among DHCP or patients (Unresolved issue).

F. Oral Surgical Procedures

1. The following apply when performing oral surgical procedures:
   a. Perform surgical and hand antisepsis using an antimicrobial product (e.g., antimicrobial soap and water or soap and water followed by alcohol-based hand scrub with persistent activity) before donning sterile surgeon's gloves (IB).
   b. Use sterile surgeon's gloves (IB).
   c. Use sterile saline or sterile water as a coolant/irrigator when performing oral surgical procedures. Use devices specifically designed for the delivery of sterile irrigating fluids (e.g., bulb syringes, single-use disposable products, and sterilizable tubing) (IB).

G. Handling of Biopsy Specimens

1. During transport, place biopsy specimens in a sturdy, leakproof container labeled with the biohazard symbol (IC).

2. If a biopsy specimen container is visibly contaminated, clean and disinfect the outside of a container, or place it in an impervious bag labeled with the biohazard symbol (IC).

H. Handling of Extracted Teeth

1. Dispose of extracted teeth as regulated medical waste unless returned to the patient (IC).

2. Do not dispose of extracted teeth containing amalgam in regulated medical waste intended for incineration (II).

3. Clean and place extracted teeth in a leakproof container labeled with a biohazard symbol and maintain hydration for transport to educational institutions or a dental laboratory (IB, IC).

4. Heat-sterilize teeth that do not contain amalgam before they are used for educational purposes (IB).

I. Dental Laboratory

1. Use personal protective equipment when handling items received in the laboratory until they have been decontaminated (IA, IC).

2. Before they are handled in a laboratory, clean, disinfect, and rinse all dental prostheses and prosthodontic materials (e.g., impressions, bite registrations, occlusal rims, extracted teeth) using an EPA-registered hospital disinfectant having at least an intermediate level (i.e., tuberculocidal claim) activity (IB).

3. Consult with manufacturers regarding the stability of specific materials (e.g., impression materials) relative to disinfection procedures (II).

4. Include specific information regarding disinfection technique used (e.g., solution used and duration), when laboratory cases are sent off-site and upon their return (II).

5. Clean and heat-sterilize heat-tolerant items used in the mouth (e.g., metal impression trays, face-bow forks) (IB).

6. Follow the manufacturer's instructions for cleaning and sterilizing or disinfecting items that become contaminated, but that do not normally contact the patient (e.g., burs, polishing points, rag wheels, articulators, case pans, lathes). If manufacturer instructions are not available, clean and heat-sterilize heat-tolerant items or clean and disinfect with an EPA-registered hospital disinfectant with low- (HIV, HBV effectiveness claim) to intermediate-level (tuberculocidal claim) activity, depending on the degree of contamination (II).

J. Laser/Electrosurgery Plumes/Surgical Smoke

1. No recommendation is offered regarding practices to reduce DHCP exposure to laser plumes/surgical smoke when using lasers in dental practice. Practices to reduce [health care personnel] HCP exposure to laser plumes/surgical smoke have been suggested, including use of a) standard precautions (e.g., high-filtration surgical masks and possibly full face shields); b) central room suction units with in-line filters to collect particulate matter from minimal plumes; and c) dedicated mechanical smoke exhaust systems with a high-efficiency filter to remove substantial amounts of laser-plume particles. The effect of the exposure (e.g., disease transmission or adverse respiratory effects) on DHCP from dental applications of lasers has not been adequately evaluated (Unresolved issue).

K. *Mycobacterium tuberculosis*

1. General Recommendations

a. Educate all DHCP regarding the recognition of signs, symptoms, and transmission of tuberculosis (IB).

b. Conduct a baseline TST, preferably by using a two-step test, for all DHCP who may have contact with persons with suspected or confirmed infectious TB, regardless of the risk classification of the setting (IB).

c. Assess each patient for a history of TB as well as symptoms suggestive of TB and document on the medical history form (IB).

d. Follow current CDC recommendations for (1) developing, maintaining, and implementing a written TB infection control plan; (2) managing a patient with suspected or active TB; (3) completing a community risk-assessment to guide employee TSTs and follow-up; and (4) managing DHCP with TB disease (IB).

2. The following apply for patients known or suspected to have active TB:

a. Evaluate the patient away from other patients and DHCP. When not being evaluated, the patient should wear a surgical mask or be instructed to cover his or her mouth and nose when coughing or sneezing (IB).

b. Defer elective dental treatment until the patient is noninfectious (IB).

c. Refer patients requiring urgent dental treatment to a previously identified facility that has TB engineering controls and a respiratory protection program (IB).

L. Creutzfeldt-Jakob Disease (CJD) and Other Prion Diseases

1. No recommendation is offered regarding use of special precautions in addition to standard precautions when treating CJD or [variant] vCJD patients. Potential infectivity of oral tissues in CJD or vCJD patients is an unresolved issue. Scientific data indicate the risk, if any, of sporadic CJD transmission during dental and oral surgical procedures is low to nil. Until additional information exists regarding the transmissibility of CJD or vCJD during dental procedures, special precautions in addition to standard precautions might be indicated when treating known CJD or vCJD patients; a list of such precautions is provided for consideration without recommendation (Unresolved issue).

M. Program Evaluation

1. Establish routine evaluation of the infection control program, including evaluation of performance indicators at an established frequency (II).

Appendix C

Centers for Disease Control and Prevention Guidelines for Prevention of Tuberculosis in Dental Settings

The Centers for Disease Control and Prevention published "Guidelines for preventing the transmission of *Mycobacterium tuberculosis* in health-care settings, 2005" in *Morbidity and Mortality Weekly Report Recommendations and Reports*, volume 54, No. RR 17, December 30, 2005. All of the details are in that publication, but the information related to dental setting is presented in this appendix. A link to the original publication can be found at http://www.cdc.gov/mmwr/pdf/rr/rr5417.pdf. Further information related to tuberculosis prevention in the dental office can be found in the May 1995* and September 2009† issues of the *Journal of the American Dental Association*.

In general, the symptoms for which patients seek treatment in a dental care setting are not likely to be caused by infectious tuberculosis. Unless a patient requiring dental care coincidentally has tuberculosis, the dental professional is not likely to encounter infectious tuberculosis in the dental setting. Furthermore, generation of droplet nuclei containing *Mycobacterium tuberculosis* during dental procedures has not been demonstrated.‡ Therefore the risk of transmission of *M. tuberculosis* in most dental settings is probably low. Nevertheless, during dental procedures, patients and dental workers share the same air for varying periods of time. Coughing may be stimulated occasionally by oral manipulations, although no specific dental procedures have been classified as "cough-inducing."

In some instances, the population served by a dental care facility, or the health care workers in the facility, may be at relatively high risk for tuberculosis. Because the potential exists for transmission of *M. tuberculosis* in dental settings, the following recommendations should be followed:

- A risk assessment (Table C-1) should be done periodically, and tuberculosis infection control policies for each dental setting should be based on the risk assessment.

The policies should include provisions for detection and referral of patients who may have undiagnosed active tuberculosis; management of patients with active tuberculosis, relative to provision of urgent dental care; and employer-sponsored health care worker education, counseling, and screening (Box C-1).

- While taking patients' initial medical histories and at periodic updates, dental health care workers routinely should ask all patients whether they have a history of tuberculosis disease and symptoms suggestive of tuberculosis.
- Patients with a medical history or symptoms suggestive of undiagnosed active tuberculosis should be referred promptly for medical evaluation of possible infectiousness. Such patients should not remain in the dental care facility any longer than required to arrange a referral. While in the dental care facility, the patients should wear surgical masks and should be instructed to cover their mouths and noses when coughing or sneezing.
- Elective dental treatment should be deferred until a physician confirms that the patient does not have infectious tuberculosis. If the patient is diagnosed as having active tuberculosis, elective dental treatment should be deferred until the patient is no longer infectious.
- If urgent dental care must be provided for a patient who has or is strongly suspected of having infectious tuberculosis, such care should be provided in facilities that can provide tuberculosis isolation (see Section II, E and G of the original publication for details). Dental health care workers should use respiratory protection while performing procedures on such patients.
- Any dental health care worker who has a persistent cough (i.e., a cough lasting 3 weeks or more), especially in the presence of other signs or symptoms compatible with active tuberculosis (e.g., weight loss, night sweats, bloody sputum, anorexia, and fever), should be evaluated promptly for tuberculosis. The health care worker should not return to the workplace until a diagnosis of tuberculosis is excluded or until the health care worker is receiving therapy and a determination is made that the health care worker is noninfectious.

---

*Cleveland JT, Gooch BF, Bolyard EA, et al: TB infection control recommendations from the CDC, 1994: considerations for dentistry, *J Am Dent Assoc* 126:593-600, 1995.

†Cleveland JF, Robison, VA and Pamlilio AL. *J Am Dent Assoc* 140:1092-1099, 2009.

‡Dueli RC, Madden RN: Droplet nuclei produced during dental treatment of tubercular patients, *Oral Surg* 30:711-716, 1970.

TABLE C-1   Conducting a Tuberculosis Risk Assessment in a Dental Setting

Assessments and Results	Risk Category
Review the community tuberculosis profile from public health records and determine the number of patients with active tuberculosis seen in the office in the last year. If patients with active tuberculosis have been in the office, skin test (PPD*) office staff.	
Patients with active tuberculosis were not treated in office, and none were reported in the community.	Minimal risk
Patients with active tuberculosis were not treated in office, but some were reported in the community. Plan to screen and refer known or suspected patients with tuberculosis to a collaborating facility for evaluation and management if treatment is required.	Very low risk
Office provided treatment to fewer than six patients with active tuberculosis, and no evidence of PPD skin test conversions was found among office staff.	Low risk
Office provided treatment to six or more patients with active tuberculosis, and no evidence of PPD skin test conversions was found among office staff.	Intermediate risk
Evidence was found of transmission of tuberculosis in the office based on skin testing data.	High risk

*PPD, Purified protein derivative from *Mycobacterium* used in skin testing.

- In dental care facilities that provide care to populations at high risk for active tuberculosis, use of engineering controls similar to those used in general-use areas (e.g., waiting rooms) of medical facilities that have a similar risk profile may be appropriate.

GUIDELINES FOR PREVENTING THE TRANSMISSION OF *MYCOBACTERIUM* TUBERCULOSIS IN HEALTH-CARE SETTINGS, 2005‡

Dental-Care Settings—Excerpt

Note: A link to the original publication can be found at http://www.cdc.gov/mmwr/pdf/rr/rr5417.pdf.

‡Prepared by Paul A. Jensen, PhD, Lauren A. Lambert, MPH, Michael F. Iademarco, MD, Renee Ridzon, MD, Division of Tuberculosis Elimination, National Center for HIV, STD, and TB Prevention. Guidelines for preventing the transmission of *Mycobacterium tuberculosis* in health-care settings, 2005 *MMWR Recomm Rep* 54(RR-17);1-141, 2005.

BOX C-1

Tuberculosis Prevention Program for the Dental Office*

For Offices in Minimal-Risk Category

- Assign specific person responsibility for the tuberculosis infection control program in the office.
- Conduct a baseline risk assessment (see Table C-1) for the office and reassess annually.
- Develop a written tuberculosis infection control plan.
- Develop and implement protocols for identifying and referring patients who may have active tuberculosis for evaluation, management, or urgent dental treatment.
- Educate, train, and counsel the office staff regarding tuberculosis.
- Develop a protocol for identifying and referring dental workers who may have active tuberculosis or positive purified protein derivative skin tests.
- Develop a protocol for investigating unprotected occupational exposure to tuberculosis.

For Offices in Low-Risk Category

- Perform all activities in the minimal- and very-low-risk categories.
- Provide tuberculosis isolation when treating patients with known or suspected active tuberculosis (see details in original *Morbidity and Mortality Weekly Report Recommendations and Reports* article).
- Perform engineering controls in the general use areas such as the waiting room to include general ventilation, high-efficiency particulate air filtration, or ultraviolet light germicidal irradiation.

For Offices in Very-Low-Risk Category

- Perform all activities in the minimal-risk category.
- As an optional activity, develop protocols and implement engineering controls in general use areas of the office such as the waiting room that may include general ventilation, high-efficiency particulate air filtration, or ultraviolet light germicidal irradiation.

*Only minimal-, very-low-, and low-risk categories are considered because these include essentially all private dental offices. Consult the original *Morbidity and Mortality Weekly Report Recommendations and Reports* article for prevention related to intermediate- or high-risk categories, Centers for Disease Control and Prevention: Guidelines for preventing the transmission of *Mycobacterium tuberculosis* in health-care facilities, 1994, *MMWR Recomm Rep* 43(RR-13), 1994.

The generation of droplet nuclei containing *M. tuberculosis* as a result of dental procedures has not been demonstrated. Nonetheless, oral manipulations during dental procedures could stimulate coughing and dispersal of infectious particles. Patients and dental health care workers (HCWs) share the same air space for varying periods, which contributes to the potential for transmission of *M. tuberculosis* in dental settings or example, during primarily routine dental procedures in a dental setting, multiple drug-resistant (MDR) TB might have been transmitted between two dental workers.

To prevent the transmission of *M. tuberculosis* in dental-care settings, certain recommendations should be followed. Infection control policies for each dental health-care setting should be developed, based on the community TB risk assessment (see Table C-1), and the policies should be reviewed annually, if possible. The policies should include appropriate screening for [latent tuberculosis infection] LTBI and TB disease for dental HCWs, education on the risk for transmission to the dental HCWs, and provisions for detection and management of patients who have suspected or confirmed TB disease.

When taking a patient's initial medical history and at periodic updates, dental HCWs should routinely document whether the patient has symptoms or signs of TB disease.

If urgent dental care must be provided for a patient who has suspected or confirmed infectious TB disease, dental care should be provided in a setting that meets the requirements for airborne infection isolation (AII). An AII room is under negative pressure with the room air preferably exhausted to the outside. Respiratory protection (at least N95 disposable respirator) should be used while performing procedures on such patients.

In dental health-care settings that routinely provide care to populations at high risk for TB disease, using engineering controls (e.g., portable high-efficiency particulate air [HEPA] units) similar to those used in waiting rooms or clinic areas of health-care settings with a comparable community-risk profile might be beneficial.

During clinical assessment and evaluation, a patient with suspected or confirmed TB disease should be instructed to observe strict respiratory hygiene and cough etiquette procedures. The patient should also wear a surgical or procedure mask, if possible. Nonurgent dental treatment should be postponed, and these patients should be promptly referred to an appropriate medical setting for evaluation of possible infectiousness. In addition, these patients should be kept in the dental health-care setting no longer than required to arrange a referral.

Appendix D

Organization for Safety, Asepsis and Prevention

(http://www.osap.org)
PO Box 6297
Annapolis, MD 21401
(800) 298-OSAP (6727) or (410) 571-0003
Since its inception in 1984, the Organization for Safety, Asepsis and Prevention (OSAP) has focused on advocacy and education to help ensure the safe delivery of oral health care. As a result of the unique cooperation between member academics, policy makers, scientists, consultants, clinicians, as well as manufacturers and distributors, OSAP integrates cutting-edge information and educational resources to an increasing number of partners throughout the dental profession. The organization is considered "the resource" for infection prevention and control and occupational safety and health in dentistry and features a robust website, educational conferences, courses, and products, and answers to the sometimes difficult questions and challenges of compliance.

The organization is comprised of two complementary entities—an association and a charitable educational foundation (OSAP Foundation). The association promotes evidence-based policies and practices for infection prevention, safety, and health in health care settings. The overall goal is to improve the safety and health of dental patients and practitioners worldwide. The foundation supports the activities of the association through the identification of funds from a wide variety of sources.

MISSION STATEMENT

OSAP's mission is to be the world's leading advocate for the safe and infection-free delivery of oral health care. Its vision is for "safe oral healthcare for people everywhere."

PURPOSES AND COMMITMENTS

The purposes and commitments of OSAP are as follows:
- Provide educational forums for dental health care professionals and the entire dental industry.
- Provide and monitor practical guidelines in infection control and human health and safety.
- Interact with regulatory agencies, professional associations, product manufacturers and distributors, and other organizations.
- Promote quality research relating to infection control and safety issues.

MEMBERSHIP

The OSAP community includes dental practitioners (dentists, hygienists, assistants, and dental laboratory technicians), allied health care workers, researchers, educators, dental manufacturers, dental distributors, sales personnel, and public health officials. Members work in private and public dental practices, industry, academic facilities, military installations, and federal agencies such as the Centers for Disease Control and Prevention, Environmental Protection Agency, Food and Drug Administration, and Occupational Safety and Health Administration. The common link is a strong commitment and interest in infection prevention and control, and patient/provider safety in dentistry. The diverse membership shares a vision of a proactive organization that encourages the unbiased, open exchange of information on science, products, and technology in the dental setting.

Interested individuals are invited to obtain many resources by joining OSAP. Members receive full online access to all current and past OSAP publications, hard copies by mail, email alerts and news summaries, and discounts on OSAP meetings and products, including all training programs and materials, texts, CDs, audiotapes, and videotapes. Enrollment information is available at http://www.osap.org.

If membership is not an option, individuals can subscribe to the OSAP newsletter, which allows dental health care workers to keep informed concerning what is required to comply with safety and infection control regulations and guidelines. *Infection Control in Practice* is published six times per year and provides opportunities to earn continuing education credits.

The Organization for Safety, Asepsis and Prevention has approximately 50 corporate members that participate fully in all OSAP activities.

PROGRAMS AND PRODUCTS

The following are examples of what is available from OSAP:

- *If Saliva Were Red* video training program: A powerful and informative visual lesson on infection control. The program includes a trainer's guide to facilitate discussion and a highly effective video on VHS and CD-ROM. Continuing education credit is available.
- *OSAP Interact Program:* A comprehensive system for in-office training that uses a workbook and videos to explain infection control concepts and offers step-by-step protocols for minimizing the risk of disease transmission in dental health care settings. Continuing education credit is available.
- *Traveler's Guide to Safe Dental Care:* A handy brochure on how to receive safe dental care when traveling outside the United States. The guide is a cooperative effort of OSAP and the Centers for Disease Control and Prevention. The guide is appropriate for all audiences: patients, dental clinicians, and other travelers.
- *From Policy to Practice: OSAP's Guide to the Guidelines:* A workbook supported by the U.S. Centers for Disease Control and Prevention to help strip away the stress and confusion of implementing the infection control and safety recommendations from the Centers for Disease Control and Prevention. The workbook addresses terms one should know, the rationale behind the guidelines, step-by-step instructions, charts and checklists, common questions and answers, exercises in understanding, and more. Continuing education credit is available.
- *Educators and Trainers Toolkit:* Available on CD-ROM, this new toolkit is a coaching workbook designed to assist with the development, planning, and promotion of successful, high-impact infection control and safety programs and presentations.
- *OSAP's Website* contains dental infection control news that is updated daily to ensure dental industry workers are aware of important events, breakthroughs, and announcements. A special section, Frequently Asked Questions, provides 24-7 access to organized responses to an increasing number of common inquiries. The Web site also contains the official OSAP position papers and sets of guidelines.
- *Annual symposium:* Includes a 3-day program of cutting-edge information and extensive networking with the experts in dental asepsis, occupational health and safety, and regulatory issues. A must-attend symposium for infection control educators, lecturers, and consultants.
- *Annual Train-the-Trainer Seminar:* An intense 4-day seminar that provides the education, resources, and training tips on infection control and human safety and health trainers' need. The seminar is cosponsored by OSAP and the U.S. Federal Services.
- *Written and spoken content:* OSAP members provide extensive written content concerning infection control and human safety and health to many dental publications. The organization also helps sponsor speakers at many important dental association meetings and conventions.
- *Strategic liaisons:* The OSAP has established formal relationships with numerous dental organizations and associations and has ties to groups both in the United States and throughout the world.

The OSAP is an objective, trusted resource for infection prevention and control and safety in dentistry. Obviously, readers of this textbook have genuine interest in infection control and human safety and health. Membership in the OSAP is necessary to remain current and to interact with others with the same interests.

Appendix E

Exposure Incident Report

Name of Exposed Person: _____

Job Classification: _____

Name of Employer: _____

Date of Exposure: _____ Time: _____

Description of the Incident: _____

_____

What barriers were used by exposed person during the incident? _____

_____

Describe corrective measures to minimize possible recurrence: _____

_____

Was source (patient) sent for medical evaluation? Yes _____ No _____ _____

_____

Patient's name: _____ Comments: _____

_____

_____

_____

Was exposed person sent for medical evaluation? Yes _____ No _____

Comments: _____

_____

Was the exposed person informed by the evaluating physician of the results of the medical evaluation as required by OSHA?

Yes _____ No _____

Was the employer informed by the evaluating physician that the exposed person was evaluated medically as required by

OSHA? Yes _____ No _____

_____

Signature of exposed person   Date

_____

Signature of employer   Date

Appendix F

Infection Control and the American Dental Association (ADA)

Twenty-five years ago, the ADA Foundation's Health Screening Program helped identify [hepatitis B virus] HBV as an occupational hazard in dentistry. The ADA responded by being the first to recommend that dentists follow standard infection control procedures. The ADA subsequently worked with the Centers for Disease Control and Prevention (CDC) to develop CDC's own infection control recommendations for dentistry, which were issued in 1993. Since then, both the ADA and CDC have updated and supplemented their recommendations from time to time to reflect new scientific knowledge and growing understanding of the principles of infection control.

In December 2003, the CDC published a major consolidation and update of its infection control recommendations for dentistry.[†] Although the procedures recommended in the 2003 document are for the most part unchanged, the new document does incorporate relevant recommendations that were previously scattered throughout several other CDC publications and contains an extensive review of the science related to dental infection control.

The 2003 CDC Guidelines (see Appendix B) are a comprehensive and evidence-based source for infection control practices relevant to the dental office that have been developed for the protection of dental care workers and their patients. The ADA urges all practicing dentists, dental auxiliaries, and dental laboratories to employ appropriate infection control procedures as described in the 2003 CDC Guidelines, and to keep up to date as scientific information leads to improvements in infection control, risk assessment, and disease management in oral health care.

The ADA has long advocated the use of infection control procedures in dental practice and provided dentists with resources to help them understand and implement them. In addition to the online resources available at www.ADA.org, the Association has a number of publications that provide detailed information about infection control and treatment of patients with infectious diseases. These include ADA catalog products, including the *Effective Infection Control* training DVD, the ADA *Regulatory Compliance Manual,* and the OSHA *Training for Dental Professionals* DVD.

---

*ADA Statement on Infection Control in Dentistry, http://www.ada.org/prof/resources/positions/statements/infectionconrol.asp. Accessed January, 2008.

†Kohn WG, Collins AS, Cleveland JL, et al; Centers for Disease Control and Prevention. Guidelines for infection control in dental health-care settings–2003. *MMWR Recomm Rep* 52(RR-17):1-61, 2003.

Appendix G

The Occupational Safety and Health Administration Bloodborne Pathogens Standard*

XI. The Standard

General Industry

Part 1910 of title 29 of the Code of Federal Regulations is amended as follows:

PART 1910-[AMENDED]

Subpart Z-[Amended]

1. The general authority citation for subpart Z of 29 CFR part 1910 continues to read as follows and a new citation for 1910.1030 is added:

Authority: Secs. 6 and 8. Occupational Safety and Health Act. 29 U.S.C. 655, 657, Secretary of Labor's Orders Nos. 12-71 (36 FR 8754). 8-76 (41 FR 25059), or 9-83 (48 FR 35736), as applicable; and 20 CFR part 1911.

Section 1910.1030 also issued under 29 U.S.C. 653.

2. Section 1910.1030 is added to read as follows:

(Note: The 2001 needlestick prevention additions to this standard are underlined.)

1910.1030 Bloodborne Pathogens

(a) *Scope and Application.* This section applies to all occupational exposure to blood or other potentially infectious materials as defined by paragraph (b) of this section.

(b) *Definitions.* For purposes of this section, the following shall apply:

Assistant Secretary means the Assistant Secretary of Labor for Occupational Safety and Health, or designated representative.

Blood means human blood, human blood components, and products made from human blood.

Bloodborne Pathogens means pathogenic microorganisms that are present in human blood and can cause disease in humans. These pathogens include, but are not limited to, hepatitis B virus (HBV) and human immunodeficiency virus (HIV).

Clinical Laboratory means a workplace where diagnostic or other screening procedures are performed on blood or other potentially infectious materials.

Contaminated means the presence or the reasonably anticipated presence of blood or other potentially infectious materials on an item or surface.

Contaminated Laundry means laundry that has been soiled with blood or other potentially infectious materials or may contain sharps.

Contaminated Sharps means any contaminated object that can penetrate the skin, including, but not limited to, needles, scalpels, broken glass, broken capillary tubes, and exposed ends of dental wires.

Decontamination means the use of physical or chemical means to remove, inactivate, or destroy bloodborne pathogens on a surface or item to the point where they are no longer capable of transmitting infectious particles and the surface or item is rendered safe for handling, use, or disposal.

Director means the Director of the National Institute for Occupational Safety and Health, U.S. Department of Health and Human Services, or designated representative.

Engineering Controls means controls (e.g., sharps disposal containers, self-sheathing needles, safer medical devices, such as sharps with engineered sharps injury protections and needleless systems) that isolate or remove the bloodborne pathogens hazard from the workplace.

Exposure Incident means a specific eye, mouth, other mucous membrane, non-intact skin, or parenteral contact with blood or other potentially infectious materials that results from the performance of an employee's duties.

Handwashing Facilities means a facility providing an adequate supply of running potable water, soap, and single use towels or hot air drying machines.

Licensed Healthcare Professional is a person whose legally permitted scope of practice allows him or her to independently perform the activities required by paragraph (f) Hepatitis B Vaccination and Post-exposure Evaluation and Follow-up.

HBV means hepatitis B virus.

HIV means human immunodeficiency virus.

---

*Reprinted from Department of Labor, Occupational Safety and Health Administration: 29 CFR Part 1910.1030. Occupational exposure to bloodborne pathogens; final rule, *Fed Regist* 56(235):645175-645182, 1991; with needlestick prevention update of 2001 added.

Needleless Systems means a device that does not use needles for (1) the collection of bodily fluids or withdrawal of body fluids after initial venous or arterial access is established; (2) the administration of medication or fluids; or (3) any other procedure involving the potential for occupational exposure to bloodborne pathogens due to percutaneous injuries from contaminated sharps.

Occupational Exposure means reasonably anticipated skin, eye, mucous membrane, or parenteral contact with blood or other potentially infectious materials that may result from the performance of an employee's duties.

Other Potentially Infectious Materials means (1) The following human body fluids: semen, vaginal secretions, cerebrospinal fluid, synovial fluid, pleural fluid, pericardial fluid, peritoneal fluid, amniotic fluid, saliva in dental procedures, any body fluid that is visibly contaminated with blood, and all body fluids in situations where it is difficult or impossible to differentiate between body fluids; (2) Any unfixed tissue or organ (other than intact skin) from a human (living or dead), and (3) HIV-containing cell or tissue cultures, organ cultures, and HIV- or HBV-containing culture medium or other solutions; and blood, organs, or other tissues from experimental animals infected with HIV or HBV.

Parenteral means piercing mucous membranes or the skin barrier through such events as needlesticks, human bites, cuts, and abrasions.

Personal Protective Equipment is specialized clothing or equipment worn by an employee for protection against a hazard. General work clothes (e.g., uniforms, pants, shirts, or blouses) not intended to function as protection against a hazard are not considered to be personal protective equipment.

Production Facility means a facility engaged in industrial-scale, large-volume, or high-concentration production of HIV or HBV.

Regulated Waste means liquid or semi-liquid blood or other potentially infectious materials; contaminated items that would release blood or other potentially infectious materials in a liquid or semi-liquid state if compressed; items that are caked with dried blood or other potentially infectious materials and are capable of releasing these materials during handling; contaminated sharps; and pathological and microbiological wastes containing blood or other potentially infectious materials.

Research Laboratory means a laboratory producing or using research-laboratory-scale amounts of HIV or HBV. Research laboratories may produce high concentrations of HIV or HBV but not in the volume found in production facilities.

Sharps with engineered sharps injury protections means nonneedle sharp or a needle device used for withdrawing body fluids accessing a vein or artery, or administering medications or other fluids, with a built-in safety feature or mechanism, that effectively reduces the risk of an exposure incident.

Source Individual means any individual, living or dead, whose blood or other potentially infectious materials may be a source of occupational exposure to the employee. Examples include, but are not limited to, hospital and clinic patients; clients in institutions for the developmentally disabled; trauma victims; clients of drug and alcohol treatment facilities; residents of hospices and nursing homes; human remains; and individuals who donate or sell blood or blood components.

Sterilize means the use of a physical or chemical procedure to destroy all microbial life, including highly resistant bacterial endospores.

Universal Precautions is an approach to infection control. According to the concept of Universal Precautions, all human blood and certain human body fluids are treated as if known to be infectious for HIV, HBV, and other bloodborne pathogens.

Work Practice Controls means controls that reduce the likelihood of exposure by altering the manner in which a task is performed (e.g., prohibiting recapping of needles by a two-handed technique).

(c) *Exposure Control–*

(1) *Exposure Control Plan.*

(i) Each employer having an employee(s) with occupational exposure as defined by paragraph (b) of this section shall establish a written Exposure Control Plan designed to eliminate or minimize employee exposure.

(ii) The Exposure Control Plan shall contain at least the following elements:

(A) The exposure determination required by paragraph (c)(2).

(B) The schedule and method of implementation for paragraphs (d) Methods of Compliance, (e) HIV and HBV Research Laboratories and Production Facilities, (f) Hepatitis B Vaccination and Post-Exposure Evaluation and Follow-up, (g) Communication of Hazards to Employees, and (h) Recordkeeping, of this standard, and

(C) The procedure for the evaluation of circumstances surrounding exposure incidents as required by paragraph (f)(3)(i) of this standard.

(iii) Each employer shall ensure that a copy of the Exposure Control Plan is accessible to employees in accordance with 29 CFR 1910.20(e).

(iv) The Exposure Control Plan shall be reviewed and updated at least annually and whenever necessary to reflect new or modified tasks and procedures that affect occupational exposure and to reflect new or revised employee positions with occupational exposure. The review and update of such plan shall also:

  (A) reflect changes in technology that eliminate or reduce exposure to bloodborne pathogens; and

  (B) document annually consideration and implementation of appropriate commercially available and effective safer medical devices designed to eliminate or minimize occupational exposure.

(v) An employer, who is required to establish an exposure control plan shall solicit input from non-managerial employees responsible for direct patient care who are potentially exposed to injuries from contaminated sharps in the identification, evaluation, and selection of effective engineering and work practice controls and shall document the solicitation in the Exposure Control Plan.

(vi) The Exposure Control Plan shall be made available to the Assistant Secretary and the Director upon request for examination and copying.

(2) *Exposure Determination.*

(i) Each employer who has an employee(s) with occupational exposure as defined by paragraph (b) of this section shall prepare an exposure determination. This exposure determination shall contain the following:

  (A) A list of all job classifications in which all employees in those job classifications have occupational exposure;

  (B) A list of job classifications in which some employees have occupational exposure; and

  (C) A list of all tasks and procedures or groups of closely related tasks and procedures in which occupational exposure occurs and that are performed by employees in job classifications listed in accordance with the provisions of paragraph (c)(2)(i)(B) of this standard.

(ii) This exposure determination shall be made without regard to the use of personal protective equipment.

(d) *Methods of Compliance—*

(1) General. Universal precautions shall be observed to prevent contact with blood or other potentially infectious materials. Under circumstances in which differentiation between body fluid types is difficult or impossible, all body fluids shall be considered potentially infectious materials.

(2) *Engineering and Work Practice Controls.*

(i) Engineering and work practice controls shall be used to eliminate or minimize employee exposure. Where occupational exposure remains after institution of these controls, personal protective equipment shall also be used.

(ii) Engineering controls shall be examined and maintained or replaced on a regular schedule to ensure their effectiveness.

(iii) Employers shall provide handwashing facilities that are readily accessible to employees.

(iv) When provision of handwashing facilities is not feasible, the employer shall provide either an appropriate antiseptic hand cleanser in conjunction with clean cloth/paper towels or antiseptic towelettes. When antiseptic hand cleansers or towelettes are used, hands shall be washed with soap and running water as soon as feasible.

(v) Employers shall ensure that employees wash their hands immediately or as soon as feasible after removal of gloves or other personal protective equipment.

(vi) Employers shall ensure that employees wash hands and any other skin with soap and water, or flush mucous membranes with water immediately or as soon as feasible following contact of such body areas with blood or other potentially infectious materials.

(vii) Contaminated needles and other contaminated sharps shall not be bent, recapped, or removed except as noted in paragraphs (d)(2)(vii)(A) and (d)(2)(vii)(B) below. Shearing or breaking of contaminated needles is prohibited.

  (A) Contaminated needles and other contaminated sharps shall not be recapped or removed unless the employer can demonstrate that no alternative is feasible or that such action is required by a specific medical procedure.

  (B) Such bending, recapping, or needle removal must be accomplished through the use of a mechanical device or a one-handed technique.

(viii) Immediately or as soon as possible after use, contaminated reusable sharps shall be placed in appropriate containers until properly reprocessed. These containers shall be:

  (A) Puncture resistant;

  (B) Labeled or color-coded in accordance with this standard;

  (C) Leakproof on the sides and bottom; and

  (D) In accordance with the requirements set forth in paragraph (d)(4)(ii)(E) for reusable sharps.

(ix) Eating, drinking, smoking, applying cosmetics or lip balm, and handling contact lenses are prohibited in work areas where there is a reasonable likelihood of occupational exposure.

(x) Food and drink shall not be kept in refrigerators, freezers, shelves, cabinets, or on countertops or bench tops where blood or other potentially infectious materials are present.

(xi) All procedures involving blood or other potentially infectious materials shall be performed in such a manner as to minimize splashing, spraying, spattering, and generation of droplets of these substances.

(xii) Mouth pipetting/suctioning of blood or other potentially infectious materials is prohibited.

(xiii) Specimens of blood or other potentially infectious materials shall be placed in a container which prevents leakage during collection, handling, processing, storage, transport, or shipping.

    (A) The container for storage, transport, or shipping shall be labeled or color-coded according to paragraph (g)(1)(i) and closed prior to being stored, transported, or shipped. When a facility utilizes Universal Precautions in the handling of all specimens, the labeling/color-coding of specimens is not necessary provided containers are recognizable as containing specimens. This exemption only applies while such specimens/containers remain within the facility. Labeling or color-coding in accordance with paragraph (g)(1)(i) is required when such specimens/containers leave the facility.

    (B) If outside contamination of the primary container occurs, the primary container shall be placed within a second container that prevents leakage during handling, processing, storage, transport, or shipping and is labeled or color-coded according to the requirements of this standard.

    (C) If the specimen could puncture the primary container, the primary container shall be placed within a secondary container that is puncture-resistant in addition to the above characteristics.

(xiv) Equipment that may become contaminated with blood or other potentially infectious materials shall be examined prior to servicing or shipping and shall be decontaminated as necessary, unless the employer can demonstrate that decontamination of such equipment or portions of such equipment is not feasible.

    (A) A readily observable label in accordance with paragraph (g)(1)(i)(H) shall be attached to the equipment stating which portions remain contaminated.

    (B) The employer shall ensure that this information is conveyed to all affected employees, the servicing representative, and/or the manufacturer, as appropriate, prior to handling, servicing, or shipping so that appropriate precautions will be taken.

(3) *Personal Protective Equipment*—

    (i) *Provision.* When there is occupational exposure, the employer shall provide, at no cost to the employee, appropriate personal protective equipment such as, but not limited to, gloves, gowns, laboratory coats, face shields or masks and eye protection, and mouthpieces, resuscitation bags, pocket masks, or other ventilation devices. Personal protective equipment will be considered "appropriate" only if it does not permit blood or other potentially infectious materials to pass through to or reach the employee's work clothes, street clothes, undergarments, skin, eyes, mouth, or other mucous membranes under normal conditions of use and for the duration of time which the protective equipment will be used.

    (ii) *Use.* The employer shall ensure that the employee uses appropriate personal protective equipment unless the employer shows that the employee temporarily and briefly declined to use personal protective equipment when, under rare and extraordinary circumstances, it was the employee's professional judgment that in the specific instance its use would have prevented the delivery of health care or public safety services or would have posed an increased hazard to the safety of the worker or co-worker. When the employee makes this judgment, the circumstances shall be investigated and documented in order to determine whether changes can be instituted to prevent such occurrences in the future.

    (iii) *Accessibility.* The employer shall ensure that appropriate personal protective equipment in the appropriate sizes is readily accessible at the worksite or is issued to employees. Hypoallergenic gloves, glove liners, powderless gloves, or other similar alternatives shall be readily accessible to those employees who are allergic to the gloves normally provided.

    (iv) *Cleaning, Laundering, and Disposal.* The employer shall clean, launder, and dispose of personal protective equipment required by paragraphs (d) and (e) of this standard, at no cost to the employee.

    (v) *Repair and Replacement.* The employer shall repair or replace personal protective equipment as needed to maintain its effectiveness, at no cost to the employee.

    (vi) If a garment(s) is penetrated by blood or other potentially infectious materials, the garment(s) shall be removed immediately or as soon as feasible.

    (vii) All personal protective equipment shall be removed prior to leaving the work area.

(viii) When personal protective equipment is removed it shall be placed in an appropriately designated area or container for storage, washing, decontamination or disposal.

(ix) *Gloves.* Gloves shall be worn when it can be reasonably anticipated that the employee may have hand contact with blood, other potentially infectious materials, mucous membranes, and non-intact skin; when performing vascular access procedures except as specified in paragraph (d)(3)(ix)(D); and when handling or touching contaminated items or surfaces.

    (A) Disposable (single use) gloves such as surgical or examination gloves shall be replaced as soon as practical when contaminated or as soon as feasible if they are torn, punctured, or when their ability to function as a barrier is compromised.

    (B) Disposable (single use) gloves shall not be washed or decontaminated for re-use.

    (C) Utility gloves may be decontaminated for re-use if the integrity of the glove is not compromised. However, they must be discarded if they are cracked, peeling, torn, punctured, or exhibit other signs of deterioration or when their ability to function as a barrier is compromised.

    (D) If an employer in a volunteer blood donation center judges that routine gloving for all phlebotomies is not necessary then the employer shall:

        (1) Periodically reevaluate this policy;

        (2) Make gloves available to all employees who wish to use them for phlebotomy;

        (3) Not discourage the use of gloves for phlebotomy; and

        (4) Require that gloves be used for phlebotomy in the following circumstances:

            (i) When the employee has cuts, scratches, or other breaks in his or her skin;

            (ii) When the employee judges that hand contamination with blood may occur, for example, when performing phlebotomy on an uncooperative source individual; and

            (iii) When the employee is receiving training in phlebotomy.

(x) *Masks, Eye Protection, and Face Shields.* Masks in combination with eye protection devices, such as goggles or glasses with solid side shields, or chin-length face shields, shall be worn whenever splashes, spray, spatter, or droplets of blood or other potentially infectious materials may be generated and eye, nose, or mouth contamination can be reasonably anticipated.

(xi) *Gowns, Aprons, and Other Protective Body Clothing.* Appropriate protective clothing such as, but not limited to, gowns, aprons, lab coats, clinic jackets, or similar outer garments shall be worn in occupational exposure situations. The type and characteristics will depend upon the task and degree of exposure anticipated.

(xii) Surgical caps or hoods and/or shoe covers or boots shall be worn in instances when gross contamination can reasonably be anticipated (e.g., autopsies, orthopaedic surgery).

(4) *Housekeeping—*

  (i) *General.* Employers shall ensure that the worksite is maintained in a clean and sanitary condition. The employer shall determine and implement an appropriate written schedule for cleaning and method of decontamination based upon the location within the facility, type of surface to be cleaned, type of soil present, and tasks or procedures being performed in the area.

 (ii) All equipment and environmental and working surfaces shall be cleaned and decontaminated after contact with blood or other potentially infectious materials.

    (A) Contaminated work surfaces shall be decontaminated with an appropriate disinfectant after completion of procedures; immediately or as soon as feasible when surfaces are overtly contaminated or after any spill of blood or other potentially infectious materials; and at the end of the work shift if the surface may have become contaminated since the last cleaning.

    (B) Protective coverings, such as plastic wrap, aluminum foil, or imperviously-backed absorbent paper used to cover equipment and environmental surfaces, shall be removed and replaced as soon as feasible when they become overtly contaminated or at the end of the work shift if they may have become contaminated during the shift.

    (C) All bins, pails, cans, and similar receptacles intended for reuse which have a reasonable likelihood for becoming contaminated with blood or other potentially infectious materials shall be inspected and decontaminated on a regularly scheduled basis and cleaned and decontaminated immediately or as soon as feasible upon visible contamination.

    (D) Broken glassware that may be contaminated shall not be picked up directly with the hands. It shall be cleaned up using mechanical means, such as a brush and dust pan, tongs, or forceps.

    (E) Reusable sharps that are contaminated with blood or other potentially infectious materials shall not be stored or processed in a manner that requires employees to reach by hand into the containers where these sharps have been placed.

(iii) *Regulated Waste.*

(A) *Contaminated Sharps Discarding and Containment.*

(1) Contaminated sharps shall be discarded immediately or as soon as feasible in containers that are:

(i) Closable;

(ii) Puncture resistant;

(iii) Leakproof on sides and bottom; and

(iv) Labeled or color-coded in accordance with paragraph (g)(1)(i) of this standard.

(2) During use, containers for contaminated sharps shall be:

(i) Easily accessible to personnel and located as close as is feasible to the immediate area where sharps are used or can be reasonably anticipated to be found (e.g., laundries);

(ii) Maintained upright throughout use; and

(iii) Replaced routinely and not be allowed to overfill.

(3) When moving containers of contaminated sharps from the area of use, the containers shall be:

(i) Closed immediately prior to removal or replacement to prevent spillage or protrusion of contents during handling, storage, transport, or shipping;

(ii) Placed in a secondary container if leakage is possible. The second container shall be:

(A) Closable;

(B) Constructed to contain all contents and prevent leakage during handling, storage, transport, or shipping; and

(C) Labeled or color-coded according to paragraph (g)(1)(i) of this standard.

(4) Reusable containers shall not be opened, emptied, or cleaned manually or in any other manner which would expose employees to the risk of percutaneous injury.

(B) *Other Regulated Waste Containment.*

(1) Regulated waste shall be placed in containers which are:

(i) Closable;

(ii) Constructed to contain all contents and prevent leakage of fluids during handling, storage, transport or shipping;

(iii) Labeled or color-coded in accordance with paragraph (g)(1)(i) of this standard; and

(iv) Closed prior to removal to prevent spillage or protrusion of contents during handling, storage, transport, or shipping.

(2) If outside contamination of the regulated waste container occurs, it shall be placed in a second container. The second container shall be:

(i) Closable;

(ii) Constructed to contain all contents and prevent leakage of fluids during handling, storage, transport or shipping;

(iii) Labeled or color-coded in accordance with paragraph (g)(1)(i) of this standard; and

(iv) Closed prior to removal to prevent spillage or protrusion of contents during handling, storage, transport, or shipping.

(C) Disposal of all regulated waste shall be in accordance with applicable regulations of the United States, States and Territories, and political subdivisions of States and Territories.

(iv) *Laundry.*

(A) Contaminated laundry shall be handled as little as possible with a minimum of agitation.

(1) Contaminated laundry shall be bagged or containerized at the location where it was used and shall not be sorted or rinsed in the location of use.

(2) Contaminated laundry shall be placed and transported in bags or containers labeled or color-coded in accordance with paragraph (g)(1)(i) of this standard. When a facility utilizes Universal Precautions in the handling of all soiled laundry, alternative labeling, or color-coding is sufficient if it permits all employees to recognize the containers as requiring compliance with Universal Precautions.

(3) Whenever contaminated laundry is wet and presents a reasonable likelihood of soak-through or leakage from the bag or container, the laundry shall be placed and transported in bags or containers which prevent soak-through and/or leakage of fluids to the exterior.

(B) The employer shall ensure that employees who have contact with contaminated laundry wear protective gloves and other appropriate personal protective equipment.

(C) When a facility ships contaminated laundry off-site to a second facility which does not utilize Universal Precautions in the handling of all laundry, the facility generating the contaminated laundry must place such laundry in bags or containers which are labeled or color-coded in accordance with paragraph (g)(1)(i).

(e) *HIV and HBV Research Laboratories and Production Facilities.* See original publication for this information.

(f) *Hepatitis B Vaccination and Post-exposure Evaluation and Follow-up—*

(1) *General.*

(i) The employer shall make available the hepatitis B vaccine and vaccination series to all employees who have occupational exposure, and post-exposure evaluation and follow-up to all employees who have had an exposure incident.

(ii) The employer shall ensure that all medical evaluations and procedures, including the hepatitis B vaccine and vaccination series and post-exposure evaluation and follow-up, including prophylaxis are:

(A) Made available at no cost to the employee;

(B) Made available to the employee at a reasonable time and place;

(C) Performed by or under the supervision of a licensed physician or by or under the supervision of another licensed healthcare professional; and

(D) Provided according to recommendations of the U.S. Public Health Service current at the time these evaluations and procedures take place, except as specified by this paragraph (f).

(iii) The employer shall ensure that all laboratory tests are conducted by an accredited laboratory at no cost to the employee.

(2) *Hepatitis B Vaccination.*

(i) Hepatitis B vaccination shall be made available after the employee has received the training required in paragraph (g)(2)(vii)(I) and within 10 working days of initial assignment to all employees who have occupational exposure unless the employee has previously received the complete hepatitis B vaccination series, antibody testing has revealed that the employee is immune, or the vaccine is contraindicated for medical reasons.

(ii) The employer shall not make participation in a prescreening program a prerequisite for receiving hepatitis B vaccination.

(iii) If the employee initially declines hepatitis B vaccination but at a later date while still covered under the standard decides to accept the vaccination, the employer shall make available hepatitis B vaccination at that time.

(iv) The employer shall assure that employees who decline to accept hepatitis B vaccination offered by the employer sign the statement (Box H-1).

(v) If a routine booster dose(s) of hepatitis B vaccine is recommended by the U.S. Public Health Service at a future date, such booster dose(s) shall be made available in accordance with section (f)(1)(ii).

(3) *Post-exposure Evaluation and Follow-up.* Following a report of an exposure incident, the employer shall make immediately available to the exposed employee a confidential medical evaluation and follow-up, including at least the following elements:

(i) Documentation of the route(s) of exposure, and the circumstances under which the exposure incident occurred;

(ii) Identification and documentation of the source individual, unless the employer can establish that identification is infeasible or prohibited by state or local law;

(A) The source individual's blood shall be tested as soon as feasible and after consent is obtained in order to determine HBV and HIV infectivity. If consent is not obtained, the employer shall establish that legally required consent cannot be obtained. When the source individual's consent is not required by law, the source individual's blood, if available, shall be tested and the results documented.

BOX H-1

Appendix A to Section 1910.1030-Hepatitis B Vaccine Declination (Mandatory)

I understand that due to my occupational exposure to blood or other potentially infectious materials I may be at risk of acquiring hepatitis B virus (HBV) infection. I have been given the opportunity to be vaccinated with hepatitis B vaccine, at no charge to myself. However, I decline hepatitis B vaccination at this time. I understand that by declining this vaccine, I continue to be at risk of acquiring hepatitis B, a serious disease. If in the future I continue to have occupational exposure to blood or other potentially infectious materials and I want to be vaccinated with hepatitis B vaccine, I can receive the vaccination series at no charge to me.

Name _____

Date _____

(B) When the source individual is already known to be infected with HBV or HIV, testing for the source individual's known HBV or HIV status need not be repeated.

(C) Results of the source individual's testing shall be made available to the exposed employee, and the employee shall be informed of applicable laws and regulations concerning disclosure of the identity and infectious status of the source individual.

(iii) Collection and testing of blood for HBV and HIV serological status;

(A) The exposed employee's blood shall be collected as soon as feasible and tested after consent is obtained.

(B) If the employee consents to baseline blood collection, but does not give consent at that time for HIV serologic testing, the sample shall be preserved for at least 90 days. If, within 90 days of the exposure incident, the employee elects to have the baseline sample tested, such testing shall be done as soon as feasible.

(iv) Post-exposure prophylaxis, when medically indicated, as recommended by the U.S. Public Health Service;

(v) Counseling; and

(vi) Evaluation of reported illnesses.

(4) *Information Provided to the Healthcare Professional.*

(i) The employer shall ensure that the healthcare professional responsible for the employee's hepatitis B vaccination is provided a copy of this regulation.

(ii) The employer shall ensure that the healthcare professional evaluating an employee after an exposure incident is provided the following information:

(A) A copy of this regulation;

(B) A description of the exposed employee's duties as they relate to the exposure incident;

(C) Documentation of the route(s) of exposure and circumstances under which exposure occurred;

(D) Results of the source individual's blood testing, if available; and

(E) All medical records relevant to the appropriate treatment of the employee, including vaccination status, which are the employer's responsibility to maintain.

(5) *Healthcare Professional's Written Opinion.* The employer shall obtain and provide the employee with a copy of the evaluating healthcare professional's written opinion within 15 days of the completion of the evaluation.

(i) The healthcare professional's written opinion for hepatitis B vaccination shall be limited to whether hepatitis B vaccination is indicated for an employee, and if the employee has received such vaccination.

(ii) The healthcare professional's written opinion for post-exposure evaluation and follow-up shall be limited to the following information:

(A) That the employee has been informed of the results of the evaluation; and

(B) That the employee has been told about any medical conditions resulting from exposure to blood or other potentially infectious materials that require further evaluation or treatment.

(iii) All other findings or diagnoses shall remain confidential and shall not be included in the written report.

(6) *Medical Recordkeeping.* Medical records required by this standard shall be maintained in accordance with paragraph (h)(1) of this section.

(g)*Communication of Hazards to Employees—*

(1) *Labels and Signs.*

(i) *Labels.*

(A) Warning labels shall be affixed to containers of regulated waste, refrigerators and freezers containing blood or other potentially infectious material; and other containers used to store, transport or ship blood or other potentially infectious materials, except as provided in paragraph (g)(1)(i) (E), (F) and (G).

(B) Labels required by this section shall include the following legend:
BIOHAZARD (see Figure 8-1, p. 89)

(C) These labels shall be fluorescent orange or orange-red or predominantly so, with lettering or symbols in a contrasting color.

(D) Labels required be affixed as close as feasible to the container by string, wire, adhesive, or other method that prevents their loss or unintentional removal.

(E) Red bags or red containers may be substituted for labels.

(F) Containers of blood, blood components, or blood products that are labeled as to their contents and have been released for transfusion or other clinical use are exempted from the labeling requirements of paragraph (g).

(G) Individual containers of blood or other potentially infectious materials that are placed in a labeled container during storage, transport, shipment or disposal are exempted from the labeling requirement.

(H) Labels required for contaminated equipment shall be in accordance with this paragraph and shall also state which portions of the equipment remain contaminated.

   (I) Regulated waste that has been decontaminated need not be labeled or color-coded.

 (ii) *Signs.*

   (A) The employer shall post signs at the entrance to work areas specified in paragraph (e), HIV and HBV Research Laboratory and Production Facilities, which shall bear the following legend:

BIOHAZARD

(Name of the Infectious Agent)

(Special requirements for entering the area)

(Name, telephone number of the laboratory director or other responsible person.)

   (B) These signs shall be fluorescent orange-red or predominantly so, with lettering or symbols in a contrasting color.

(2) *Information and Training.*

 (i) Employers shall ensure that all employees with occupational exposure participate in a training program that must be provided at no cost to the employee and during working hours.

 (ii) Training shall be provided as follows:

   (A) At the time of initial assignment to tasks where occupational exposure may take place;

   (B) Within 90 days after the effective date of the standard; and

   (C) At least annually thereafter.

(iii) For employees who have received training on bloodborne pathogens in the year preceding the effective date of the standard, only training with respect to the provisions of the standard that were not included need be provided.

(iv) Annual training for all employees shall be provided within one year of their previous training.

 (v) Employers shall provide additional training when changes such as modification of tasks or procedures or institution of new tasks or procedures affect the employee's occupational exposure. The additional training may be limited to addressing the new exposures created.

(vi) Material appropriate in content and vocabulary to educational level, literacy, and language of employees shall be used.

(vii) The training program shall contain at a minimum the following elements:

   (A) An accessible copy of the regulatory text of this standard and an explanation of its contents;

   (B) A general explanation of the epidemiology and symptoms of bloodborne diseases;

   (C) An explanation of the modes of transmission of bloodborne pathogens;

   (D) An explanation of the employer's exposure control plan and the means by which the employee can obtain a copy of the written plan;

   (E) An explanation of the appropriate methods for recognizing tasks and other activities that may involve exposure to blood and other potentially infectious materials;

   (F) An explanation of the use and limitations of methods that will prevent or reduce exposure, including appropriate engineering controls, work practices, and personal protective equipment;

   (G) Information on the types, proper use, location, removal, handling, decontamination and disposal of personal protective equipment;

   (H) An explanation of the basis for selection of personal protective equipment;

   (I) Information on the hepatitis B vaccine, including information on its efficacy, safety, method of administration, the benefits of being vaccinated, and that the vaccine and vaccination will be offered free of charge;

   (J) Information on the appropriate actions to take and persons to contact in an emergency involving blood or other potentially infectious materials;

   (K) An explanation of the procedure to follow if an exposure incident occurs, including the method of reporting the incident and the medical follow-up that will be made available;

   (L) Information on the post-exposure evaluation and follow-up that the employer is required to provide for the employee following an exposure incident;

   (M) An explanation of the signs and labels and/or color coding required by paragraph (g)(1); and

   (N) An opportunity for interactive questions and answers with the person conducting the training session.

(viii) The person conducting the training shall be knowledgeable in the subject matter covered by the elements contained in the training program as it relates to the workplace that the training will address.

(ix) Additional Initial Training for Employees in HIV and HBV Laboratories and Production Facilities, Employees in HIV or HBV research laboratories and HIV or HBV production facilities shall receive the following initial training in addition to the above training requirements.

(A) The employer shall assure that employees demonstrate proficiency in standard microbiological practices and techniques and in the practices and operations specific to the facility before being allowed to work with HIV or HBV.

(B) The employer shall assure that employees have prior experience in the handling of human pathogens or tissue cultures before working with HIV or HBV.

(C) The employer shall provide a training program to employees who have no prior experience in handling human pathogens. Initial work activities shall not include the handling of infectious agents. A progression of work activities shall be assigned as techniques are learned and proficiency is developed. The employer shall assure that employees participate in work activities involving infectious agents only after proficiency has been demonstrated.

(h) *Recordkeeping*—

(1) *Medical Records.*

(i) The employer shall establish and maintain an accurate record for each employee with occupational exposure, in accordance with 29 CFR 1910.20.

(ii) This record shall include:

(A) The name and social security number of the employee;

(B) A copy of the employee's hepatitis B vaccination status including the dates of all the hepatitis B vaccinations and any medical records relative to the employee's ability to receive vaccination as required by paragraph (f)(2);

(C) A copy of all results of examinations, medical testing, and follow-up procedures as required by paragraph (f)(3);

(D) The employer's copy of the healthcare professional's written opinion as required by paragraph (f)(5); and

(E) A copy of the information provided to the healthcare professional as required by paragraphs (f)(4)(ii)(B)(C) and (D).

(iii) Confidentiality. The employer shall ensure that employee medical records required by paragraph (h)(1) are:

(A) Kept confidential; and

(B) Are not disclosed or reported without the employee's express written consent to any person within or outside the workplace except as required by this section or as may be required by law.

(iv) The employer shall maintain the records required by paragraph (h) for at least the duration of employment plus 30 years in accordance with 29 CFR 1910.20.

(2) *Training Records.*

(i) Training records shall include the following information:

(A) The dates of the training sessions;

(B) The contents or a summary of the training sessions;

(C) The names and qualifications of persons conducting the training; and

(D) The names and job titles of all persons attending the training sessions.

(ii) Training records shall be maintained for 3 years from the date on which the training occurred.

(3) *Availability.*

(i) The employer shall ensure that all records required to be maintained by this section shall be made available upon request to the Assistant Secretary and the Director for examination and copying.

(ii) Employee training records required by this paragraph shall be provided upon request for examination and copying to employees, to employee representatives, to the Director, and to the Assistant Secretary in accordance with 29 CFR 1910.20.

(Employee medical records required by this paragraph shall be provided upon request for examination and copying to the subject employee, to anyone having written consent of the subject employee, to the Director, and to the Assistant Secretary in accordance with 29 CFR 1910.20.

(4) *Transfer of Records.*

(i) The employer shall comply with the requirements involving transfer of records set forth in 29 CFR 1910.20(h).

(ii) If the employer ceases to do business and there is no successor employer to receive and retain the records for the prescribed period, the employer shall notify the Director, at least three months prior to their disposal and transmit them to the Director, if required by the Director to do s o, within that three month period.

(5) *Sharps injury log* (Note: Dentistry is exempt from this portion rule and need not keep a sharps injury log unless an incident results in a death or hospitalization of three or more employees. This part of the Standard is included here only for completeness).

(i) The employer shall establish and maintain a sharps injury log for the recording of percutaneous injuries from contaminated sharps. The information in the sharps injury log shall be recorded and maintained in such a manner as to protect the confidentiality of the injured employee. The sharps injury log shall contain, at a minimum:

(A) The type and brand of device involved in the incident,

(B) The department or work area where the exposure incident occurred, and

(C) An explanation of how the incident occurred.

(ii) The requirement to establish and maintain a sharps injury log shall apply to any employer who is required to maintain a log of occupational injuries and illnesses under 29 CFR 1904.6 [Note: Dentistry is excluded as noted previously.

(iii) The sharps injury log shall be maintained for the period required by 29 CFR 1904.6.

(i) *Dates—*

(1) *Effective Date.* The standard shall become effective on March 6, 1992.

(2) The Exposure Control Plan required by paragraph (c)(2) of this section shall be completed on or before May 5, 1992.

(3) Paragraph (g)(2) Information and Training and (h) Recordkeeping shall take effect on or before June 4, 1992.

(4) Paragraphs (d)(2) Engineering and Work Practice Controls, (d)(3) Personal Protective Equipment, (d)(4) Housekeeping, (e) HIV and HBV Research Laboratories and Production Facilities, (f) Hepatitis B Vaccination and Post-Exposure Evaluation and Follow-up, and (g)(1) Labels and Signs, shall take effect July 6, 1992.

Appendix H

Occupational Safety and Health Administration Hazard Communication/Globally Harmonized System Regulatory Text - 2012*

(a) Purpose.

(a)(1) The purpose of this section is to ensure that the hazards of all chemicals produced or imported are classified, and that information concerning the classified hazards is transmitted to employers and employees. The requirements of this section are intended to be consistent with the provisions of the United Nations Globally Harmonized System of Classification and Labeling of Chemicals (GHS), Revision 3. The transmittal of information is to be accomplished by means of comprehensive hazard communication programs, which are to include container labeling and other forms of warning, safety data sheets and employee training.

(a)(2) This occupational safety and health standard is intended to address comprehensively the issue of classifying the potential hazards of chemicals, and communicating information concerning hazards and appropriate protective measures to employees, and to preempt any legislative or regulatory enactments of a state, or political subdivision of a state, pertaining to this subject. Classifying the potential hazards of chemicals and communicating information concerning hazards and appropriate protective measures to employees, may include, for example, but is not limited to, provisions for: developing and maintaining a written hazard communication program for the workplace, including lists of hazardous chemicals present; labeling of containers of chemicals in the workplace, as well as of containers of chemicals being shipped to other workplaces; preparation and distribution of safety data sheets to employees and downstream employers; and development

and implementation of employee training programs regarding hazards of chemicals and protective measures. Under section 18 of the Act, no state or political subdivision of a state may adopt or enforce any requirement relating to the issue addressed by this Federal standard, except pursuant to a Federally-approved state plan.

(b) Scope and application.

(b)(1) This section requires chemical manufacturers or importers to classify the hazards of chemicals which they produce or import, and all employers to provide information to their employees about the hazardous chemicals to which they are exposed, by means of a hazard communication program, labels and other forms of warning, safety data sheets, and information and training. In addition, this section requires distributors to transmit the required information to employers. (Employers who do not produce or import chemicals need only focus on those parts of this rule that deal with establishing a workplace program and communicating information to their workers.)

(b)(2) This section applies to any chemical which is known to be present in the workplace in such a manner that employees may be exposed under normal conditions of use or in a foreseeable emergency.

(b)(3) This section applies to laboratories only as follows:

(i) Employers shall ensure that labels on incoming containers of hazardous chemicals are not removed or defaced;

(ii) Employers shall maintain any safety data sheets that are received with incoming shipments of hazardous chemicals, and ensure that they are readily accessible during each work shift to laboratory employees when they are in their work areas;

*United States Department of Labor, Occupational Safety and Health Administration: *29 CFR Part 1910.2000. Hazard Communication Standard*, http://www.osha.gov/dsg/hazcom/HCSFinalRegTxt.html, accessed April 2012.

(iii) Employers shall ensure that laboratory employees are provided information and training in accordance with paragraph (h) of this section, except for the location and availability of the written hazard communication program under paragraph (h)(2)(iii) of this section; and,

(iv) Laboratory employers that ship hazardous chemicals are considered to be either a chemical manufacturer or a distributor under this rule, and thus must ensure that any containers of hazardous chemicals leaving the laboratory are labeled in accordance with paragraph (f) of this section, and that a safety data sheet is provided to distributors and other employers in accordance with paragraphs (g)(6) and (g)(7) of this section.

(b)(4) In work operations where employees only handle chemicals in sealed containers which are not opened under normal conditions of use (such as are found in marine cargo handling, warehousing, or retail sales), this section applies to these operations only as follows:

(i) Employers shall ensure that labels on incoming containers of hazardous chemicals are not removed or defaced;

(ii) Employers shall maintain copies of any safety data sheets that are received with incoming shipments of the sealed containers of hazardous chemicals, shall obtain a safety data sheet as soon as possible for sealed containers of hazardous chemicals received without a safety data sheet if an employee requests the safety data sheet, and shall ensure that the safety data sheets are readily accessible during each work shift to employees when they are in their work area(s); and,

(iii) Employers shall ensure that employees are provided with information and training in accordance with paragraph (h) of this section (except for the location and availability of the written hazard communication program under paragraph (h)(2)(iii) of this section), to the extent necessary to protect them in the event of a spill or leak of a hazardous chemical from a sealed container.

(b)(5) This section does not require labeling of the following chemicals:

(i) Any pesticide as such term is defined in the Federal Insecticide, Fungicide, and Rodenticide Act (7 U.S.C. 136 et seq.), when subject to the labeling requirements of that Act and labeling regulations issued under that Act by the Environmental Protection Agency;

(ii) Any chemical substance or mixture as such terms are defined in the Toxic Substances Control Act (15 U.S.C. 2601 et seq.), when subject to the labeling requirements of that Act and labeling regulations issued under that Act by the Environmental Protection Agency;

(iii) Any food, food additive, color additive, drug, cosmetic, or medical or veterinary device or product, including materials intended for use as ingredients in such products (e.g., flavors and fragrances), as such terms are defined in the Federal Food, Drug, and Cosmetic Act (21 U.S.C. 301 et seq.) or the Virus-Serum-Toxin Act of 1913 (21 U.S.C. 151 et seq.), and regulations issued under those Acts, when they are subject to the labeling requirements under those Acts by either the Food and Drug Administration or the Department of Agriculture;

(iv) Any distilled spirits (beverage alcohols), wine, or malt beverage intended for non-industrial use, as such terms are defined in the Federal Alcohol Administration Act (27 U.S.C. 201 et seq.) and regulations issued under that Act, when subject to the labeling requirements of that Act and labeling regulations issued under that Act by the Bureau of Alcohol, Tobacco, Firearms and Explosives;

(v) Any consumer product or hazardous substance as those terms are defined in the Consumer Product Safety Act (15 U.S.C. 2051 et seq.) and Federal Hazardous Substances Act (15 U.S.C. 1261 et seq.) respectively, when subject to a consumer product safety standard or labeling requirement of those Acts, or regulations issued under those Acts by the Consumer Product Safety Commission; and,

(vi) Agricultural or vegetable seed treated with pesticides and labeled in accordance with the Federal Seed Act (7 U.S.C. 1551 et seq.) and the labeling regulations issued under that Act by the Department of Agriculture.

(b)(6) This section does not apply to:

(i) Any hazardous waste as such term is defined by the Solid Waste Disposal Act, as amended by the Resource Conservation and Recovery Act of 1976, as amended (42 U.S.C. 6901 et seq.), when subject to regulations issued under that Act by the Environmental Protection Agency;

(ii) Any hazardous substance as such term is defined by the Comprehensive Environmental Response, Compensation and Liability Act (CERCLA) (42 U.S.C. 9601 et seq.) when the hazardous substance is the focus of remedial or removal action being conducted under CERCLA in accordance with Environmental Protection Agency regulations.

(iii) Tobacco or tobacco products;

(iv) Wood or wood products, including lumber which will not be processed, where the chemical manufacturer or importer can establish that the only hazard they pose to employees is the potential for flammability or combustibility (wood or wood products which have been treated with a hazardous chemical covered by this standard, and wood which may be subsequently sawed or cut, generating dust, are not exempted);

(v) Articles (as that term is defined in paragraph (c) of this section);

(vi) Food or alcoholic beverages which are sold, used, or prepared in a retail establishment (such as a grocery store, restaurant, or drinking place), and foods intended for personal consumption by employees while in the workplace;

(vii) Any drug, as that term is defined in the Federal Food, Drug, and Cosmetic Act (21 U.S.C. 301 et seq.), when it is in solid, final form for direct administration to the patient (e.g., tablets or pills); drugs which are packaged by the chemical manufacturer for sale to consumers in a retail establishment (e.g., over-the-counter drugs); and drugs intended for personal consumption by employees while in the workplace (e.g., first aid supplies);

(viii) Cosmetics which are packaged for sale to consumers in a retail establishment, and cosmetics intended for personal consumption by employees while in the workplace;

(ix) Any consumer product or hazardous substance, as those terms are defined in the Consumer Product Safety Act (15 U.S.C. 2051 et seq.) and Federal Hazardous Substances Act (15 U.S.C. 1261 et seq.) respectively, where the employer can show that it is used in the workplace for the purpose intended by the chemical manufacturer or importer of the product, and the use results in a duration and frequency of exposure which is not greater than the range of exposures that could reasonably be experienced by consumers when used for the purpose intended;

(x) Nuisance particulates where the chemical manufacturer or importer can establish that they do not pose any physical or health hazard covered under this section;

(xi) Ionizing and nonionizing radiation; and,

(xii) Biological hazards.

(c) Definitions.

"Article" means a manufactured item other than a fluid or particle: (i) which is formed to a specific shape or design during manufacture; (ii) which has end use function(s) dependent in whole or in part upon its shape or design during end use; and (iii) which under normal conditions of use does not release more than very small quantities (e.g., minute or trace amounts of a hazardous chemical [as determined under paragraph (d) of this section]), and does not pose a physical hazard or health risk to employees.

"Assistant Secretary" means the Assistant Secretary of Labor for Occupational Safety and Health, U.S. Department of Labor, or designee.

"Chemical" means any substance, or mixture of substances.

"Chemical manufacturer" means an employer with a workplace where chemical(s) are produced for use or distribution.

"Chemical name" means the scientific designation of a chemical in accordance with the nomenclature system developed by the International Union of Pure and Applied Chemistry (IUPAC) or the Chemical Abstracts Service (CAS) rules of nomenclature, or a name that will clearly identify the chemical for the purpose of conducting a hazard classification.

"Classification" means to identify the relevant data regarding the hazards of a chemical; review those data to ascertain the hazards associated with the chemical; and decide whether the chemical will be classified as hazardous according to the definition of hazardous chemical in this section. In addition, classification for health and physical hazards includes the determination of the degree of hazard, where appropriate, by comparing the data with the criteria for health and physical hazards.

"Commercial account" means an arrangement whereby a retail distributor sells hazardous chemicals to an employer, generally in large quantities over time and/or at costs that are below the regular retail price.

"Common name" means any designation or identification such as code name, code number, trade name, brand name or generic name used to identify a chemical other than by its chemical name.

"Container" means any bag, barrel, bottle, box, can, cylinder, drum, reaction vessel, storage tank, or the like that contains a hazardous chemical. For purposes of this section, pipes or piping systems, and engines, fuel tanks, or other operating systems in a vehicle, are not considered to be containers.

"Designated representative" means any individual or organization to whom an employee gives written authorization to exercise such employee's rights under this section. A recognized or certified collective bargaining agent shall be treated automatically as a designated representative without regard to written employee authorization.

"Director" means the Director, National Institute for Occupational Safety and Health, U.S. Department of Health and Human Services, or designee.

"Distributor" means a business, other than a chemical manufacturer or importer, which supplies hazardous chemicals to other distributors or to employers.

"Employee" means a worker who may be exposed to hazardous chemicals under normal operating conditions or in foreseeable emergencies. Workers such as office workers or bank tellers who encounter hazardous chemicals only in non-routine, isolated instances are not covered.

"Employer" means a person engaged in a business where chemicals are either used, distributed, or are produced for use or distribution, including a contractor or subcontractor.

"Exposure or exposed" means that an employee is subjected in the course of employment to a chemical that is a physical or health hazard, and includes potential (e.g., accidental or possible) exposure. "Subjected" in terms of health hazards includes any route of entry (e.g., inhalation, ingestion, skin contact or absorption.)

"Foreseeable emergency" means any potential occurrence such as, but not limited to, equipment failure, rupture of containers, or failure of control equipment which could result in an uncontrolled release of a hazardous chemical into the workplace.

"Hazard category" means the division of criteria within each hazard class e.g., (oral acute toxicity and flammable liquids include four hazard categories). These categories compare hazard severity within a hazard class and should not be taken as a comparison of hazard categories more generally.

"Hazard class" means the nature of the physical or health hazards (e.g., flammable solid, carcinogen, oral acute toxicity).

"Hazard not otherwise classified (HNOC)" means an adverse physical or health effect identified through evaluation of scientific evidence during the classification process that does not meet the specified criteria for the physical and health hazard classes addressed in this section. This does not extend coverage to adverse physical and health effects for which there is a hazard class addressed in this section, but the effect either falls below the cut-off value/concentration limit of the hazard class or is under a GHS hazard category that has not been adopted by OSHA (e.g., acute toxicity Category 5).

"Hazard statement" means a statement assigned to a hazard class and category that describes the nature of the hazard(s) of a chemical, including, where appropriate, the degree of hazard.

"Hazardous chemical" means any chemical which is classified as a physical hazard or a health hazard, a simple asphyxiant, combustible dust, pyrophoric gas, or hazard not otherwise classified.

"Health hazard" means a chemical which is classified as posing one of the following hazardous effects: acute toxicity (any route of exposure); skin corrosion or irritation; serious eye damage or eye irritation; respiratory or skin sensitization; germ cell mutagenicity; carcinogenicity; reproductive toxicity; specific target organ toxicity (single or repeated exposure); or aspiration hazard. The criteria for determining whether a chemical is classified as a health hazard are detailed in Appendix A to §1910.1200 -- Health Hazard Criteria.

"Immediate use" means that the hazardous chemical will be under the control of and used only by the person who transfers it from a labeled container and only within the work shift in which it is transferred.

"Importer" means the first business with employees within the Customs Territory of the United States which receives hazardous chemicals produced in other countries for the purpose of supplying them to distributors or employers within the United States.

"Label" means an appropriate group of written, printed or graphic information elements concerning a hazardous chemical that is affixed to, printed on, or attached to the immediate container of a hazardous chemical, or to the outside packaging.

"Label elements" means the specified pictogram, hazard statement, signal word and precautionary statement for each hazard class and category.

"Mixture" means a combination or a solution composed of two or more substances in which they do not react.

"Physical hazard" means a chemical that is classified as posing one of the following hazardous effects: explosive; flammable (gases, aerosols, liquids, or solids); oxidizer (liquid, solid or gas); self-reactive; pyrophoric (liquid or solid); self-heating; organic peroxide; corrosive to metal; gas under pressure; or in contact with water emits flammable gas. See Appendix B to §1910.1200 -- Physical Hazard Criteria.

"Pictogram" means a composition that may include a symbol plus other graphic elements, such as a border, background pattern, or color, that is intended to convey specific information about the hazards of a chemical. Eight pictograms are designated under this standard for application to a hazard category.

"Precautionary statement" means a phrase that describes recommended measures that should be taken to minimize or prevent adverse effects resulting from exposure to a hazardous chemical, or improper storage or handling.

"Product identifier" means the name or number used for a hazardous chemical on a label or in the SDS. It provides a unique means by which the user can identify the chemical. The product identifier used shall permit cross-references to be made among the list of hazardous chemicals required in the written hazard communication program, the label and the SDS.

"Produce" means to manufacture, process, formulate, blend, extract, generate, emit, or repackage.

"Pyrophoric gas" means a chemical in a gaseous state that will ignite spontaneously in air at a temperature of 130 degrees F (54.4 degrees C) or below.

"Responsible party" means someone who can provide additional information on the hazardous chemical and appropriate emergency procedures, if necessary.

"Safety data sheet (SDS)" means written or printed material concerning a hazardous chemical that is prepared in accordance with paragraph (g) of this section.

"Signal word" means a word used to indicate the relative level of severity of hazard and alert the reader to a potential hazard on the label. The signal words used in this section are "danger" and "warning." "Danger" is used for the more severe hazards, while "warning" is used for the less severe.

"Simple asphyxiant" means a substance or mixture that displaces oxygen in the ambient atmosphere, and can thus cause oxygen deprivation in those who are exposed, leading to unconsciousness and death.

"Specific chemical identity" means the chemical name, Chemical Abstracts Service (CAS) Registry Number, or any other information that reveals the precise chemical designation of the substance.

"Substance" means chemical elements and their compounds in the natural state or obtained by any production process, including any additive necessary to preserve the stability of the product and any impurities deriving from the process used, but excluding any solvent which may be separated without affecting the stability of the substance or changing its composition.

"Trade secret" means any confidential formula, pattern, process, device, information or compilation of information that is used in an employer's business, and that gives the employer an opportunity to obtain an advantage over competitors who do not know or use it. Appendix E to §1910.1200—Definition of Trade Secret, sets out the criteria to be used in evaluating trade secrets.

"Use" means to package, handle, react, emit, extract, generate as a byproduct, or transfer.

"Work area" means a room or defined space in a workplace where hazardous chemicals are produced or used, and where employees are present.

"Workplace" means an establishment, job site, or project, at one geographical location containing one or more work areas.

(d) **Hazard classification.**

(d)(1) Chemical manufacturers and importers shall evaluate chemicals produced in their workplaces or imported by them to classify the chemicals in accordance with this section. For each chemical, the chemical manufacturer or importer shall determine the hazard classes, and where appropriate, the category of each class that apply to the chemical being classified. Employers are not required to classify chemicals unless they choose not to rely on the classification performed by the chemical manufacturer or importer for the chemical to satisfy this requirement.

(d)(2) Chemical manufacturers, importers or employers classifying chemicals shall identify and consider the full range of available scientific literature and other evidence concerning the potential hazards. There is no requirement to test the chemical to determine how to classify its hazards. Appendix A to §1910.1200 shall be consulted for classification of health hazards, and Appendix B to §1910.1200

shall be consulted for the classification of physical hazards.

(d)(3) Mixtures.

(i) Chemical manufacturers, importers, or employers evaluating chemicals shall follow the procedures described in Appendices A and B to §1910.1200 to classify the hazards of the chemicals, including determinations regarding when mixtures of the classified chemicals are covered by this section.

(ii) When classifying mixtures they produce or import, chemical manufacturers and importers of mixtures may rely on the information provided on the current safety data sheets of the individual ingredients, except where the chemical manufacturer or importer knows, or in the exercise of reasonable diligence should know, that the safety data sheet misstates or omits information required by this section.

(e) Written hazard communication program.

(e)(1) Employers shall develop, implement, and maintain at each workplace, a written hazard communication program which at least describes how the criteria specified in paragraphs (f), (g), and (h) of this section for labels and other forms of warning, safety data sheets, and employee information and training will be met, and which also includes the following:

(i) A list of the hazardous chemicals known to be present using a product identifier that is referenced on the appropriate safety data sheet (the list may be compiled for the workplace as a whole or for individual work areas); and,

(ii) The methods the employer will use to inform employees of the hazards of non-routine tasks (for example, the cleaning of reactor vessels), and the hazards associated with chemicals contained in unlabeled pipes in their work areas.

(e)(2) "Multi-employer workplaces." Employers who produce, use, or store hazardous chemicals at a workplace in such a way that the employees of other employer(s) may be exposed (for example, employees of a construction contractor working on-site) shall additionally ensure that the hazard communication programs developed and implemented under this paragraph (e) include the following:

(i) The methods the employer will use to provide the other employer(s) on-site access to safety data sheets for each hazardous chemical the other employer(s)' employees may be exposed to while working;

(ii) The methods the employer will use to inform the other employer(s) of any precautionary measures that need to be taken to protect employees during the workplace's normal operating conditions and in foreseeable emergencies; and,

(iii) The methods the employer will use to inform the other employer(s) of the labeling system used in the workplace.

(e)(3) The employer may rely on an existing hazard communication program to comply with these requirements, provided that it meets the criteria established in this paragraph (e).

(e)(4) The employer shall make the written hazard communication program available, upon request, to employees, their designated representatives, the Assistant Secretary and the Director, in accordance with the requirements of 29 CFR 1910.1020 (e).

(e)(5) Where employees must travel between workplaces during a work shift, i.e., their work is carried out at more than one geographical location, the written hazard communication program may be kept at the primary workplace facility.

(f) Labels and other forms of warning.

(f)(1) **Labels on shipped containers.** The chemical manufacturer, importer, or distributor shall ensure that each container of hazardous chemicals leaving the workplace is labeled, tagged or marked. Hazards not otherwise classified do not have to be addressed on the container. Where the chemical manufacturer or importer is required to label, tag or mark the following shall be provided:

(i) Product identifier;

(ii) Signal word;

(iii) Hazard statement(s);

(iv) Pictogram(s);

(v) Precautionary statement(s); and,

(vi) Name, address, and telephone number of the chemical manufacturer, importer, or other responsible party.

(f)(2) The chemical manufacturer, importer, or distributor shall ensure that the information provided under paragraphs (f)(1)(i) through (v) is in accordance with Appendix C, Allocation of Label Elements, for each hazard class and associated hazard category for the hazardous chemical, prominently displayed, and in English (other languages may also be included if appropriate).

(f)(3) The chemical manufacturer, importer, or distributor shall ensure that the information provided under paragraphs (f)(1)(ii) through (iv) is located together on the label, tag, or mark.

(f)(4) **Solid materials**

(i) For solid metal (such as a steel beam or a metal casting), solid wood, or plastic items that are not exempted as articles due to their downstream use, or shipments of whole grain, the required label may be transmitted to the customer at the time of the initial shipment, and need not be included with subsequent shipments to the same employer unless the information on the label changes;

(ii) The label may be transmitted with the initial shipment itself, or with the safety data sheet that is to be provided prior to or at the time of the first shipment; and,

(iii) This exception to requiring labels on every container of hazardous chemicals is only for the solid material itself, and does not apply to hazardous chemicals used in conjunction with, or known to be present with, the material and to which employees handling the items in transit may be exposed (for example, cutting fluids or pesticides in grains).

(f)(5) Chemical manufacturers, importers, or distributors shall ensure that each container of hazardous chemicals leaving the workplace is labeled, tagged, or marked in accordance with this section in a manner which does not conflict with the requirements of the Hazardous Materials Transportation Act (49 U.S.C. 1801 et seq.) and regulations issued under that Act by the Department of Transportation.

(f)(6) Workplace labeling. Except as provided in paragraphs (f)(7) and (f)(8) of this section, the employer shall ensure that each container of hazardous chemicals in the workplace is labeled, tagged or marked with either:

(i) The information specified under paragraphs (f)(1)(i) through (v) for labels on shipped containers; or,

(ii) Product identifier and words, pictures, symbols, or combination thereof, which provide at least general information regarding the hazards of the chemicals, and which, in conjunction with the other information immediately available to employees under the hazard communication program, will provide employees with the specific information regarding the physical and health hazards of the hazardous chemical.

(f)(7) The employer may use signs, placards, process sheets, batch tickets, operating procedures, or other such written materials in lieu of affixing labels to individual stationary process containers, as long as the alternative method identifies the containers to which it is applicable and conveys the information required by paragraph (f)(6) of this section to be on a label. The employer shall ensure the written materials are readily accessible to the employees in their work area throughout each work shift.

(f)(8) The employer is not required to label portable containers into which hazardous chemicals are transferred from labeled containers, and which are intended only for the immediate use of the employee who performs the transfer. For purposes of this section, drugs which are dispensed by a pharmacy to a health care provider for direct administration to a patient are exempted from labeling.

(f)(9) The employer shall not remove or deface existing labels on incoming containers of hazardous chemicals, unless the container is immediately marked with the required information.

(f)(10) The employer shall ensure that workplace labels or other forms of warning are legible, in English, and prominently displayed on the container, or readily available in the work area throughout each work shift. Employers having employees who speak other languages may add the information in their language to the material presented, as long as the information is presented in English as well.

(f)(11) Chemical manufacturers, importers, distributors, or employers who become newly aware of any significant information regarding the hazards of a chemical shall revise the labels for the chemical within six months of becoming aware of the new information, and shall ensure that labels on containers of hazardous chemicals shipped after that time contain the new information. If the chemical is not currently produced or imported, the chemical manufacturer, importer, distributor, or employer shall add the information to the label before the chemical is shipped or introduced into the workplace again.

(g) **Safety data sheets.**

(g)(1) Chemical manufacturers and importers shall obtain or develop a safety data sheet for each hazardous chemical they produce or import. Employers shall have a safety data sheet in the workplace for each hazardous chemical which they use.

(g)(2) The chemical manufacturer or importer preparing the safety data sheet shall ensure that it is in English (although the employer may maintain copies in other languages as well), and includes at least the following section numbers and headings, and associated information under each heading, in the order listed (See Appendix D to §1910.1200--Safety Data Sheets, for the specific content of each section of the safety data sheet):

(i) Section 1, Identification;

(ii) Section 2, Hazard(s) identification;

(iii) Section 3, Composition/information on ingredients;

(iv) Section 4, First-aid measures;

(v) Section 5, Fire-fighting measures;

(vi) Section 6, Accidental release measures;

(vii) Section 7, Handling and storage;

(viii) Section 8, Exposure controls/personal protection;

(ix) Section 9, Physical and chemical properties;

(x) Section 10, Stability and reactivity;

(xi) Section 11, Toxicological information.

Note 1 to paragraph (g)(2): To be consistent with the GHS, an SDS must also include the following headings in this order:

(xii) Section 12, Ecological information;

(xiii) Section 13, Disposal considerations;

(xiv) Section 14, Transport information; and

(xv) Section 15, Regulatory information.

Note 2 to paragraph (g)(2): OSHA will not be enforcing information requirements in sections 12 through 15, as these areas are not under its jurisdiction.

(xvi) Section 16, Other information, including date of preparation or last revision.

(g)(3) If no relevant information is found for any subheading within a section on the safety data sheet, the chemical manufacturer, importer or employer preparing the safety data sheet shall mark it to indicate that no applicable information was found.

(g)(4) Where complex mixtures have similar hazards and contents (i.e. the chemical ingredients are essentially the same, but the specific composition varies from mixture to mixture), the chemical manufacturer, importer or employer may prepare one safety data sheet to apply to all of these similar mixtures.

(g)(5) The chemical manufacturer, importer or employer preparing the safety data sheet shall ensure that the information provided accurately reflects the scientific evidence used in making the hazard classification. If the chemical manufacturer, importer or employer preparing the safety data sheet becomes newly aware of any significant information regarding the hazards of a chemical, or ways to protect against the hazards, this new information shall be added to the safety data sheet within three months. If the chemical is not currently being produced or imported the chemical manufacturer or importer shall add the information to the safety data sheet before the chemical is introduced into the workplace again.

(g)(6)(i) Chemical manufacturers or importers shall ensure that distributors and employers are provided an appropriate safety data sheet with their initial shipment, and with the first shipment after a safety data sheet is updated;

(ii) The chemical manufacturer or importer shall either provide safety data sheets with the shipped containers or send them to the distributor or employer prior to or at the time of the shipment;

(iii) If the safety data sheet is not provided with a shipment that has been labeled as a hazardous chemical, the distributor or employer shall obtain one from the chemical manufacturer or importer as soon as possible; and,

(iv) The chemical manufacturer or importer shall also provide distributors or employers with a safety data sheet upon request.

(g)(7)(i) Distributors shall ensure that safety data sheets, and updated information, are provided to other distributors and employers with their initial shipment and with the first shipment after a safety data sheet is updated;

(ii) The distributor shall either provide safety data sheets with the shipped containers, or send them to the other distributor or employer prior to or at the time of the shipment;

(iii) Retail distributors selling hazardous chemicals to employers having a commercial account shall provide a safety data sheet to such employers upon request, and shall post a sign or otherwise inform them that a safety data sheet is available;

(iv) Wholesale distributors selling hazardous chemicals to employers over-the-counter may also provide safety data sheets upon the request of the employer at the time of the over-the-counter purchase, and shall post a sign or otherwise inform such employers that a safety data sheet is available;

(v) If an employer without a commercial account purchases a hazardous chemical from a retail distributor not required to have safety data sheets on file (i.e., the retail distributor does not have commercial accounts and does not use the materials), the retail distributor shall provide the employer, upon request, with the name, address, and telephone number of the chemical manufacturer, importer, or distributor from which a safety data sheet can be obtained;

(vi) Wholesale distributors shall also provide safety data sheets to employers or other distributors upon request; and,

(vii) Chemical manufacturers, importers, and distributors need not provide safety data sheets to retail distributors that have informed them that the retail distributor does not sell the product to commercial accounts or open the sealed container to use it in their own workplaces.

(g)(8) The employer shall maintain in the workplace copies of the required safety data sheets for each hazardous chemical, and shall ensure that they are readily accessible during each work shift to employees when they are in their work area(s). (Electronic access and other alternatives to maintaining paper copies of the safety data sheets are permitted as long as no barriers to immediate employee access in each workplace are created by such options.)

(g)(9) Where employees must travel between workplaces during a work shift, i.e., their work is carried out at more than one geographical location, the safety data sheets may be kept at the primary workplace facility. In this situation, the employer shall ensure that employees can immediately obtain the required information in an emergency.

(g)(10) Safety data sheets may be kept in any form, including operating procedures, and may be designed to cover groups of hazardous chemicals in a work area where it may be more appropriate to address the hazards of a process rather than individual hazardous chemicals. However, the employer shall ensure that in all cases the required information is provided for each hazardous chemical, and is readily accessible during each work shift to employees when they are in their work area(s).

(g)(11) Safety data sheets shall also be made readily available, upon request, to designated representatives, the Assistant Secretary, and the Director, in accordance with the requirements of 29 CFR 1910.1020(e).

(h) Employee information and training.

(h)(1) Employers shall provide employees with effective information and training on hazardous chemicals in their work area at the time of their initial assignment, and whenever a new chemical hazard the employees have not previously been trained about is introduced into their work area. Information and training may be designed to cover categories of hazards (e.g., flammability, carcinogenicity) or specific chemicals. Chemical-specific information must always be available through labels and safety data sheets.

(h)(2) Information. Employees shall be informed of:

(i) The requirements of this section;

(ii) Any operations in their work area where hazardous chemicals are present; and,

(iii) The location and availability of the written hazard communication program, including the required list(s) of hazardous chemicals, and safety data sheets required by this section.

(h)(3) Training. Employee training shall include at least:

(i) Methods and observations that may be used to detect the presence or release of a hazardous chemical in the work area (such as monitoring conducted by the employer, continuous monitoring devices, visual appearance or odor of hazardous chemicals when being released, etc.);

(ii) The physical, health, simple asphyxiation, combustible dust, and pyrophoric gas hazards, as well as hazards not otherwise classified, of the chemicals in the work area;

(iii) The measures employees can take to protect themselves from these hazards, including specific procedures the employer has implemented to protect employees from exposure to hazardous chemicals, such as appropriate work practices, emergency procedures, and personal protective equipment to be used; and,

(iv) The details of the hazard communication program developed by the employer, including an explanation of the labels received on shipped containers and the workplace labeling system used by their employer; the safety data sheet, including the order of information and how employees can obtain and use the appropriate hazard information.

(i) Trade secrets.

(1) The chemical manufacturer, importer, or employer may withhold the specific chemical identity, including the chemical name, other specific identification of a hazardous chemical, or the exact percentage (concentration) of the substance in a mixture, from the safety data sheet, provided that:

(i) The claim that the information withheld is a trade secret can be supported;

(ii) Information contained in the safety data sheet concerning the properties and effects of the hazardous chemical is disclosed;

(iii) The safety data sheet indicates that the specific chemical identity and/or percentage of composition is being withheld as a trade secret; and,

(iv) The specific chemical identity and percentage is made available to health professionals, employees, and designated representatives in accordance with the applicable provisions of this paragraph.

(i)(2) Where a treating physician or nurse determines that a medical emergency exists and the specific chemical identity and/or specific percentage of composition of a hazardous chemical is necessary for emergency or first-aid treatment, the chemical manufacturer, importer, or employer shall immediately disclose the specific chemical identity or percentage composition of a trade secret chemical to that treating physician or nurse, regardless of the existence of a written statement of need or a confidentiality agreement. The chemical manufacturer, importer, or employer may require a written statement of need and confidentiality agreement, in accordance with the provisions of paragraphs (i)(3) and (4) of this section, as soon as circumstances permit.

(i)(3) In non-emergency situations, a chemical manufacturer, importer, or employer shall, upon request, disclose a specific chemical identity or percentage composition, otherwise permitted to be withheld under paragraph (i)(1) of this section, to a health professional (i.e. physician, industrial hygienist, toxicologist, epidemiologist, or occupational health nurse) providing medical or other occupational health services to exposed employee(s), and to employees or designated representatives, if:

(i) The request is in writing;

(ii) The request describes with reasonable detail one or more of the following occupational health needs for the information:

(A) To assess the hazards of the chemicals to which employees will be exposed;

(B) To conduct or assess sampling of the workplace atmosphere to determine employee exposure levels;

(C) To conduct pre-assignment or periodic medical surveillance of exposed employees;

(D) To provide medical treatment to exposed employees;

(E) To select or assess appropriate personal protective equipment for exposed employees;

(F) To design or assess engineering controls or other protective measures for exposed employees; and,

(G) To conduct studies to determine the health effects of exposure.

(iii) The request explains in detail why the disclosure of the specific chemical identity or percentage composition is essential and that, in lieu thereof, the disclosure of the following information to the health professional, employee, or designated representative, would not satisfy the purposes described in paragraph (i)(3)(ii) of this section:

(A) The properties and effects of the chemical;

(B) Measures for controlling workers' exposure to the chemical;

(C) Methods of monitoring and analyzing worker exposure to the chemical; and,

(D) Methods of diagnosing and treating harmful exposures to the chemical;

(iv) The request includes a description of the procedures to be used to maintain the confidentiality of the disclosed information; and,

(v) The health professional, and the employer or contractor of the services of the health professional (i.e. downstream employer, labor organization, or individual employee),

employee, or designated representative, agree in a written confidentiality agreement that the health professional, employee, or designated representative, will not use the trade secret information for any purpose other than the health need(s) asserted and agree not to release the information under any circumstances other than to OSHA, as provided in paragraph (i)(6) of this section, except as authorized by the terms of the agreement or by the chemical manufacturer, importer, or employer.

(i)(4) The confidentiality agreement authorized by paragraph (i)(3)(iv) of this section:

  (i) May restrict the use of the information to the health purposes indicated in the written statement of need;

  (ii) May provide for appropriate legal remedies in the event of a breach of the agreement, including stipulation of a reasonable pre-estimate of likely damages; and,

  (iii) May not include requirements for the posting of a penalty bond.

(i)(5) Nothing in this standard is meant to preclude the parties from pursuing non-contractual remedies to the extent permitted by law.

(i)(6) If the health professional, employee, or designated representative receiving the trade secret information decides that there is a need to disclose it to OSHA, the chemical manufacturer, importer, or employer who provided the information shall be informed by the health professional, employee, or designated representative prior to, or at the same time as, such disclosure.

(i)(7) If the chemical manufacturer, importer, or employer denies a written request for disclosure of a specific chemical identity or percentage composition, the denial must:

  (i) Be provided to the health professional, employee, or designated representative, within thirty days of the request;

  (ii) Be in writing;

  (iii) Include evidence to support the claim that the specific chemical identity or percent of composition is a trade secret;

  (iv) State the specific reasons why the request is being denied; and,

  (v) Explain in detail how alternative information may satisfy the specific medical or occupational health need without revealing the trade secret.

(i)(8) The health professional, employee, or designated representative whose request for information is denied under paragraph (i)(3) of this section may refer the request and the written denial of the request to OSHA for consideration.

(i)(9) When a health professional, employee, or designated representative refers the denial to OSHA under paragraph (i)(8) of this section, OSHA shall consider the evidence to determine if:

  (i) The chemical manufacturer, importer, or employer has supported the claim that the specific chemical identity or percentage composition is a trade secret;

  (ii) The health professional, employee, or designated representative has supported the claim that there is a medical or occupational health need for the information; and,

  (iii) The health professional, employee or designated representative has demonstrated adequate means to protect the confidentiality.

(i)(10)(i) If OSHA determines that the specific chemical identity or percentage composition requested under paragraph (i)(3) of this section is not a "bona fide" trade secret, or that it is a trade secret, but the requesting health professional, employee, or designated representative has a legitimate medical or occupational health need for the information, has executed a written confidentiality agreement, and has shown adequate means to protect the confidentiality of the information, the chemical manufacturer, importer, or employer will be subject to citation by OSHA.

  (ii) If a chemical manufacturer, importer, or employer demonstrates to OSHA that the execution of a confidentiality agreement would not provide sufficient protection against the potential harm from the unauthorized disclosure of a trade secret, the Assistant Secretary may issue such orders or impose such additional limitations or conditions upon the disclosure of the requested chemical information as may be appropriate to assure that the occupational health services are provided without an undue risk of harm to the chemical manufacturer, importer, or employer.

(i)(11) If a citation for a failure to release trade secret information is contested by the chemical manufacturer, importer, or employer, the matter will be adjudicated before the Occupational Safety and Health Review Commission in accordance with the Act's enforcement scheme and the applicable Commission rules of procedure. In accordance with the Commission rules, when a chemical manufacturer, importer, or employer continues to withhold the information during the contest, the Administrative Law Judge may review the citation and supporting documentation "in camera" or issue appropriate orders to protect the confidentiality of such matters.

(i)(12) Notwithstanding the existence of a trade secret claim, a chemical manufacturer, importer, or employer shall, upon request, disclose to the Assistant Secretary any information which this section requires the chemical manufacturer, importer, or employer to make available. Where there is a trade secret claim, such claim shall be made no later than at the time the information is provided to the Assistant Secretary so that suitable determinations of trade secret status can be made and the necessary protections can be implemented.

(i)(13) Nothing in this paragraph shall be construed as requiring the disclosure under any circumstances of process information which is a trade secret.

(j) Effective dates.

(1) Employers shall train employees regarding the new label elements and safety data sheets format by December 1, 2013.

(2) Chemical manufacturers, importers, distributors, and employers shall be in compliance with all modified provisions of this section no later than June 1, 2015, except:

(i) After December 1, 2015, the distributor shall not ship containers labeled by the chemical manufacturer or importer unless the label has been modified to comply with paragraph (f)(1) of this section.

(ii) All employers shall, as necessary, update any alternative workplace labeling used under paragraph (f)(6), update the hazard communication program required by paragraph (h)(1), and provide any additional employee training in accordance with paragraph (h)(3) for newly identified physical or health hazards no later than June 1, 2016.

(3) Chemical manufacturers, importers, distributors, and employers may comply with either §1910.1200 revised as of October 1, 2011, or the current version of this standard, or both during the transition period.

The Appendices referred to are located at http://www.osha.gov/dsg/hazcom/ghs-final-rule.html.

Glossary

abatement Process of correcting, putting an end to, eliminating a harmful situation

acidic Condition caused by an abundance of hydrogen ions (H+) resulting in a pH of less than 7.0

acidogenic An organism that produces acids during growth

aciduric An organism that survives in acidic environments less than pH 5.5

acquired defenses In contrast to innate defenses (immunity), immunity obtained in some manner other than by heredity

acquired immunodeficiency syndrome (AIDS) An infectious disease caused by the human immunodeficiency virus, which destroys the lymphocyte cells that provide immunity

actinomycosis Infection with endogenous oral *Actinomyces* species resulting in nodular lesions that may form abscesses; cervical facial actinomycosis occurs in the neck–jaw area

acute retroviral syndrome The symptoms of initial infection with human immunodeficiency virus (fever, rash, muscle/joint pains, sore throat, swollen glands, diarrhea)

acute stage In a disease, the period when symptoms are the greatest

adherence The attachment of a microorganism to a host cell or other surface

agar A polysaccharide extracted from seaweed and used as the basic component for semisolid bacterial growth media

alcohol-based hand rubs Hand hygiene preparations containing alcohol and emollients used as a rub without rinsing

allergen A foreign substance (e.g., pollen) that acts as an antigen but stimulates an allergic response

allergic contact dermatitis A type IV hypersensitivity resulting from contact with a chemical allergen (e.g., poison ivy, certain reactions to patient care gloves); the cell-mediated reaction occurs only where contact with the allergen has been made

allergy Disorder in which the immune system reacts inappropriately, usually by responding to an antigen it normally ignores (also called hypersensitivity)

American Dental Assistants Association (ADAA) A national professional organization for dental assistants (see Appendix A)

American Dental Association (ADA) A nonprofit professional association the membership of which is made up of dentists in the United States. Its purpose is to assist its members in providing the highest professional and ethical care to citizens of the United States and to serve as an advocate for the advancement of the profession (see Appendix A)

American Dental Hygienists Association (ADHA) The largest national organization representing the professional interests of the more than 135,000 registered dental hygienists in the United States. The mission of the association is to advance the art and science of dental hygiene by ensuring access to quality oral health care; increasing awareness of the cost-effective benefits of prevention; promoting the highest standards of dental hygiene education, licensure, practice, and research; and representing and promoting the interests of dental hygienists (see Appendix A)

American Society of Testing and Materials (ASTM) A nonprofit organization that provides a global forum for the development and publication of voluntary consensus standards for materials, products, systems, and services. The society provides standards that are accepted and used in research and development, product testing, quality systems, and commercial transactions around the globe

amino acid An organic acid containing an amino group and a carboxyl group; the building blocks of protein

anabolism The synthesis of large molecules from simpler components

anaphylactic shock An immunoglobulin E-mediated allergic reaction giving a systemic response that can be life-threatening

anion A negatively charged ion

antibiotics Chemical substances produced by microorganisms that can inhibit the growth of or destroy other microorganisms

antibodies Proteins produced in response to an antigen that are capable of binding specifically to that antigen

antigens Substances or cells that the body identifies as foreign and toward which it mounts an immune response

antimicrobial mouth rinse A mouth rinse possessing germicidal properties

antiseptics Chemical agents that can be used safely externally on tissues to destroy microorganisms or to inhibit their growth

AOAC International A worldwide provider and facilitator in the development, use, and harmonization of validated analytic methods and laboratory quality assurance programs and services

asepsis The absence of infection or infectious materials or agents

aseptic retrieval Retrieving a single item from a container without contaminating other items in the container

aseptic techniques Procedures that reduce or eliminate the spread of microbes

Association for the Advancement of Medical Instrumentation (AAMI) An association dedicated to increasing the understanding, safety, and efficacy of medical instrumentation (see Appendix A)

asthma Respiratory distress caused by inhaled or ingested allergens or by hypersensitivity to endogenous microorganisms

asymptomatic carriers Persons infected with a pathogen but who have no symptoms of the infection

autoclave An instrument for sterilization by means of moist heat under pressure

bacilli (singular: bacillus) Rodlike bacteria

bacteremia The presence of bacteria in the blood

bacteria All prokaryotic organisms

bacterial endocarditis A life-threatening infection and inflammation of the lining and valves of the heart

bacterial growth An increase in the number of bacterial cells of one type (also called bacterial multiplication)

bactericidal Lethal to bacteria

bacteriology The study of bacteria

bacteriophages Viruses that infect bacteria

bacteriostatic Stopping the growth of bacteria, but not necessarily killing the bacteria

binary fission The process by which bacteria multiply; the cell divides into two cells

binomial nomenclature The system of taxonomy in which each organism is assigned a genus and species name

bioburden The microbial or organic material on a surface or object before decontamination

biodegradation The breakdown of materials by microbes in the environment

biofilm A mass or layer of live microorganisms attached to a surface

biologic indicators (BIs) Paper strips or vials containing bacterial spores used to monitor the use and functioning of heat and gas sterilizers

biologic monitoring The use of biologic indicators (e.g., spore strips) to test the use and functioning of sterilizers (same as spore testing)

bloodborne diseases Infectious diseases that are spread through contact with infected blood and other body fluids

bloodborne pathogens Disease-producing microorganisms that are spread by contact with blood or other body fluids from an infected person

bloodborne pathogens standard A law developed by the OSHA and passed by Congress that directs employers to protect employees from occupational exposure to blood and other potentially infectious material

body-substance isolation Procedures designed to reduce the risk of transmission of pathogens from moist body surfaces

boil-water notice A notice to boil municipal water before using it for drinking, bathing, or health care

bulk blood Amounts of blood removed during surgery or drawn for analysis or transfusion

calculus Plaque that has mineralized (accumulated calcium) forming a hardened material on the tooth's surface; also known as tartar

candidiasis A fungal infection caused by *Candida albicans* that appears as thrush or denture stomatitis in the mouth

capsid The protein coating of a virus that protects the nucleic acid core from the environment and determines the shape of the virus

capsule A structure outside the bacterial cell wall that is antiphagocytic and protects the cell from drying

carbohydrates Compounds composed of carbon, hydrogen, and oxygen that serve as the main source of energy for most living things

caries Tooth decay (see dental caries)

carbon footprint The footprint left by the production or consumption of an item

carrier state A stage of an infectious disease in which the host carries the infectious agent, usually in the absence of symptoms

catabolism The chemical breakdown of molecules in which energy is released

catalase An enzyme that converts hydrogen peroxide to water and molecular oxygen

catastrophes and fatal accidents Second priority of an OSHA inspection and involves investigations of fatalities and accidents resulting in a death or hospitalization of three or more employees

cation A positively charged ion

cell wall A layer on most bacterial and fungal cells that maintains the shape of the cell and protects against mechanical damage

cell-mediated immunity Immune response carried out at the cellular level by T lymphocytes

cellulitis Inflammation of the loose subcutaneous cellular tissue

Centers for Disease Control and Prevention (CDC) The federal facility for disease eradication, epidemiology, and education headquartered in Atlanta, Georgia (see Appendix A)

CFU/mL Colony-forming units per milliliter

chemical Any element, chemical compound, or mixture of elements and compounds

chemical distributor A business, other than a chemical manufacturer or importer, that supplies hazardous chemicals to other distributors or to an employer

chemical hygiene officer A designated employee who is qualified by training or experience to provide technical guidance in the development and implementation of a chemical hygiene plan

chemical hygiene plan A written program developed and implemented by the employer that sets forth procedures, equipment, personal protective equipment, and work practices that are capable of protecting employees from health hazards presented by hazardous chemicals used in a particular workplace and involve the application of the tenets of prudent practice

chemical importer An employer with a workplace where chemical(s) are produced for use or distribution

chemical indicators Materials containing a chemical that changes color or form with exposure to heat, steam, or ethylene oxide gas, and are used to monitor exposure of items to heat- or gas-sterilizing agents

chemical manufacturer An employer with a workplace where chemical(s) are produced for use or distribution

chemical monitoring The use of chemical indicators to test the use and functioning of sterilizers

chemical vapor sterilizer An instrument for sterilization by means of hot formaldehyde vapors under pressure (also referred to as an unsaturated chemical vapor sterilizer)

chickenpox A disease with skin lesions caused by the varicella-zoster virus

Chlamydia Group of nonmotile, spherical bacteria that are obligate intracellular parasites with a complex life cycle

chlorination The addition of chlorine to water to kill microorganisms

chlorines Active ingredients in some intermediate-level disinfectants

chronic periodontitis A slowly progressing destruction of the supporting structures of the teeth, the most common form being periodontitis

ciliary escalator The physical movement created by the action of cilia (hairlike projections) on the surface of respiratory epithelial cells that moves mucus and trapped particles up and out of the lungs

cleanliness The state of being clean; freedom from dirt, soil, or extraneous material

clinical contact surface Surface that may be touched with gloved hands during patient care or that may become contaminated with blood or other potentially infectious material, and subsequently contact instruments, devices, hands, or gloves (e.g., light handles, switches, and drawer handles)

cocci (singular: coccus) Spherical bacteria

collagenase An enzyme that degrades body protein collagen in connective tissue

colony A mass of cells that originated from one cell or one colony-forming unit

colony-forming units (CFU) The original cells that begin multiplication to form a colony

common-touch surfaces Drawers/cabinets/door knobs and latches, refrigerator/freezer/toilet handles, dishes, utensils, dials, and switches

communicable disease Infectious disease that can be spread from one host to another (also called contagious disease)

complaints and referrals Third priority of an OSHA inspection and involves formal employee complaints of unsafe or unhealthy working conditions and referrals from any source (including patients) about a workplace hazard

complement system A set of proteins present in blood that when activated form a nonspecific defense mechanism against many different microorganisms

construction The action of framing, devising, or forming by the putting together of parts; erection, building. Internal construction commonly is referred to as renovation

construction-related outbreaks Adverse health results in patients and practitioners caused by construction or renovation; often involves airborne contaminants but also may spread by contaminated water or direct and indirect touch; also can result from a construction-related deficiency, such as a lack of handwashing facilities or movement of sharps of containers

contact dermatitis A type of allergy mediated by special T lymphocytes that results in a skin reaction after skin contact with an allergen (e.g., poison ivy)

contractors Companies or persons licensed to perform certain types of construction activities

convalescent stage In a disease, that period when the symptoms are subsiding and the person is recovering

cross-contamination The spreading of microbes between persons and/or environmental surfaces

culture of safety Factors that influence overall attitudes and behavior in the office. A safety culture reflects the shared commitment of the employer and employees toward ensuring the safety of the work environment.

cytoplasm The semifluid substance inside the cytoplasmic membrane of cells

cytoplasmic membrane The structural layer of a bacterial cell immediately internal to the cell wall

cytotoxic Toxic to cells

daylight loaders Equipment that allows the developing of radiographs in regular room lighting

de minimis **violation** Violation (in regard to a complaint to OSHA) that has no direct or immediate relationship to safety or health

decontamination Removing of the bioburden from objects or surfaces

delta hepatitis Hepatitis D (See hepatitis)

demineralization Removal of minerals from tooth structures; this causes dental caries

dental aerosols Small droplets of oral fluid and water generated during use of handpieces, ultrasonic scalers, and air/water syringes

Dental Assisting National Board, Inc. The nationally recognized certification and credentialing agency for dental assistants (see Appendix A)

dental caries An infectious disease resulting in the destruction of the teeth by microbial acids

dental plaque (oral biofilm) An accumulation of bacteria on the teeth in the absence of oral hygiene

denture stomatitis An infection of the alveolar ridge caused by *Candida albicans* and producing a reddening of the tissue under dentures

deoxyribonucleic acid (DNA) Nucleic acid that carries hereditary information from one generation to the next

design A plan or scheme conceived in the mind and intended for subsequent execution; the information required to carry out engineering works; the preliminary conception of an idea that is to be carried into effect by action

digital radiographic sensors Sensors that take the place of x-ray film when taking radiographs and that send the images to computer monitors for viewing

direct contact Mode of disease transmission requiring person-to-person body contact

disinfectant An antimicrobial chemical used to kill microorganisms on inanimate surfaces

disinfection Reducing the number of pathogenic organisms on objects or in materials so that they pose no threat of disease

disposable item An item used on one patient and then discarded

droplet infection Contact transmission of disease through small liquid droplets

dry heat sterilizer An instrument for sterilizing by means of heated air

emergency action plan (EAP) A plan that describes escape routes and procedures to follow for any emergency

emerging diseases New infectious diseases that have not been recognized before or are known to be infectious diseases with changing patterns

employees Persons who perform work for pay

employers Persons who pay others for work

endemic disease A disease that is constantly present in a specific population

endogenous Arising from the inside, such as an infection caused by opportunistic microorganisms already present in the body

endospore A resistant, dormant structure formed inside some bacteria such as *Geobacillus, Bacillus,* and *Clostridium* that can survive adverse conditions

endotoxin A toxic substance in the gram-negative bacterial cell wall that is released when the bacterium dies

engineering controls Devices that reduce the risk of exposure to potentially infectious materials (e.g., a sharps container)

entry floor mats If used and maintained properly, these can eliminate dirt that is tracked into the office on people's shoes

envelope The outer lipid-rich layer of some viruses that is derived from the host cell membrane on release of the virus from the host cell

environmental airborne contaminants Unwanted airborne constituents that may reduce the acceptability of air

environmental impact A change in the environment caused by some action or material

Environmental Protection Agency (EPA) A federal agency charged with the approval and oversight of the use and disposal of hazardous materials (see Appendix A)

enzymes Protein catalysts that control the rate of chemical reactions in cells

EPA-registered disinfectant A disinfectant that has been deemed safe and effective by the Environmental Protection Agency

EPA-registered product A product that has been deemed safe and effective by the Environmental Protection Agency

epidemic A disease outbreak that has a very high incidence in a population over a relatively short period of time

epidemiology The study of factors and mechanisms involved in the spread of disease within a population

epidermis The thin outer layer of the skin

event-related storage A storage practice that recognizes that a package and its contents should remain sterile until some event causes the item(s) to become contaminated

exogenous An infection caused by microorganisms that enter the body from the environment

exotoxin A soluble toxin secreted by microorganisms into their surroundings, including host tissues

exposure control plan A written plan required by the OSHA that describes how exposure to bloodborne disease agents will be controlled in a given work site

extracellular enzymes Exoenzymes produced by bacteria that act in the environment around the organism

facultative anaerobes Bacteria that carry on aerobic metabolism when oxygen is present but shift to anaerobic metabolism when oxygen is absent

failure to abate violation Exists when the employer has not corrected a violation for which OSHA has issued a citation and the abatement date has passed or covered under the settlement agreement

FDA-cleared barrier A surface cover that has been deemed safe and effective by the Food and Drug Administration

Federal Register The official daily publication for rules, proposed rules, and notices of federal agencies and organizations, and for executive orders and other presidential documents

fimbriae Short, hairlike projections from bacterial cells that function in adherence

fire prevention plan A plan that lists major workplace fire hazards; proper use, storage, and disposal of potential ignition sources; types of fire protection equipment present; names of persons responsible for equipment maintenance; policing of flammable and combustible materials to minimize fire; and employee training

fire safety standard Regulations that are part of a facility's emergency response and that apply to fire prevention or suppression

flagella Long, thin structures of some bacteria that provide means of locomotion

flash sterilization A sterilization procedure use for emergency purposes (requires a short turnaround time) that involves unwrapped items processed in a sterilizer for short exposure times

follow-up inspections Determines if an employer has corrected previous violations cited by OSHA

fomite An object that in itself is not harmful but which is able to harbor pathogens

Food and Drug Administration (FDA) An agency of the Department of Health and Human Services responsible for ensuring the safety and effectiveness of food, drugs, cosmetics, and medical devices (see Appendix A)

food safety Activities that reduce or eliminate hazardous conditions that can cause bodily injury after consuming food

fungi Nonphotosynthetic, eukaryotic organisms

fungicidal Lethal to fungi, including molds and yeasts

general duty clause A part of the of the U.S. Occupational Safety and Health Act, which states that: "each employer shall furnish to each of his employees employment and a place of employment which are free from recognized hazards that are causing or are likely to cause death or serious physical harm to his employees; each employee shall comply with occupational safety and health standards and all rules, regulations and orders issued pursuant to this Act which are applicable to his own actions and conduct; each employer shall comply with occupational safety and health standards promulgated under this act; each employee shall comply with occupational safety and health standards, and all rules, regulations, and orders issued pursuant to this Act which are applicable which are applicable to his own actions and conduct"

genus The first name of an organism in binomial nomenclature; (e.g., *Streptococcus* in *Streptococcus mutans*)

gingivitis A periodontal disease characterized by inflammation of the soft tissue (gingiva) around the teeth

gloves Coverings for the hands worn for protection against a hazard

glucosyltransferases Enzymes produced by *Streptococcus mutans* and some other bacteria that convert sucrose to glucan and fructose

glycocalyx Term used to refer to all substances containing polysaccharides found external to the cell wall

going green To use products and procedures that have lower adverse impacts on health and the environment than do regular products and procedures

gram-negative Term for bacteria that stain pink in the differential Gram stain procedure

gram-positive Term for bacteria that stain blue in the differential Gram stain procedure

gravity displacement steam sterilizer A steam sterilizer in which the air is replaced by steam through gravity without involving a mechanical removal of the air (in contrast to a vacuum steam sterilizer)

greenhouse effect A natural occurrence that helps regulate the temperature of our planet

greenhouse gases Gases such as carbon dioxide (CO_2), methane (CH_4), nitrous oxide (N_2O), and hydrofluorocarbons (HFC)

green products Products that are supposed to be more friendly to the environment

hand hygiene Procedures (e.g., handwashing or use of hand rubs) that remove or kill microorganisms on the hands

hand-foot-and-mouth disease A rare disease producing vesicles on the palms of the hands, the soles of the feet, and inside the mouth caused by certain coxsackieviruses

handwashing A form of hand hygiene that can be divided into two categories: routine handwashing and surgical hand antisepsis. Routine handwashing is designed to remove soil and transient microorganisms. The purpose of surgical hand antisepsis is to remove or destroy transient microorganisms and reduce normal flora

hay fever Irritation of the eyes and upper respiratory tract caused by inhaled allergens

hazard communication program An OSHA standard written program that describes how exposure of employees in the office to hazardous chemicals will be prevented

hazard communication standard A standard with the goal of preventing employee exposure to hazardous chemicals. The standard also states that information from the manufacturers of hazardous chemicals must be conveyed by employers to employees and that the facilities are responsible for making sure the information is received and understood (also called HazCom Standard, HazMat Program, "Employee Right to Know")

hazardous chemical A chemical for which statistically significant evidence based on a scientifically designed and conducted study indicates the acute or chronic health effects that may occur to exposed employees; many chemicals used within dental offices/clinics are considered hazardous

HBcAg Hepatitis B core antigen. Antibodies to the core antigen occur during infection

HBeAg Hepatitis B soluble antigen. The presence of this antigen denotes high infectivity

HBsAg Hepatitis B surface antigen. The presence of this antigen denotes the presence of the hepatitis B virus

HBV vaccination Immunization against hepatitis B virus infection; for adults, vaccination involves the application of three injections: the first any time, the second 1 to 2 months later, and the third 4 to 6 months after the first injection

health hazard A chemical, physical, or microbial condition that can damage the body

HEPA High-efficiency particulate air filters; they can filter out microorganisms from air

hepatitis A virus The virus that causes liver disease in situations ranging from isolated cases of disease to widespread epidemics; good personal hygiene and proper sanitation can help prevent hepatitis A; vaccines are also available

hepatitis An inflammation of the liver usually caused by viruses but sometimes by other organisms or toxic chemicals; hepatitis A and E viruses are spread by contaminated food and water; hepatitis B, C, D, and G viruses are bloodborne disease agents

hepatitis B vaccine A synthetic vaccine against hepatitis B with indirect protection against hepatitis D

hepatitis B virus A virus that attacks the liver, causing serious disease; the virus can cause lifelong infection, cirrhosis (scarring) of the liver, liver cancer, liver failure, and death; the most important infectious occupational hazard for dentistry; a vaccine is available

hepatitis C virus A virus that causes liver disease, is found in the blood of persons who have the disease, and is spread by contact with the blood of an infected person; occupational hazard for dental personnel; chronicity occurs in more than 80% of cases

hepatitis D virus A virus that requires the presence of hepatitis B virus to reproduce and incorporates into the capsid of hepatitis B virus; infection can be acquired as a coinfection with hepatitis B virus or as a superinfection of persons with chronic hepatitis B virus infection; can cause severe acute and chronic infections

hepatitis E virus A virus that is the major causative agent of enterically transmitted non-A, non-B hepatitis worldwide

herpangina A disease producing vesicles in the posterior part of the mouth caused by certain coxsackieviruses

herpes labialis Fever blisters (cold sores) on the lips

herpetic whitlow Infection of the fingers with herpes simplex virus

high-level disinfectants Antimicrobial chemical solutions shown to kill all microorganisms, but not necessarily high numbers of bacterial spores

high-level disinfection Use of a liquid high-level disinfectant/sterilant to kill all microorganisms except high numbers of bacterial spores

high-volume evacuation (HVE) The use of a vacuum system to remove fluids and debris from patients' mouths

histolytic enzymes Enzymes that can degrade a component in tissues or cells of the body

HIV disease A disease that includes human immunodeficiency virus infection or AIDS

HIV-1 Human immunodeficiency virus type 1

HIV infection Infection with HIV-1 before the development of AIDS

hospital disinfectant An antimicrobial chemical effective against the test microbes *Staphylococcus aureus, Salmonella choleraesuis,* and *Pseudomonas aeruginosa,* as representative vegetative bacteria

hospital waste Waste generated in a hospital

housekeeping surfaces Surfaces that do not come into contact with devices used in dental procedures

human herpesviruses A group of eight related viruses, including herpes simplex viruses, varicella-zoster virus, cytomegalovirus, and Epstein-Barr virus

human immunodeficiency virus (HIV) The virus that causes AIDS/HIV disease. This virus may be passed from one person to another when infected blood, semen, or vaginal secretions come in contact with an uninfected person's broken skin or mucous membranes. In addition, infected pregnant women can pass HIV to their babies during pregnancy or delivery and through breast-feeding. Persons with HIV have what is called HIV infection. Some of these persons will develop AIDS as a result of their HIV infection

hyaluronidase Bacterially produced enzyme that digests hyaluronic acid, which holds body cells together

hydrophilic viruses Viruses without lipid envelopes such as polioviruses, adenoviruses, coxsackieviruses; these viruses are generally considered to be more difficult to kill by some germicides than are lipophilic viruses

hypersensitivity Disorder in which the immune system reacts inappropriately, usually by responding to an antigen it normally ignores (also called allergy)

imminent danger First priority in an OSHA inspection and involves a reasonable certainty that a danger exists that could cause death or serious physical harm unless eliminated

immunity The ability to defend against the damage that may be caused by a microorganism

immunization The process of inoculating the body with specific antigens with the intention of producing immunity to those antigens

immunodeficiency Disorder in which the immune system responds inadequately to an antigen because of inborn or acquired defects in B or T lymphocytes

incidence The number of new cases of a particular disease seen in a specific period of time

incubation stage In a disease, the time between infection and the appearance of signs and symptoms

independent water reservoir A container that supplies nonmunicipal water to the dental unit

indirect contact Spread of disease agents through fomites (objects or surfaces)

infection Growth and survival of a microorganism on or in the body

infection control Controlling the spread of disease agents by performing specific procedures (same as infection prevention)

infection control overkill Excessive infection control (e.g., cleaning and disinfecting and then covering surfaces between each patient)

infection prevention Controlling the spread of disease agents by performing specific procedures (same as infection control)

infectious diseases Diseases caused by microorganisms

infectious mononucleosis An infection of white blood cells caused by the Epstein-Barr virus

infectious waste Medical waste that has been shown to be capable of transmitting an infectious disease

influenza A respiratory infectious disease caused by an influenza virus

innate defenses Naturally occurring body defense mechanisms against infectious disease agents

in-office monitoring The dental facility spore-tests sterilizers without any help from outside facilities, in contrast to mail-in testing services which supply all items needed for the testing

instrument washers Mechanical washers designed to clean medical and dental instruments

interferon A small protein released from virus-infected cells that causes adjacent cells to produce a protein that interferes with viral replication

intermediate viruses Viruses without envelopes that are not as resistant to chemical killing as the hydrophilic nonenveloped viruses but which are more resistant to chemical killing than the lipophilic enveloped viruses (see Table 13-4)

intermediate-level disinfectant An antimicrobial solution that destroys vegetative bacteria, most fungi, and most viruses; inactivates *Mycobacterium tuberculosis* var. *bovis* but is not necessarily capable of killing bacterial spores

iodophors Iodine complexed with certain organic compounds and used as the active ingredients in some intermediate-level disinfectants

irritant contact dermatitis A nonimmunologic irritation of the skin by chemicals

jaundice Yellow skin color caused by excessive bilirubin in the blood from the breakdown of erythrocytes; caused by impaired liver function and common in hepatitis

juvenile periodontitis A rapidly progressing destruction of the supporting structures of the teeth that most commonly occurs in the first molar area in teenagers

kPa A metric unit for measuring pressure in kilopascals

label Written, printed, or graphic material displayed on or affixed to containers of hazardous chemicals that provides necessary information

latex A milky white fluid extracted from the rubber tree *Hevea brasiliensis* that contains the rubber material cis-1,4 polyisoprene

latex allergy A type I hypersensitivity (mediated by immunoglobulin E antibody) resulting from contact with a chemical allergen in latex materials (e.g., latex gloves) or in materials associated with latex products (e.g., airborne powder from latex gloves)

LD$_{50}$ Lethal dose 50%. A measure of toxicity; the dose of a substance that kills 50% of the test animals

Legionnaire's disease A type of pneumonia caused by *Legionella pneumophila* that lives in water supplies; this disease is not spread from person to person but by aspiration of contaminated water

lipids A diverse group of water-insoluble compounds

lipophilic viruses Viruses with an outer lipid envelope such as influenza viruses, herpes simplex viruses, and HIV-1; these viruses generally are considered to be killed more easily by some germicides than are hydrophilic and intermediate viruses (see Table 13-4)

lipopolysaccharide Part of the outer layer of the cell wall in gram-negative bacteria (also called endotoxin)

low-level disinfectant An antimicrobial solution that destroys most vegetative bacteria, some fungi, and some viruses; does not inactivate *Mycobacterium tuberculosis* var. *bovis*

lymphocytes Leukocytes (white blood cells) found in large numbers in lymphoid tissues that contribute to immunity

lymphokines Chemicals secreted by lymphocytes that help mediate the immune response

lysis The disruption of a cell

lysozyme An enzyme in saliva and some other body fluids that acts on peptidoglycan to weaken the bacterial cell walls

lytic cycle The sequence of events in which a virus infects a cell, replicates, and eventually causes rupture of the cell

macrophages Phagocytic leukocytes found in tissues

mail-in monitoring A service for dental facilities that provides all supplies and instructions needed to spore-test sterilizers, in contrast to in-office monitoring where the office performs these tests without outside help

malaise A symptom of disease in which the person "feels bad" and is usually tired and weak

mask A covering for the mouth and nose worn for protection against a hazard

material safety data sheet (MSDS) See safety data sheet

mechanical monitoring The use of readings (e.g., time, temperature, and pressure) from sterilizer gauges and readouts to determine the use and functioning of sterilizers

medical waste Waste generated during patient diagnosis, treatment, or immunization

mesophiles Organisms that grow best at 37° C (98.6° F)

mesosomes Membranous structures of bacterial cells that contain extracellular enzymes used in nutrition

metabolism The sum of all chemical reactions that occur in living organisms

microaerophiles Bacteria that grow best in the presence of a small amount of free oxygen

microbial growth Increase in the number of cells because of cell division

microbiology The study of microorganisms

micrometer (μm) Unit of measure equal to 0.000001 m or 10^{-6} m

minimum bactericidal concentration The lowest concentration of an antimicrobial agent that kills microorganisms

minimum inhibitory concentration The lowest concentration of an antimicrobial agent that prevents growth of microorganisms

mutans streptococci A group of *Streptococcus* sp. with properties similar to *S. mutans* (*S. cricetus, S. ferus, S. macacae, S. mutans, S. rattus, S. sobrinus*)

mycology The study of fungi

National Institute for Occupational Safety and Health (NIOSH) An agency in the U.S. Department of Health and Human Services that was established to help assure safe and healthful working conditions by providing research, information, education, and training in the field of occupational safety and health; it was created by the Occupational Safety and Health Act of 1970

necrotizing ulcerative gingivitis Microbial destruction of the interdental papillae involving predisposing factors such as stress (also known as "trench mouth")

neutrophils White blood cells that phagocytose bacteria early in the inflammation process

nonenveloped viruses Viruses without envelopes that are hydrophilic or intermediate in their solubility, being more resistant to chemical killing than enveloped viruses (see Table 13-4)

nonregulated medical waste Medical waste that is not shown to have a disease-producing potential and that can be disposed of along with nonmedical waste

non–self-cleansing areas The sites around the teeth that are not kept clean by contact with the tongue and cheeks

normal microbiota Microorganisms commonly found in or on the body

nosocomial infections Infections acquired in a hospital or other medical facility

Notice of Intent to Contest A written petition submitted to OSHA within 15 days of a citation with which the employer does not agree, and it must describe the disagreement with a citation, with the penalty and/or with the indicated abatement

nucleic acid core The genes of viruses

nucleoid Nuclear region in bacteria

obligate aerobes Bacteria that must have free oxygen to grow

obligate anaerobes Bacteria that are killed by free oxygen

obligate intracellular parasites Organisms that can live or multiply only inside a living host cell

Occupational Exposure to Bloodborne Pathogens; Final Rule Implemented in 1992, the Occupational Exposure to Bloodborne Pathogens; Final Rule addresses concerns of occupational transmission of human immunodeficiency virus, hepatitis B, and other bloodborne pathogens, and applies to all employees whose occupation requires exposure to human blood, human blood products, unfixed human tissue, human cell culture, and other potentially infectious material. The rule outlines procedures employers must use to prevent occupational exposure of employees to bloodborne pathogens

Occupational Safety and Health Act of 1970 (The Act) An Act created to ensure safe and healthful working conditions by authorizing enforcement of standards developed under the Act; by encouraging and assisting state governments to improve and expand their own occupational safety and health programs; and by providing for research, information, education, and training in the field of occupational health and safety. Under the Act, the Occupational Safety and Health Administration was created within the Department of Labor, and the National Institute for Occupational Safety and Health was created within the U.S. Department of Health and Human Services

Occupational Safety and Health Administration (OSHA) A federal agency charged with establishing guidelines and regulations regarding worker safety, including storage and disposal of toxic chemicals and hazardous materials and the safety and proper use of clinical and office equipment. The organization was created in 1971 by the Occupational Safety and Health Act of 1970 (see Appendix A)

office safety Practicing infection control procedures, managing hazardous materials and regulated medical waste, and ensuring safety against fire and storms

opportunistic pathogens Organisms that usually are harmless but can cause disease under certain conditions (if given the opportunity)

oral candidiasis *Candida albicans* infection of the mouth producing white cottage cheese-like lesions

Organization for Safety, Asepsis and Prevention (OSAP) A nonprofit organization comprising dental practitioners, allied health care workers, industry representatives, military personnel, and other interested persons with a collective mission to promote infection control and related science-based health and safety policies and practices (see Appendices A and D)

OSAP Traveler's Guide to Safe Dental Care Provides information for safer dental care while abroad and includes a checklist that helps readers organize their review of office infection control procedures (see http://www.osap.org/?page=TravelersGuide&hhSearchTerms=Travel+and+Guide)

OSHA General Duty Clause See general duty clause

other-than-serious violation An OSHA violation in which the most serious injury or illness that would most likely occur from the hazardous condition cannot reasonably cause death or serious illness

ozone-depleting substances (ODS) Substances such as some solvents, aerosol propellants, and coolants

pandemic An epidemic that has become worldwide

pasteurization Mild heating to destroy pathogens and other organisms that cause spoilage (e.g., 71.6° C [161° F] for 15 seconds)

pathogens Microorganisms capable of causing disease in its host

pathology waste Body fluids or tissues removed from the body (e.g., extracted teeth and biopsy specimens)

pellicle The thin, saliva-based protein layer that coats the teeth and forms the base over which dental plaque develops

peptide A short chain of amino acids

peptidoglycan A polymer in bacterial cell wall composed of a peptide and a polysaccharide

percutaneous Through the skin

performance standards Standards that monitor outcomes rather than specific procedures

periapical infection An infection of the tissue around the apex of the root of a tooth

periodontal disease An infectious disease that results in destruction of the soft tissue or bone that supports the teeth (e.g., gingivitis and periodontitis)

periodontitis An inflammation of the periodontal tissue resulting in destruction of the bone in which the teeth are set

periodontopathogen A microorganism important in causing a periodontal disease

personal protective equipment (PPE) Equipment (e.g., gloves, masks, protective eyewear, and protective clothing) that help protect the body from exposure to potentially infectious agents or hazardous chemicals

pH A means of expressing the hydrogen ion concentration (acidity) of a solution

phagocytosis Ingestion of bacteria and other small particles by white blood cells

phenolics Derivatives of phenol used as active ingredients in some intermediate-level disinfectants

physical hazard A chemical for which scientifically valid evidence indicates that it is a combustible liquid, a compressed gas, explosive, flammable, an organic peroxide and oxidizer, pyrophoric, unstable (reactive), or water reactive

pili Projections from the bacterial cell used to attach bacteria to surfaces (fimbriae) or for conjugation (sex pili)

plan ahead Consider actions to take in the future

planktonic Microorganisms that are free-floating (not attached to surfaces) in their fluid environment; this is in contrast to biofilm microorganisms that are attached to surfaces

pneumonia An inflammation of lung tissue caused by bacteria, viruses, protozoa, or fungi

polysaccharide A carbohydrate formed by the linking of many monosaccharides

portal of entry A site at which microorganisms can gain access to body tissues

portal of exit A site at which microorganisms can leave the body

positive steam flush/pressure pulse sterilizer A steam sterilizer that uses repeated sequences of steam flushes and pressure pulses to remove the air from the sterilizer chamber before the steam is generated (in contrast to a vacuum steam sterilizer and a gravity displacement steam sterilizer)

potable water Water meeting the U.S. drinking water standards

precleaning Efforts to remove the bioburden from surfaces or instruments prior to disinfection or sterilization

preconstruction Actions taken in advance of construction, commonly involving planning for future action and including securing of necessary financing, permits, and releases

preprocedure mouth rinsing Use of a mouth rinse before a dental procedure to reduce the number of microorganisms present

prepubertal periodontitis Destruction of the supporting structures around primary teeth

prevalence The number of persons infected with a particular disease at any one time

primary contractor The company or person responsible for the execution, supervision, and overall coordination of a project and that also may perform some of the individual construction tasks. Most primary contractors are not licensed to perform all specialty trades and must hire specialty contractors for such tasks (e.g., electric and plumbing)

prions A pathogenic form of a neural protein particle without any nucleic acid implicated as a cause of various neurodegenerative diseases such as scrapie, Creutzfeldt-Jakob disease, and bovine spongiform encephalopathy

probiotics Microbes that when administered in an adequate amount can confer a health benefit on a host

prodromal stage In a disease, the short period during which early nonspecific symptoms, such as malaise and headache, sometimes appear

programmed inspections OSHA inspections aimed at specific high-hazard industries, workplaces, occupations, or health substances, or other industries identified in OSHA's current inspection procedures

prokaryotes Microorganisms that lack a nucleus; all bacteria are prokaryotes

proteases Enzymes that degrade protein into peptides or amino acids

protective clothing Clothing required to shield or guard the wearer from infectious, toxic, or harmful substances while engaged in employment duties

protective eyewear Goggles or safety glasses worn to protect the worker or the patient from accidental exposure to blood or other body fluids or to prevent injury from instruments

protein A polymer of amino acids joined by peptide bonds

protozoa Single-celled, microscopic, eukaryotic organisms in the kingdom *Protista*

protozoology The study of protozoa

prudent practices A plan originally developed in 1981 by the National Research Council, also referred to as Prudent Practices for Handling Hazardous Chemicals in Laboratories, that is used in the preparation of the chemical hygiene plan of a workplace. The plan helps to organize identified hazards and provides recommendations for each type of hazard and deals with safety and chemical hazards

psi A unit for measuring pressure in pounds per square inch

psychrophiles Cold-loving bacteria that grow best at a temperature of 7° C (44.6° F)

pulpitis Inflammation of the pulp of a tooth

pure culture A culture that contains only a single species of organism

purified protein derivative A protein derived from *Mycobacterium tuberculosis* and used in the tuberculin skin test

quaternary ammonium compounds Surface active compounds used as active ingredients in some low-level disinfectants

radiographic asepsis Infection control procedures related to the handling of radiographs

rapidly progressive periodontitis A rapidly progressing destruction of the supporting structures of the teeth that occurs most commonly in young adults

recycling Reported to reduce emission of greenhouse gases and water pollutants by minimizing the manufacturing process from virgin materials. This saves energy, supplies, and valuable raw materials, and reduces the need for disposal facilities such as landfills. Recycling also may help sustain the environment for future generations

regulated medical waste Medical waste shown to have a disease-producing potential and that must he handled in a specified fashion to ensure proper containment and disposal

renovation The renewal or restoration of structure

repeated violation An OSHA violation identical to a previously cited violation but detected again on a revisit

resident skin flora Species of microorganisms that are always present on on the skin

respirator A device designed to prevent inhalation of airborne particles (e.g., the N-9 respirator meets minimum filtration performance criteria for respiratory protection in areas of tuberculosis exposure)

retrofitting To subject to a retrofit; to modify so as to incorporate in older products changes made in later products of the same type or model

retroviruses RNA viruses that use the enzyme reverse transcriptase to synthesize DNA from RNA during multiplication of the virus inside of host cells (e.g., HIV-1)

reuse life For germicides, this is the period of time a solution should remain effective as it is used and reused (for contrast, see use life)

ribonucleic acid (RNA) Nucleic acid that directs or participates in the assembly of proteins

Rickettsia Small, nonmotile, gram-negative bacteria that are obligate intracellular parasites of mammalian and arthropod cells

rubber dam A latex or silicone square used to isolate a tooth or teeth before treatment; most commonly used in the field of endodontics

safety coordinator A person identified to manage office safety

safety data sheet (SDS) OSHA's newer phrase for material safety data sheet. Written or printed material concerning the procedures for handling or working with a hazardous chemical that includes physical data, toxicity, health effects, first aid, reactivity, storage, disposal, protective equipment, and spill/leak procedures. Safety data sheets are required for each hazardous chemical listed with a facility

saliva ejector A low-volume vacuum system to remove saliva from patients' mouths

septicemia An infection caused by rapid multiplication of pathogens in the blood

serious violation An OSHA violation that exists when the workplace hazard could cause injury or illness that would most likely result in death or serious physical harm, unless the employer did not know or could have not known of the violation

seroconversion The formation of detectable antibodies after exposure to an antigen

severe acute respiratory syndrome (SARS) A disease that emerged in 2003 in China and the cities of Hong Kong, Hanoi, and Singapore. The syndrome is a pneumonialike disease caused by a previously unrecognized coronavirus from domesticated animals (possibly cats) that is spread by droplet infection or by indirect or direct contact

sharps All items that can puncture the skin

sharps containers Puncture-resistant containers for disposal of sharp items that could puncture the skin (also called sharps boxes)

shelf life The period of time a solution or products may be stored before activation or use and still be effective on activation or use

shingles The recurrent form of chickenpox causing red bumps that change into blisters in a broad band on one side of the body; associated with itching and pain

single-use device (SUD) A devise originally cleared by the Food and Drug Administration (FDA) for a single use on one patient

sodium hypochlorite NaOCl, the active ingredient in bleach and sometimes used as a disinfectant

spatter Large droplets of oral fluids generated during use of handpieces, ultrasonic scalers, and air/water syringes

species The second name of an organism in binomial nomenclature (e.g., *mutans* in *Streptococcus mutans*)

spirilla (singular: spirillum) Corkscrew-shaped bacteria

spirochete A flexible, wavy-shaped bacterium

sporadic disease A disease that is limited to a small number of isolated cases, posing no great threat to a large population

spore A form taken by some bacteria that is resistant to heat, drying, and chemicals

spore testing The use of biologic indicators (bacterial spores) to test the use and functioning of sterilizers (same as biologic monitoring)

sporicidal An agent that kills bacterial endospores and therefore can be called a sterilant

spray-wipe-spray A procedure to disinfectant a surface: spray on the disinfectant, wipe the surface to clean it, and then respray the disinfectant for disinfection (in contrast to the wipe-discard-wipe procedure)

standard precautions Consideration of blood and all body fluids, including secretions and excretions (except sweat), nonintact skin, and mucous membranes, as potentially infectious in all patients

standards In regard to OSHA, these are rules set forth to protect the workers of America (e.g., the Bloodborne Pathogens Standard)

sterilant An agent capable of killing all microorganisms

sterility assurance level The level of spores shown to be killed by a defined sterilization process (e.g., a sterility assurance level of 10^{-6} indicates only a 1 in 1 million chance an item will not be sterile)

sterility assurance The correct use of appropriate instrument packaging, sterilization, storage, and monitoring procedures to help ensure the sterility and the maintenance of sterility of the items processed through a sterilizer

sterility The state in which no living organisms are in or on a material

sterilization The killing or removal of all microorganisms in a material or on an object

streptococcal pharyngitis "Strep" throat

subacute bacterial endocarditis A bacterial infection of the inside of the heart caused by bacteria present in the blood

subclinical infection An infection that does not produce symptoms (also called asymptomatic infection)

subcontractor A person or company that enters a binding agreement, a contract, or one of several contracts for carrying out a previous contract or a part of it, often involving performance of specific or specialize activity

sucrose A sugar containing one molecule of fructose and one molecule of glucose (also called table sugar)

superoxide dismutase An enzyme that converts toxic superoxide to molecular oxygen and hydrogen peroxide

surface asepsis Procedures that prevent the involvement of environmental surfaces in spreading disease agents

surface covers Materials impervious to water (e.g., plastic sheets) used to cover surfaces and prevent their contamination

surgical procedures As defined by the Centers for Disease Control and Prevention, the "incision, excision, or reflection of tissue that exposes the normally sterile areas of the oral cavity. Examples include biopsy, periodontal surgery, apical surgery, implant surgery, and surgical extractions of teeth (e.g., removal of erupted or noneRupted tooth, requiring elevation of the mucoperiosteal flap, removal of bone and/or section of tooth, and suturing if needed...)"

systemic infection An infection that involves the entire body

tetanus An infectious neuromuscular disease caused by the bacterium *Clostridium tetani*

tetanus toxoid Inactivated tetanus toxin used to immunize against tetanus

thermophiles Heat-loving bacteria that grow best at a temperature of 56° C (132.8° F)

thrush Oral candidiasis

toxigenic diseases Diseases that are caused by the toxins produced by microorganisms

toxin A poisonous substance

toxoid An inactivated toxin that is immunogenic but not toxic

transient bacteremia Bacteria present in the blood for only a short period of time

transient skin flora Microorganisms that may be present on the body under certain conditions and for certain lengths of time

transitional days Time for passing or passage from one condition, action, or (rarely) place to another; change; time in which a facility is brought up to functioning status

tuberculocidal An agent that can kill *Mycobacterium tuberculosis* var. *bovis*

tuberculosis An infectious diseases caused by *Mycobacterium tuberculosis* that usually involves the lungs but that may involve the skin or other tissues

ultrasonic cleaners Equipment that uses ultrasonic energy to remove debris from (clean) items such as medical and dental instruments

universal precautions Consideration of all patients as being infected with bloodborne pathogens and therefore applying infection control procedures to the care of all patients

universal sterilization The sterilization of all reusable instruments between use on patients

unproven treatments Methods used to improve health that do not have scientific evidence that they work

unsaturated chemical vapor sterilizer See chemical vapor sterilizer

upper respiratory tract The nasal cavity, pharynx, larynx, trachea, bronchi, and larger bronchioles

use life For germicidal agents, this is the period of time a solution is effective after it has been activated or prepared for use (for contrast, see reuse life)

vaccines Substances that contains an antigen to which the immune system responds

vacuum pump sterilizer See vacuum steam sterilizer

vacuum steam sterilizer A steam sterilizer in which the air in the chamber is removed by drawing a vacuum on the chamber before the steam enters at the beginning of the sterilization portion of the cycle (prevacuum) or in which the steam is removed at the end of the sterilization portion of the cycle (postvacuum), in contrast to a gravity displacement steam sterilizer and a positive steam flush/pressure pulse sterilizer

volatile organic compounds Examples include some solvents, paints, benzene, gasoline vapors and compounds in automobile exhaust. These react with oxides of nitrogen and sunlight to produce ozone, the main component of smog

work restrictions In the field of infection prevention this would be infectious diseases that would exclude a worker from work to prevent the spread of their disease to co-workers or patients. Examples include measles, mumps, pertussis, rubella, chickenpox, conjunctivitis

viral hepatitis Inflammation of the liver caused by a virus

virology The study of viruses

virucidal Lethal to viruses

viruses Submicroscopic, acellular, obligate intracellular parasites composed of a nucleic acid core inside a protein coat

walk through A good way to assess the cleanliness of the office. Pretend you are a patient and periodically observe the office environment

whitlow A herpetic lesion on a finger that can result from exposure to oral, ocular, and (probably) genital herpes

wicking The drawing of microorganisms or other particles through material that is wet (e.g., bacteria contaminating the outside of wet paper instrument packs are drawn through to the inside of the pack contaminating the instruments)

willful violation An OSHA violation where the employer knew that a hazardous condition existed but made no reasonable effort to eliminate it and in which the hazardous condition violated a standard

wipe-discard-wipe A disinfection procedure in which a disinfectant wipe is used to clean the surfaces then is discarded and a second disinfectant wipe is used to disinfect the surface (in contrast to the spray-wipe-spray procedure)

work practice controls Procedures that reduce the likelihood of exposure to potentially infectious materials (e.g., not recapping needles by hand)

written hazard communication program A compliance process for the hazard communications standard that includes a written clinic/office program manual, container labeling, and other forms of information transfer and warnings, and employee training

zoonotic Involving animals

Index

Page numbers followed by a *b* indicate boxes; *f,* figures; *t,* tables.